www.fleshandbones.com

The international community for medical students and instructors. Have you joined?

For students

- Free MCQs to test your knowledge
- Online support and revision help for your favourite textbooks
- Student reviews of the books on your reading lists
- Download clinical rotation survival guides
- Win great prizes in our games and competitions

The great online resource for everybody involved in medical education

For instructors

- Download free images and buy others from our constantly growing image bank
- Preview sample chapters from new textbooks
- Request inspection copies
- Browse our reading rooms for the latest information on new books and electronic products
- Secure online ordering with prompt delivery, as well as full contact details to order by phone, fax or post

Log on and register FREE today

fleshandbones.com
– an online resource for medical instructors and students

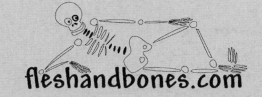
fleshandbones.com

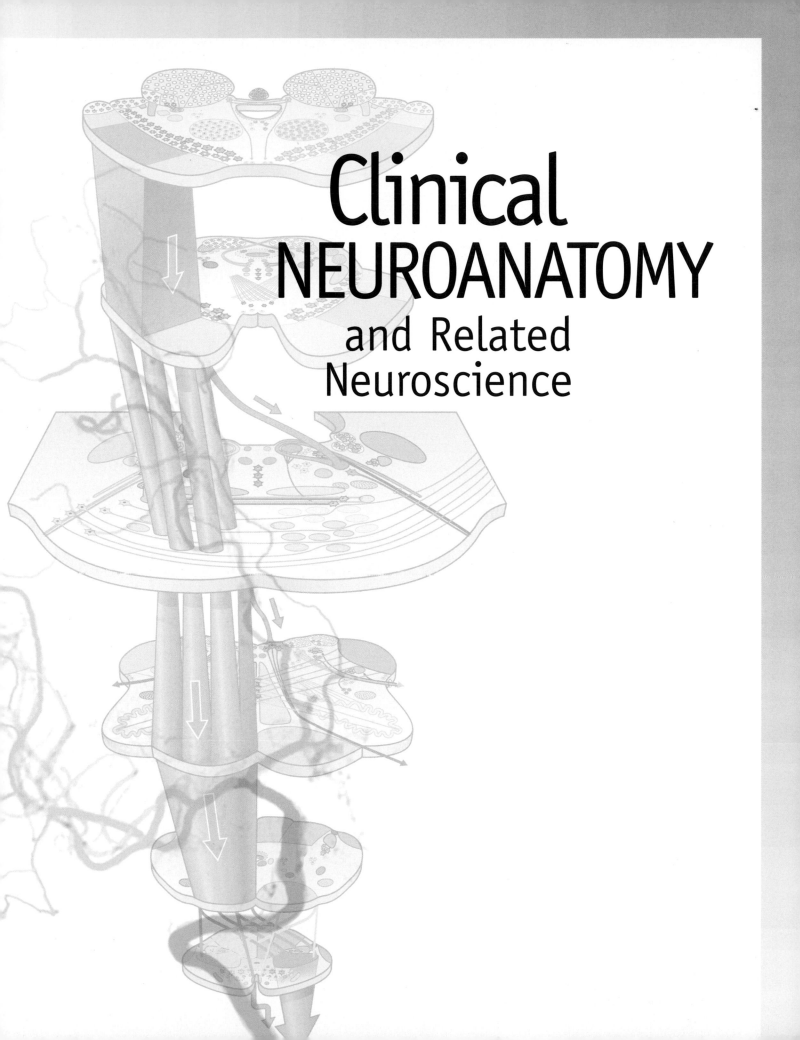

Clinical
NEUROANATOMY
and Related
Neuroscience

Commissioning Editor: Ellen Green
Project Development Manager: Barbara Simmons
Project Controller: Nancy Arnott
Designer: Judith Wright

Clinical
NEUROANATOMY
and Related Neuroscience

FOURTH EDITION

M J T FitzGerald

MD PhD DSc MRIA
Emeritus Professor
Department of Anatomy
University College
Galway
Ireland

Jean Folan-Curran

BSc MB BCh PhD
Professor
Department of Anatomy
National University of Ireland
Galway
Ireland

Illustrations by
Richard Tibbitts and **Paul Richardson**

W.B. SAUNDERS

Edinburgh • London • New York • Philadelphia • St Louis • Sydney • Toronto

W. B. Saunders
An imprint of Elsevier Science Limited

First edition 1985
Second edition 1992
Third edition 1996
Fourth edition 2002
Reprinted 2002

ISBN 0702 025585
International Student Edition 0702 025763

British Library Cataloguing in Publication Data
A catalogue record for this book is available from the British Library

Library of Congress Cataloging in Publication Data
A catalog record for this book is available from the Library of Congress

Medical knowledge is constantly changing. As new information
becomes available, changes in treatment, procedures, equipment and
the use of drugs become necessary. The authors and the publishers
have, as far as it is possible, taken care to ensure that the information
given in this text is accurate and up to date. However, readers are
strongly advised to confirm that the information, especially with
regard to drug usage, complies with the latest legislation and
standards of practice.

The
publisher's
policy is to use
**paper manufactured
from sustainable forests**

Printed in Spain

Coventry University

Preface

The new edition of this book incorporates significant changes. The term Clinical now introduces the title in order to emphasise its general orientation, and the term Related Neuroscience indicates the inclusion of abundant functional information basic to the interpretation of disordered neurological performance. We believe that this approach will be beneficial to medical students during their basic and clinical training, and to students of allied health professions including dentistry, physical therapy, speech therapy and clinical psychology.

This edition has a co-author, and an international Panel of Consultants has been added to provide advice on content.

The book is unusual in its overall structure. Most books provide an initial account of the anatomy of the nervous system as a whole and then follow with a one-by-one analysis of the sensory, motor and cognitive systems. We have tried instead to maintain an integrated approach in order to enable readers to appreciate the numerous ways in which the systems interact.

Our overall aim has been to produce a book that is up-to-date and appealing to readers. The following special features have been vital in promoting this aim:

• The 300 line illustrations of the 3rd edition have been re-rendered and 60 new ones have been added. Members of the Panel of Consultants have provided excellent photographs in the areas of 3-dimensional computer graphics, neuroangiography, functional magnetic resonance imaging and positron emission tomography.

• A novel approach has been used for complex diagrams, by provision of 'guided tours' whereby readers follow a series of arrows numbered in accordance with the usual sequence of activation of the component neurons.

• For the brainstem, the rather daunting Weigert-stained photographs have been replaced by graphic illustrations enabling a 'bottom-up' journey along sensory pathways and a 'top-down' journey along motor pathways.

• Close acquaintance with anatomy of the musculoskeletal system has provided material on various nerve root compression syndromes relevant to students of orthopedics and physical therapy. Chapters dealing with normal and abnormal cranial nerve function have also been expanded.

• Particular attention has been paid to the interface of the functional anatomy of the autonomic nervous system and pharmacology.

• The chapter on the limbic system has been expanded to incorporate recent advances provided by PET and fMRI technology.

• An exceptionally large glossary is provided, devoted in the main to definitions of functional and dysfunctional terms.

The authors wish to express sincere appreciation to those who helped bring this book to fruition. The Panel of Consultants has been highly beneficial, notably in providing information and opinions in their individual areas of special expertise. And it was a particular pleasure to receive the specialist input, and photographs, from three Panel members who are former students, namely Professors Raymond Dolan (PET), Paul Finn (fMRI) and Pearse Morris (Neuroangiography).

Richard Tibbitts of Antbits Illustration, Hertfordshire, with fellow illustrator Paul Richardson, transformed our draft diagrams, prepared in the form of pixel graphics, into elegant works art, as readers will see for themselves. In this context, the first author wishes to pay tribute to Peter FitzGerald (DPhil Psych Oxon) for patient over-the-phone initiation into the world of graphic illustration.

Finally, we thank the staff of the publishers, in particular Ellen Green and Barbara Simmons, for their constant assistance and sage advice.

TF
JF-C

Panel of Consultants

G Arjundas, Institute of Neurology, Medical University, Chennai, India

J A Armour, Department of Physiology and Biophysics, Dalhousie University School of Medicine, Halifax, Nova Scotia, Canada

N E Bharucha, Chief, Department of Neuroepidemiology, Medical Research Centre, Bombay Hospital, Mumbai, India

D Brooks, Department of Anatomy, Cornell University School of Medicine, New York, USA

J S Chopra, Department of Anatomy, Chandigarh University School of Medicine, Chandigarh, India

J Chowdhury, Department of Anatomy, Calcutta University School of Medicine, India

R J Dolan, Wellcome Department of Cognitive Neurology, Institute of Neurology, University College, London, UK

J P Finn, Director, MRI Facility, Northwestern University School of Medicine, Chicago, USA

J A Gosling, Chinese University Medical School, Hong Kong

B Hillen, Department of Anatomy, University of Utrecht School of Medicine, Holland

H-J Kretschmann, Department of Neuroanatomy, Medical University of Hannover, Germany

B E Leonard, Department of Pharmacology, National University of Ireland at Galway, Ireland

Dr P Morris, Department of Neuroradiology, Wake Forest University School of Medicine, Winston-Salem, N Carolina, USA

E Mtui, Department of Anatomy, Cornell University School of Medicine, New York, USA

Kathleen Mulligan, Department of Anatomy, University of Washington, Seattle, USA

Wei Yi Ong, Department of Anatomy, University of Singapore School of Medicine, Singapore

D Riches, Department of Anatomy, International University of Malaysia, Kuala Lumpur, Malaysia

N N Sarangi, Department of Anatomy, University of Salt Lake City, Calcutta, India

H Staunton, Chief of Neurology, Beaumont Hospital, Dublin, Ireland

Elizabeth Tancred, University of New South Wales School of Medicine, Sydney, Australia

B Ulfhake, Department of Neural Transmission, Karolinska Institutet, Stockholm, Sweden

Sashi Wadhwa, Department of Anatomy, All India Institute of Medical Sciences, Bombay, India

Contents

Embryology

SPINAL CORD

Neurulation

The entire nervous system originates from the **neural plate**, an ectodermal thickening in the floor of the amniotic sac (*Figure 1.1*). During the third week after fertilization, the plate forms paired **neural folds**, which unite to create the **neural tube** and **neural canal**. Union of the folds commences in the future neck region of the embryo* and proceeds rostrally and caudally from there. The open ends of the tube, the **neuropores**, are closed off before the end of the fourth week. The process of formation of the neural tube from the ectoderm is known as *neurulation*.

Cells at the edge of each neural fold escape from the line of union and form the **neural crest** alongside the tube. Cell types derived from the neural crest include spinal and autonomic ganglion cells and the Schwann cells of peripheral nerves.

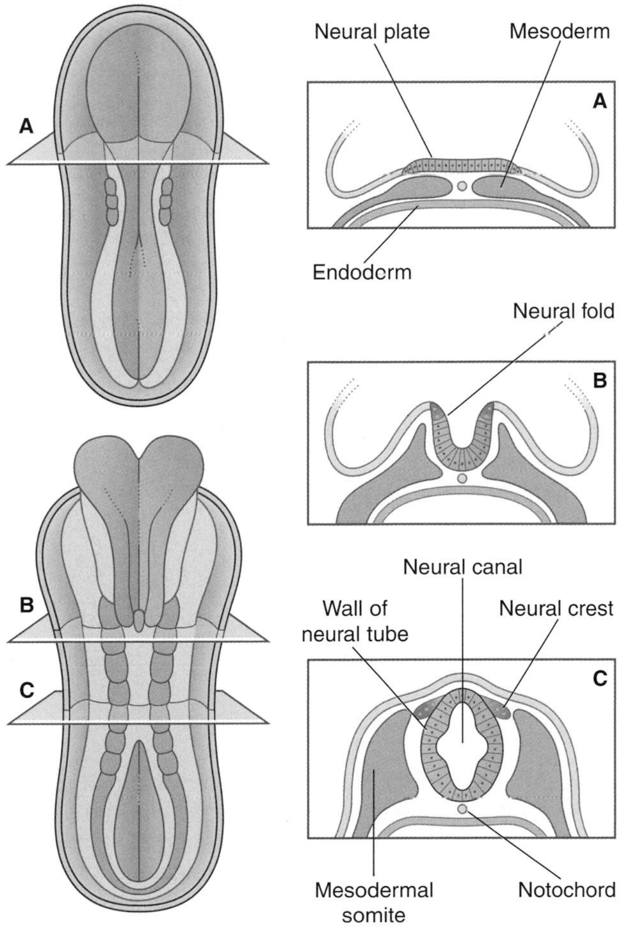

Spinal nerves

The dorsal part of the neural tube is called the **alar plate**; the ventral part is the **basal plate** (*Figure 1.2*). Neurons developing in the alar plate are predominantly sensory in function and receive dorsal nerve roots growing in from the spinal ganglia. Neurons in the basal plate are predominantly motor and give rise to ventral nerve roots. At appropriate levels of the spinal cord, the ventral roots also contain autonomic fibers. The dorsal and ventral roots unite to form the spinal nerves, which emerge from the vertebral canal in the interval between the neural arches being formed by the mesenchymal vertebrae.

The cells of the spinal (dorsal root) ganglia are initially bipolar. They become unipolar by the coalescence of their two processes at one side of the parent cells.

BRAIN

Brain vesicles

Rostrally, the closed neural tube expands in the form of three brain vesicles: the **prosencephalon** or forebrain, the **mes-**

Figure 1.1 Cross-section A is from a 3-somite (20-day) embryo. Cross-sections B and C are from an 8-somite (22-day) embryo.

* For descriptive purposes, the human embryo is in the prone (face down) position. The terms *ventral* and *dorsal* correspond to the adult *anterior* and *posterior*. The terms *rostral* and *caudal* correspond to *superior* and *inferior*.

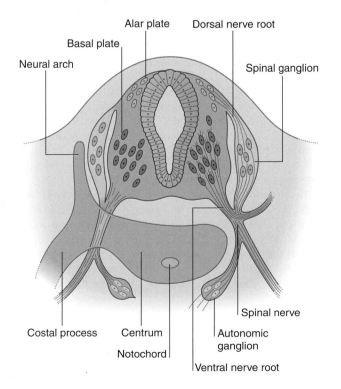

Figure 1.2 Neural tube, spinal nerve, and mesenchymal vertebra of an embryo at 6 weeks.

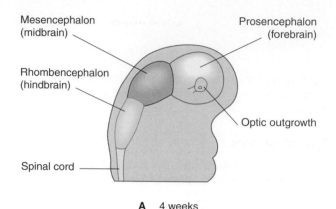

A 4 weeks

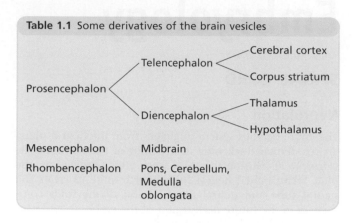

Table 1.1 Some derivatives of the brain vesicles

Prosencephalon	Telencephalon	Cerebral cortex
		Corpus striatum
	Diencephalon	Thalamus
		Hypothalamus
Mesencephalon	Midbrain	
Rhombencephalon	Pons, Cerebellum, Medulla oblongata	

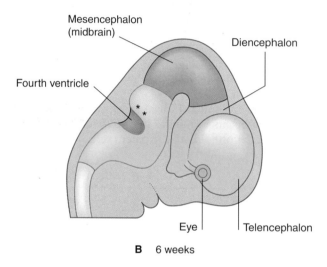

B 6 weeks

Figure 1.3 Brain vesicles, seen from the right side. Asterisks indicate the site of initial development of the cerebellum.

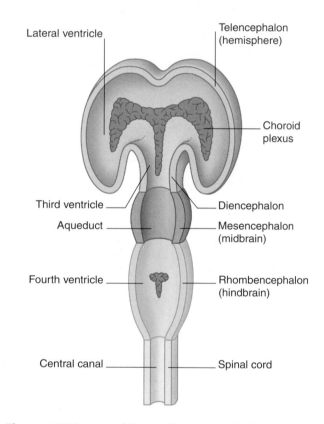

Figure 1.4 Diagram of the developing ventricular system. Choroid plexuses are shown in red.

encephalon or midbrain, and the **rhombencephalon** or hindbrain (*Figure 1.3*).

The alar plate of the prosencephalon expands on each side to form the **telencephalon**, or cerebral hemispheres. The basal plate remains in place here, as the **diencephalon**. Finally, an **optic outgrowth** from the diencephalon is the forerunner of the retina and optic nerve.

The diencephalon, mesencephalon and rhombencephalon constitute the embryonic brainstem.

The brainstem buckles as development proceeds. As a result, the mesencephalon is carried to the summit of the brain. The rhombencephalon folds upon itself, causing the alar plates to flare and creating the rhomboid (diamond-shaped) fourth ventricle of the brain. The rostral part of the rhombencephalon gives rise to the pons and cerebellum. The caudal part gives rise to the medulla oblongata (*Table 1.1*).

Ventricular system and choroid plexuses

The neural canal dilates within the cerebral hemispheres, forming the lateral ventricles; these communicate with the third ventricle contained within the diencephalon. The third and fourth ventricles communicate through the aqueduct of the midbrain (*Figure 1.4*).

The thin roofs of the forebrain and hindbrain are invaginated by tufts of capillaries which form the choroid plexuses of the four ventricles. The choroid plexuses secrete cerebrospinal fluid (CSF) which flows through the ventricular system. The fluid leaves the fourth ventricle through three apertures in its roof (*Figure 1.5*).

Cranial nerves

Figure 1.6 illustrates the state of development of the cranial nerves during the sixth week after fertilization.

- The olfactory nerve (I) forms from bipolar neurons developing in the epithelium lining the olfactory pit.

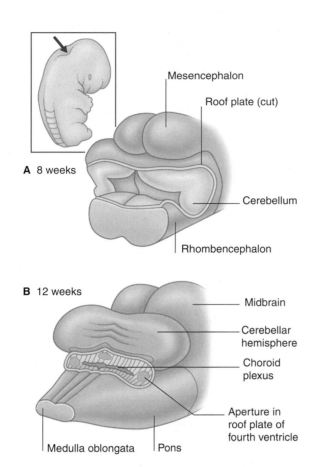

A 8 weeks

Mesencephalon

Roof plate (cut)

Cerebellum

Rhombencephalon

B 12 weeks

Midbrain

Cerebellar hemisphere

Choroid plexus

Aperture in roof plate of fourth ventricle

Medulla oblongata   Pons

Figure 1.5 Dorsal views of the developing hindbrain (see arrow in inset). **(A)** At 8 weeks, the cerebellum is emerging from the fourth ventricle. **(B)** At 12 weeks, the ventricle is becoming hidden by the cerebellum and three apertures have appeared in the roof plate.

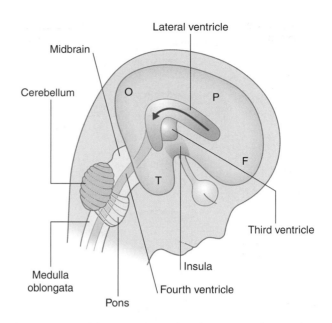

Lateral ventricle

Midbrain

Cerebellum

O   P

T   F

Third ventricle

Insula

Medulla oblongata

Fourth ventricle

Pons

Figure 1.7 Fetal brain at 14 weeks. The arrow indicates the C-shaped growth of the hemisphere around the insula. F, P, O, T, frontal, parietal, occipital, temporal lobes.

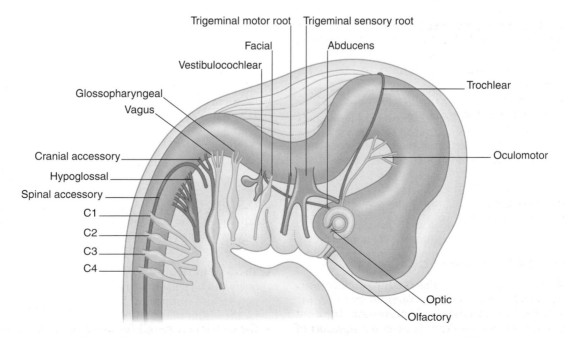

Trigeminal motor root   Trigeminal sensory root

Facial   Abducens

Vestibulocochlear

Glossopharyngeal   Trochlear

Vagus

Cranial accessory   Oculomotor

Hypoglossal

Spinal accessory

C1

C2

C3

C4

Optic

Olfactory

Figure 1.6 Cranial nerves of a 6-week embryo. (Adapted from Bossy et al., 1990.)

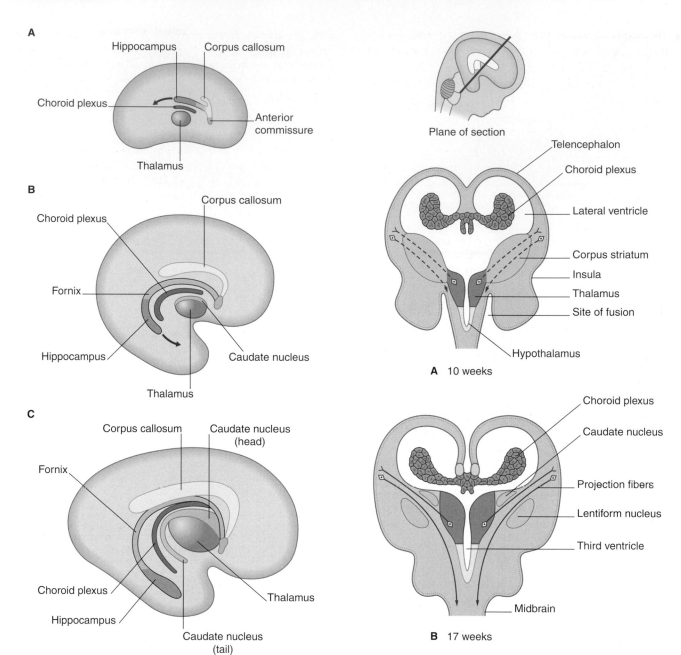

A
Hippocampus   Corpus callosum
Choroid plexus
Anterior commissure
Thalamus

B
Corpus callosum
Choroid plexus
Fornix
Hippocampus
Caudate nucleus
Thalamus

C
Corpus callosum   Caudate nucleus (head)
Fornix
Choroid plexus
Thalamus
Hippocampus
Caudate nucleus (tail)

Plane of section

Telencephalon
Choroid plexus
Lateral ventricle
Corpus striatum
Insula
Thalamus
Site of fusion
Hypothalamus

A 10 weeks

Choroid plexus
Caudate nucleus
Projection fibers
Lentiform nucleus
Third ventricle
Midbrain

B 17 weeks

Figure 1.8 Medial aspect of developing left hemisphere. The hippocampus, initially dorsal to the thalamus, migrates into the temporal lobe (arrows in **A** and **B**), leaving the fornix in its wake. The concavity of the arch so formed contains the choroid fissure (the line of insertion of the choroid plexus into the lateral ventricle) and the tail of the caudate nucleus.

Figure 1.9 Coronal sections of the developing cerebrum. In **A**, the corpus striatum is traversed by fibers projecting from thalamus to cerebral cortex and from cerebral cortex to spinal cord. In **B**, the corpus striatum has been divided, to form the caudate and lentiform nuclei (fusion persists at the anterior end, not shown here).

- The optic nerve (II) is growing centrally from the retina.
- The oculomotor (III) and trochlear (IV) nerves arise from the midbrain, and the abducens (VI) nerve arises from the pons; all three will supply extrinsic muscles of the eye.
- The three divisions of the trigeminal (V) nerve will be sensory to the skin of the face and scalp, to the mucous membranes of the oronasal cavity and to the teeth. A motor root will supply the muscles of mastication (chewing).

- The facial (VII) nerve will supply the muscles of facial expression. The vestibulocochlear (VIII) nerve will supply the organs of hearing and balance, which develop from the otocyst.
- The glossopharyngeal (IX) nerve is composite. Most of its fibers will be sensory to the oropharynx. The vagus (X) nerve is also composite; it contains a large sensory element for the supply of the mucous membranes of the digestive system, and a large motor (parasympathetic) element for the supply of the heart and gastrointestinal tract.

- The cranial accessory (XIc) nerve will be distributed by the vagus to the muscles of the larynx and pharynx.
- The spinal accessory (XIs) nerve will supply the sternomastoid and trapezius muscles. The hypoglossal (XII) nerve will supply the muscles of the tongue.

Cerebral hemispheres

In the telencephalon, mitotic activity takes place in the **ventricular zone**, just outside the lateral ventricle. Daughter cells migrate to the outer surface of the expanding hemisphere and form the cerebral cortex.

Expansion of the cerebral hemispheres is not uniform. A region on the lateral surface, the insula, is relatively quiescent and forms a pivot around which the expanding hemisphere rotates. Frontal, parietal, occipital, and temporal lobes can be identified at 14 weeks' gestational age (*Figure 1.7*).

On the medial surface of the hemisphere, a patch of cerebral cortex, the hippocampus, belongs to a fifth, limbic lobe of the brain. The hippocampus is drawn into the temporal lobe, leaving in its wake a strand of fibers called the fornix. Within the concavity of this arc is the choroid fissure, through which the choroid plexus invaginates the lateral ventricle (*Figure 1.8*).

The anterior commissure develops as a connection linking olfactory (smell) regions of the left and right sides. Above this, a much larger commissure, the corpus callosum, links matching areas of the cerebral cortex of the two sides. It extends backward above the fornix.

Coronal sections of the telencephalon reveal a mass of gray matter in the base of each hemisphere which is the forerunner of the corpus striatum. Beside the third ventricle, the diencephalon gives rise to the thalamus and hypothalamus (*Figure 1.9*).

The expanding cerebral hemispheres come into contact with the diencephalon and they fuse with it (see 'site of fusion' in (*Figure 1.9A*). One consequence is that the term 'brainstem' is restricted thereafter to the remaining, free parts: midbrain, pons, and medulla oblongata. A second consequence is that the cerebral cortex is able to project fibers direct to the brainstem. Together with fibers projecting from thalamus to cortex, they split the corpus striatum into caudate and lentiform nuclei (*Figure 1.9B*).

By the 28th week of development, several sulci (fissures) have appeared on the surface of the brain, notably the lateral, central, and calcarine sulci (*Figure 1.10*).

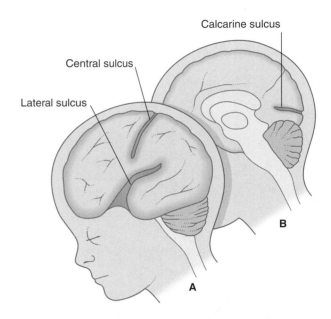

Figure 1.10 Three major cortical sulci in a fetus of 28 weeks. **(A)** Lateral surface of left hemisphere; **(B)** medial surface.

Core Information

The nervous system takes the initial form of a cellular neural tube derived from the ectoderm and enclosing a neural canal. A ribbon of cells escapes along each side of the tube to form the neural crest. The more caudal part of the tube forms the spinal cord. The neural crest forms spinal ganglion cells that send dorsal nerve roots into the sensory, alar plate of the cord. The basal plate of the cord contains motor neurons that emit ventral roots to complete the spinal nerves by joining the dorsal roots.

The more rostral part of the tube forms three brain vesicles. Of these, the prosencephalon (forebrain) gives rise to the cerebral hemispheres (telencephalon) dorsally and the diencephalon ventrally; the mesencephalon becomes the midbrain; and the rhombencephalon becomes the hindbrain (pons, medulla oblongata, cerebellum).

The neural tube expands rostrally to create the ventricular system of the brain. CSF is secreted by a choroid capillary plexus that invaginates the roof plates of the ventricles.

The cerebral hemispheres develop frontal, parietal, temporal, occipital and limbic lobes. The hemispheres are cross-linked by the corpus callosum and anterior commissure. Gray matter in the base of each hemisphere is the forerunner of the corpus striatum. The hemispheres fuse with the side walls of the diencephalon, whereupon the mesencephalon and rhombencephalon are all that remain of the embryonic brainstem.

REFERENCES

Bossy, J., O'Rahilly, R. and Müller, F. (1990) Ontogenese du systeme nerveux. In *Anatomie Clinique: Neuroanatomie* (Bossy, J., ed.), pp. 357–388. Paris: Springer-Verlag.

Cabana, T. (1993) Development of the nervous system. In *Neuroscience for Rehabilitation* (Cohen, M., ed.), pp. 357–387. Philadelphia: Lippincott.

FitzGerald, M.J.T. and FitzGerald, M. (1994) *Human Embryology*. London: Baillière Tindall.

Larsen, W.J. (1993) *Human Embryology*. New York: Churchill Livingstone.

O'Rahilly, R. and Gardner, E. (1979) The initial development of the human brain. *Acta Anat.* **104**: 123–133.

O'Rahilly, R. and Müller, F. (1987) The developmental anatomy and histology of the human central nervous system. In *Handbook of Clinical Neurology*, Vol. 6, Malformations (Myrianthopoulos, N.C., ed.), pp. 1–17. Amsterdam: Elsevier.

Sadler, T.W. (1990) *Langman's Medical Embryology*, 6th edn. Baltimore: Williams & Wilkins.

Cerebral topography

Box 2.1 Brain planes

Figure Box 2.1.1 (A) Planes of reference for the CNS as a whole. In this presentation only the brainstem (owing to its obliquity) differs from the standard for gross anatomy. However, some authors use the terms 'ventral' and 'dorsal' instead of 'anterior' and 'posterior' with respect to the spinal cord and some use the terms 'rostral' and 'caudal' to signify 'superior' and 'inferior' with respect to spinal cord and/or brainstem.

The horizontal line represents the bicommissural plane. AC, PC, anterior and posterior commissures.

 (B) The brain sectioned in the bicommissural plane. (Adapted from Kretschmann, H-J. and Weinrich, W. (1998) *Neurofunctional Systems: 3D Reconstructions with Correlated Neuroimaging: Text and CD-ROM*. New York: Thieme, with kind permission of the authors and the publisher.)

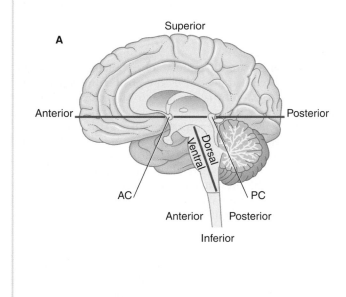

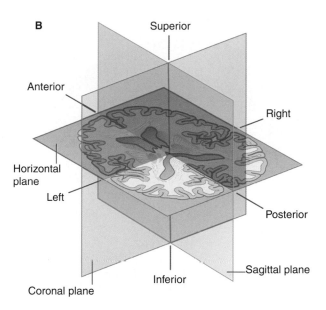

SURFACE FEATURES

Lobes

The surfaces of the two cerebral hemispheres are furrowed by **sulci**, the intervening ridges being called **gyri**. Most of the cerebral cortex is concealed from view in the walls of the sulci. Although the patterns of the various sulci vary from brain to brain, some are sufficiently constant to serve as descriptive landmarks.

The deepest sulci are the **lateral sulcus** (*Sylvian fissure*) and the **central sulcus** (*Rolandic fissure*) (*Figure 2.1A*). These two serve to divide the hemisphere into four **lobes**, with the aid of two imaginary lines: one line extends back from the lateral sulcus; the other reaches from the upper end of the **parieto-occipital sulcus** (*Figure 2.1B*) to a blunt **pre-occipital notch** at the lower border of the hemi-

sphere. The lobes are called **frontal**, **parietal**, **occipital**, and **temporal**.

The blunt tips of the frontal, occipital, and temporal lobes are the respective **poles** of the hemispheres.

The lips (**opercula**) of the lateral sulcus can be pulled apart to expose the **insula** (*Figure 2.2*). The insula was mentioned in Chapter 1 as being relatively quiescent during prenatal expansion of the telencephalon.

The medial surface of the hemisphere is exposed by cutting the **corpus callosum**, a massive band of white matter connecting matching areas of the cortex of the two hemispheres. The corpus callosum consists of a main part or **trunk**, a posterior end or **splenium**, an anterior end or **genu** ('knee'), and a narrow **rostrum** reaching from the genu to the **anterior commissure** (*Figure 2.3B*). The frontal lobe lies anterior to a line drawn from the upper end of the central sulcus to the trunk of the corpus callosum (*Figure 2.3B*). The

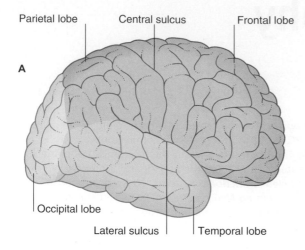

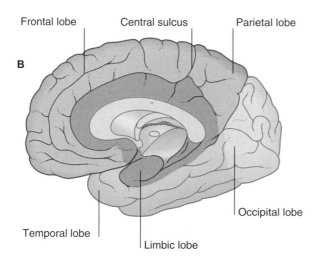

Figure 2.1 The five lobes of the brain. **(A)** Lateral surface of right cerebral hemisphere. **(B)** Medial surface of right hemisphere.

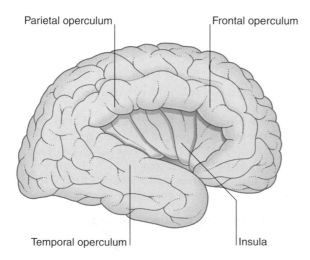

Figure 2.2 Insula, seen upon retraction of the opercula.

parietal lobe lies behind this line, and it is separated from the occipital lobe by the parieto-occipital sulcus. The temporal lobe lies in front of a line drawn from the pre-occipital notch to the splenium.

Figures 2.3 to *2.6* should be consulted along with the following description of surface features of the lobes of the brain.

Frontal lobe

The lateral surface of the **frontal lobe** contains the **precentral gyrus** bounded in front by the **precentral sulcus**. Further forward, **superior, middle,** and **inferior frontal gyri** are separated by **superior** and **inferior frontal sulci**. On the medial surface, the superior frontal gyrus is separated from the **cingulate gyrus** by the **cingulate sulcus**. The inferior or orbital surface is marked by several **orbital gyri**. In contact with this surface are the **olfactory bulb** and **olfactory tract**.

Parietal lobe

The anterior part of the parietal lobe contains the **postcentral gyrus** bounded behind by the **postcentral sulcus**. The posterior parietal lobe is divided into **superior** and **inferior parietal lobules** by an **intraparietal sulcus**. The inferior parietal lobule shows a **supramarginal gyrus**, capping the upturned end of the lateral sulcus, and an **angular gyrus** capping the superior temporal sulcus. The medial surface contains the posterior part of the **paracentral lobule** and, behind this, the **precuneus**. The paracentral lobule (partly contained in the frontal lobe) is so called because of its relationship to the central sulcus.

Occipital lobe

The lateral surface of the occipital lobe is marked by several **lateral occipital gyri**. The medial surface contains the **cuneus** ('wedge') between the parieto-occipital sulcus and the important **calcarine sulcus**. The inferior surface shows three gyri and three sulci. The **lateral** and **medial occipitotemporal gyri** are separated by the **occipitotemporal sulcus**. The **lingual gyrus** lies between the collateral sulcus and the anterior end of the calcarine sulcus.

Temporal lobe

The lateral surface of the temporal lobe displays **superior, middle,** and **inferior temporal gyri** separated by **superior and inferior temporal sulci**. The inferior surface shows the anterior parts of the occipitotemporal gyri. The lingual gyrus continues forward as the **parahippocampal gyrus** which ends in a blunt medial projection, the **uncus**. As will be seen later in views of the sectioned brain, the parahippocampal gyrus underlies a rolled-in part of the cortex, the **hippocampus**.

Limbic lobe

A fifth, **limbic lobe** of the brain surrounds the medial margin of the hemisphere. Surface contributors to the limbic lobe include the cingulate and parahippocampal gyri. It is more usual to speak of the *limbic system*, which includes the hippocampus, fornix, amygdala, and other elements (Ch. 29).

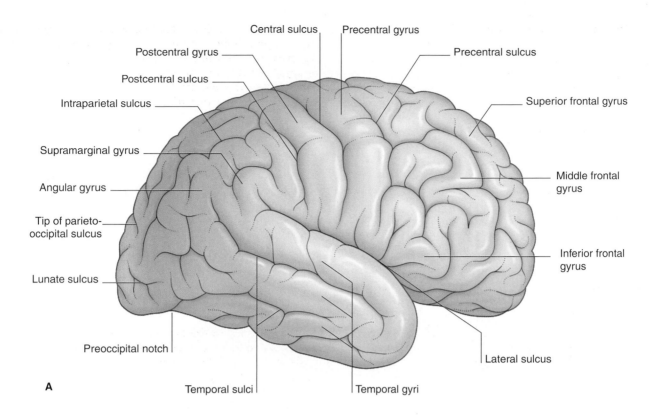

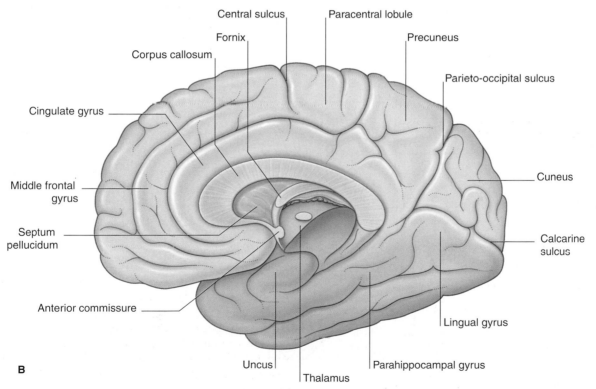

Figure 2.3 (A) Lateral and **(B)** medial views of the right cerebral hemisphere, depicting the main gyri and sulci.

Diencephalon

The largest components of the diencephalon are the **thalamus** and the **hypothalamus** (*Figures 2.6, 2.7*). These nuclear groups form the side walls of the third ventricle.

Between them is a shallow **hypothalamic sulcus**, which represents the rostral limit of the embryonic sulcus limitans. The hypothalamus forms the floor of the third ventricle as well.

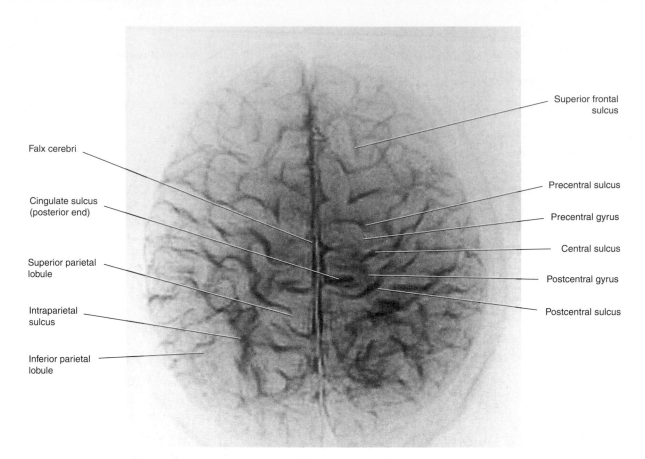

Figure 2.4 'Thick slice' surface anatomy brain MRI scan from a healthy volunteer. (Reproduced from Neuroradiology (1990) 32: 439–448 with kind permission of Professor K. Katada and the publisher.)

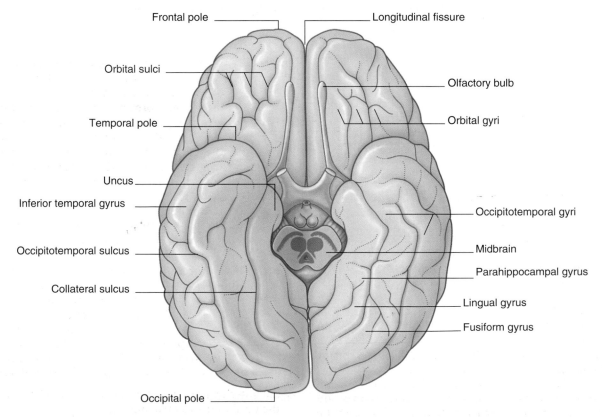

Figure 2.5 Cerebrum viewed from below, depicting the main gyri and sulci.

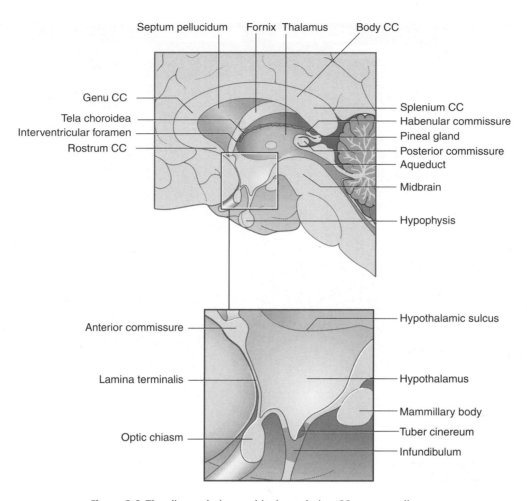

Figure 2.6 The diencephalon and its boundaries. CC, corpus callosum.

INTERNAL ANATOMY OF THE CEREBRUM

The arrangement of the following structures will now be described: thalamus, caudate, and lentiform nuclei, internal capsule; hippocampus and fornix; association and commissural fibers; lateral and third ventricles.

Thalamus, caudate and lentiform nuclei, internal capsule

The two thalami face one another across the slot-like third ventricle. More often than not, they kiss, creating an **inter-thalamic adhesion** (*Figure 2.8*). In *Figure 2.9*, the thalamus and related structures are assembled in a mediolateral sequence. In contact with the upper surface of the thalamus are the **head** and **body** of the **caudate nucleus**. The **tail** of the caudate nucleus passes forward below the thalamus, but not in contact with it.

The thalamus is separated from the lentiform nucleus by the **internal capsule**, which is a common site for a *stroke* resulting from local arterial hemorrhage. The internal capsule contains fibers running from thalamus to cortex and from cortex to thalamus, brainstem, and spinal cord. In the interval between cortex and internal capsule, these ascend-ing and descending fibers form the **corona radiata**. Below the internal capsule, the **crus** of the midbrain receives descending fibers continuing into the brainstem.

The lens-shaped **lentiform nucleus** is composed of two parts, **putamen** and **globus pallidus**. The putamen and caudate nucleus are of similar structure and their anterior ends are fused. Behind this, they are linked by strands of gray matter which traverse the internal capsule: hence the term **corpus striatum** (or, simply, **striatum**) used to include the putamen and caudate nucleus. The term **pallidum** refers to the globus pallidus.

The caudate and lentiform nuclei belong to the **basal ganglia**, a term originally applied to a half-dozen masses of gray matter located near the base of the hemisphere. In current usage, the term designates four nuclei known to be involved in motor control: the caudate and lentiform nuclei, the subthalamic nucleus in the diencephalon, and the substantia nigra in the midbrain (*Table 2.1*).

In horizontal section, the internal capsule has a dog-leg shape (see photograph of a fixed-brain section in *Figure 2.10*, and living-brain MRI 'slice' in *Figure 2.11*). The internal capsule has four named parts in horizontal sections:

1 the **anterior limb**, between the lentiform nucleus and the head of the caudate nucleus;

2 the **genu**;

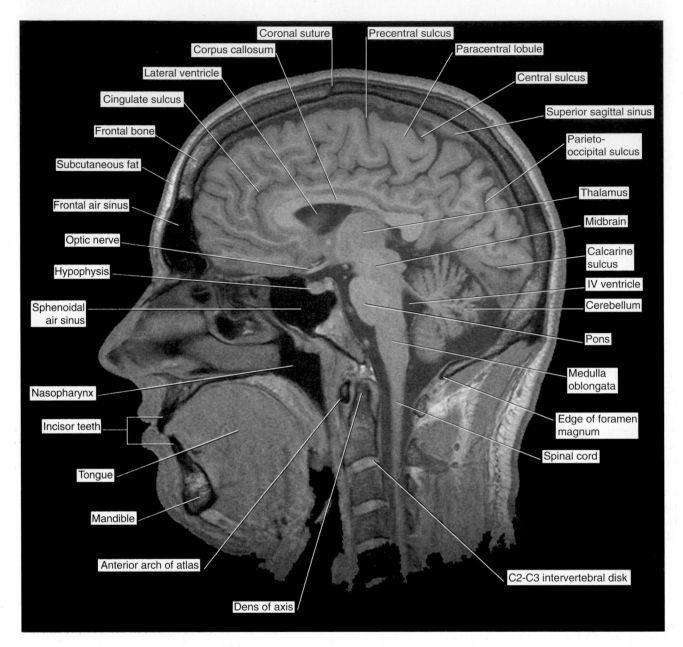

Figure 2.7 Sagittal MRI 'slice' of the living brain. (From a series kindly provided by Professor J. Paul Finn, Director, MRI Facility, Northwestern University Medical School, Chicago.)

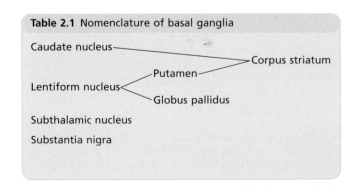

Table 2.1 Nomenclature of basal ganglia

Caudate nucleus ⎤
⎟ Corpus striatum
Putamen ⎦

Lentiform nucleus ⎤
⎟
Globus pallidus ⎦

Subthalamic nucleus

Substantia nigra

3 the **posterior limb**, between the lentiform nucleus and the thalamus;

4 the **retrolentiform part**, behind the lentiform nucleus and lateral to the thalamus.

The **corticospinal tract** (CST) descends in the posterior limb of the internal capsule. It is also called the **pyramidal tract**, a *tract* being a bundle of fibers serving a common function. The CST originates mainly from the *motor cortex* within the precentral gyrus. It descends through the corona radiata, internal capsule, and crus of midbrain and continues to the lower end of the brainstem before crossing to the opposite side of the spinal cord.

From a clinical standpoint, *the CST is the most important pathway in the entire central nervous system (CNS)* for two

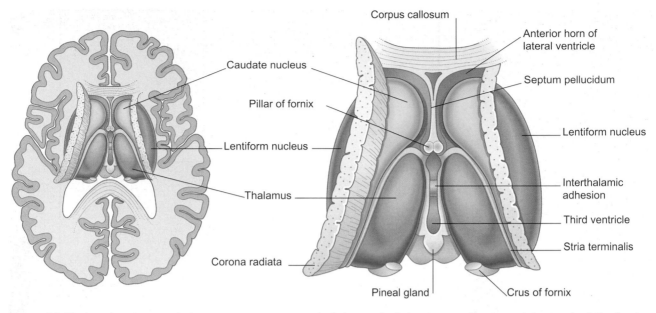

Figure 2.8 Thalamus and corpus striatum, seen upon removal of the trunk of the corpus callosum and the trunk of the fornix.

reasons. First, it mediates voluntary movements of all kinds, and interruption of the tract by disease leads to motor weakness (called *paresis*) or motor paralysis. Second, it extends the entire vertical length of the CNS, rendering it vulnerable to disease or trauma in the cerebral hemisphere or brainstem on one side, and to spinal cord disease or trauma on the other side.

A coronal section through the anterior limb is represented in *Figure 2.12*; a corresponding MRI view is shown in *Figure 2.13*. A coronal section through the posterior limb from a fixed brain is shown in *Figure 2.14*; a corresponding MRI 'slice' is shown in *Figure 2.15*.

Lateral to the lentiform nucleus are the **external capsule**, **claustrum**, and **extreme capsule**.

Hippocampus and fornix

The **hippocampus** is first seen in embryonic life above the corpus callosum. The bulk of it remains in that position in lower mammals, including rodents. In primates, it retreats into the temporal lobe as this develops, leaving a tract of white matter, the **fornix**, in its wake. The mature hippocampus stretches the full length of the floor of the inferior (temporal) horn of the lateral ventricle (*Figure 2.16*). The mature fornix comprises a **body** beneath the trunk of the corpus callosum, a **crus** which enters it from each hippocampus, and two **pillars (columns)** which leave it to enter the diencephalon. Intimately related to the crus and body is the **choroid fissure**, through which the choroid plexus is inserted into the lateral ventricle.

Association and commissural fibers

Fibers leaving the cerebral cortex fall into three groups:

- **association fibers**, which pass from one part of a single hemisphere to another;
- **commissural fibers**, which link matching areas of the two hemispheres;

- **projection fibers**, which run to subcortical nuclei in the cerebral hemisphere, brainstem, and spinal cord.

Association fibers (*Figure 2.17*)

Short association fibers pass from one gyrus to another within a lobe.

Long association fibers link one lobe with another. Bundles of long association fibers include:

- the **superior longitudinal fasciculus**, linking the frontal and occipital lobes;
- the **inferior longitudinal fasciculus**, linking the occipital and temporal lobes;
- the **arcuate fasciculus**, linking the frontal lobe with the occipitotemporal cortex;
- the **uncinate fasciculus**, linking the frontal and anterior temporal lobes;
- the **cingulum**, underlying the cortex of the cingulate gyrus.

Cerebral commissures

Corpus callosum

The **corpus callosum** is much the largest of the commissures linking matching areas of the left and right cerebral cortex (*Figure 2.17*). From the **body**, some fibers pass laterally and upward, intersecting the corona radiata. Other fibers pass laterally and then bend downward as the **tapetum** to reach the lower parts of the temporal and occipital lobes. Fibers traveling to the medial wall of the occipital lobe emerge from the splenium on each side and form the **occipital (major) forceps**. The **frontal (minor) forceps** emerges from each side of the genu to reach the medial wall of the frontal lobe.

Minor commissures

The **anterior commissure** interconnects the anterior parts of the temporal lobes, as well as the two olfactory tracts.

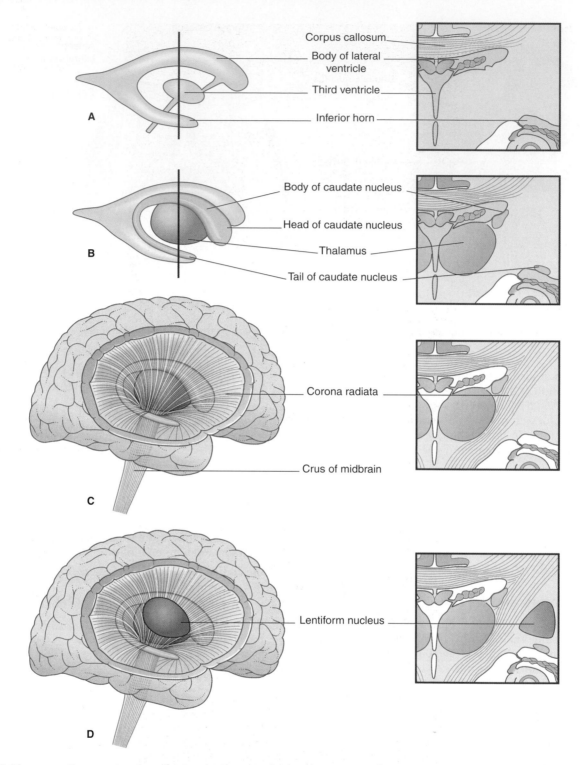

A

- Corpus callosum
- Body of lateral ventricle
- Third ventricle
- Inferior horn

B

- Body of caudate nucleus
- Head of caudate nucleus
- Thalamus
- Tail of caudate nucleus

C

- Corona radiata
- Crus of midbrain

D

- Lentiform nucleus

Figure 2.9 Diagrammatic reconstruction of corpus striatum and related structures. The vertical lines on the left in **A** and **B** indicate the level of the coronal sections on the right. **(A)** Ventricular system. **(B)** Thalamus and caudate nucleus in place. **(C)** Addition of projections to and from cerebral cortex. **(D)** Lentiform nucleus in place.

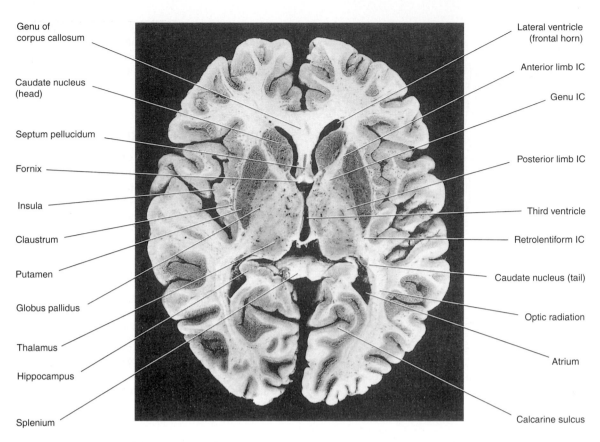

Genu of
corpus callosum

Caudate nucleus
(head)

Septum pellucidum

Fornix

Insula

Claustrum

Putamen

Globus pallidus

Thalamus

Hippocampus

Splenium

Lateral ventricle
(frontal horn)

Anterior limb IC

Genu IC

Posterior limb IC

Third ventricle

Retrolentiform IC

Caudate nucleus (tail)

Optic radiation

Atrium

Calcarine sulcus

Figure 2.10 Horizontal section of fixed brain in the plane indicated at top. IC, internal capsule. (Photograph reproduced from Gluhbegovic and Williams (1980) with kind permission of the authors and J.B. Lippincott, Inc.)

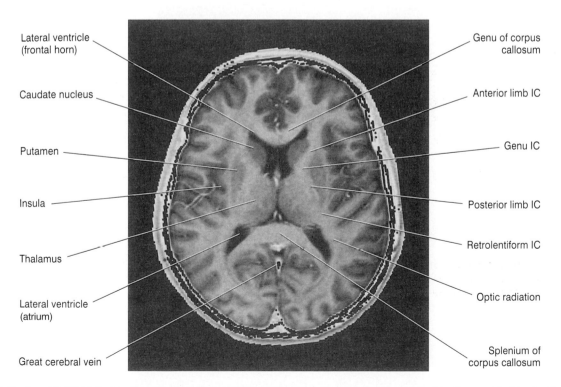

Lateral ventricle
(frontal horn)

Caudate nucleus

Putamen

Insula

Thalamus

Lateral ventricle
(atrium)

Great cerebral vein

Genu of corpus
callosum

Anterior limb IC

Genu IC

Posterior limb IC

Retrolentiform IC

Optic radiation

Splenium of
corpus callosum

Figure 2.11 Horizontal MRI 'slice' in the plane of Figure 2.10. IC, internal capsule. (From a series kindly provided by Professor J. Paul Finn, Director, MRI Facility, Northwestern University Medical School, Chicago.) *Note:* Horizontal 'slices' are viewed from below as a rule.

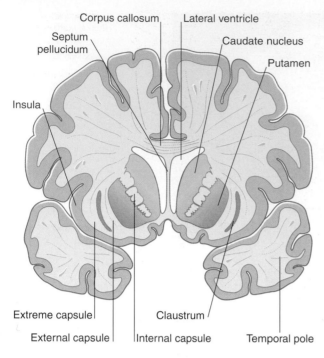

Figure 2.12 Drawing of a coronal section through the anterior limb of the internal capsule.

The **posterior commissure** and the **habenular commissure** lie directly in front of the pineal gland.

The **commissure of the fornix** contains some fibers traveling from one hippocampus to the other by way of the two crura.

Lateral and third ventricles

The **lateral ventricle** consists of a **body** (central part) within the parietal lobe, and **anterior** (frontal), **posterior** (occipital), and **inferior** (temporal) **horns** (*Figure 2.20*). The anterior limit of the central part is the **interventricular foramen**, located between thalamus and anterior pillar of the fornix, through which it communicates with the third ventricle. The central part joins the occipital and temporal horns at the **atrium** (*Figure 2.21*).

The relationships of the lateral ventricle are listed below:

- *Anterior horn:* lies between head of caudate nucleus and septum pellucidum. Its other boundaries are formed by the corpus callosum: trunk above, genu in front, rostrum below.
- *Body:* lies below the trunk of the corpus callosum and above the thalamus and anterior part of the body of the fornix. Medially is the septum pellucidum, which tapers

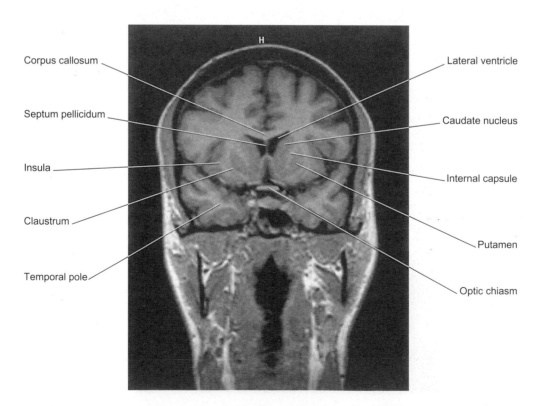

Figure 2.13 Coronal MRI 'slice' at the level indicated at top. (From a series kindly provided by Professor J. Paul Finn, Director, MRI Facility, Northwestern University Medical School, Chicago.) *Note:* Coronal 'slices' are viewed from the front.

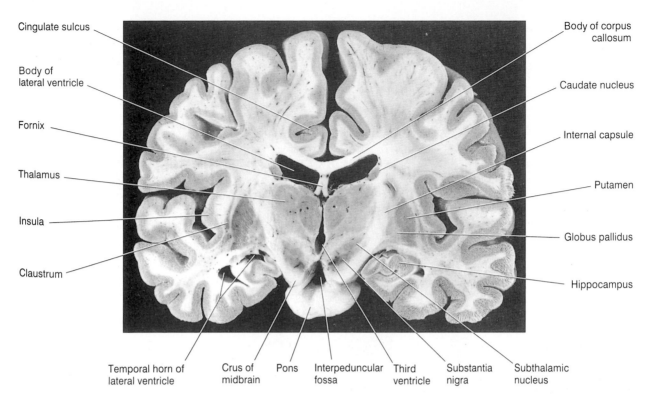

Figure 2.14 Coronal section of fixed brain at the level indicated at top. (Photograph reproduced from Gluhbegovic and Williams (1980) with kind permission of the authors and J.B. Lippincott, Inc.)

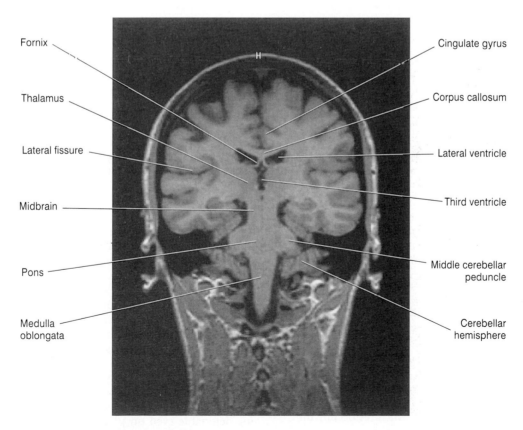

Figure 2.15 Coronal MRI 'slice' at the level indicated at top. (From a series kindly provided by Professor J. Paul Finn, Director, MRI Facility, Northwestern University Medical School, Chicago.)

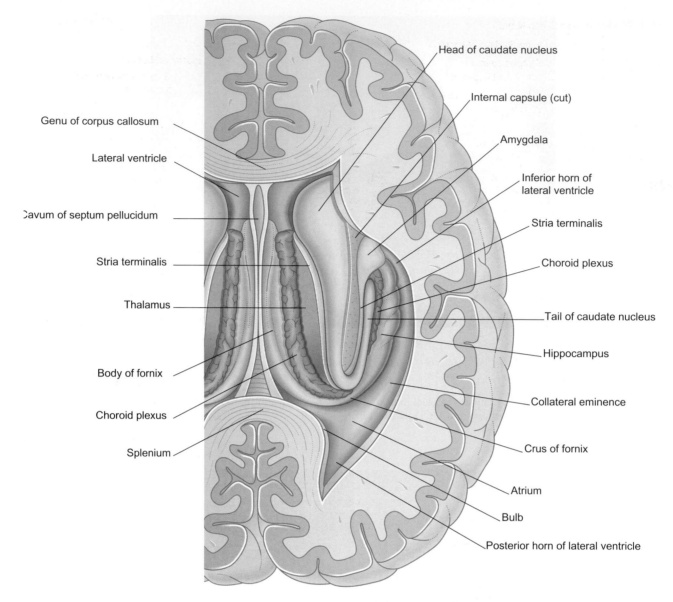

Figure 2.16 Tilted view of the ventricular system showing the continuity of structures in the body and inferior horn of the lateral ventricle. *Note:* The amygdala, stria terminalis, and tail of caudate nucleus occupy the roof of the inferior horn; the hippocampus occupies the floor. (The choroid plexus is 'reduced' in order to show related structures.)

away posteriorly where the fornix rises to meet the corpus callosum. The **septum pellucidum** is formed of the thinned-out walls of the two cerebral hemispheres. Its bilateral origin may be indicated by a central cavity (**cavum**).

- *Posterior horn:* lies below the splenium and medial to the tapetum of the corpus callosum. On the medial side, the forceps major forms the **bulb** of the posterior horn.

- *Inferior horn:* lies below the tail of the caudate nucleus and, at the anterior end, the **amygdala** (*Figure 2.16*), a nucleus belonging to the limbic system. The hippocampus and its associated structures occupy the full length of the floor.

- Outside these is the **collateral eminence**, created by the collateral sulcus.

The **third ventricle** is the cavity of the diencephalon. Its boundaries are shown in *Figure 2.6*. A **choroid plexus** hangs from its roof, which is formed of a double layer of pia mater called the **tela choroidea**. Above this are the fornix and corpus callosum. In each side wall are the thalamus and hypothalamus. The anterior wall is formed by the anterior commissure, the **lamina terminalis**, and the **optic chiasm**. In the floor are the **infundibulum**, the **tuber cinereum**, the **mammillary bodies** (also spelt 'mamillary'), and the upper end of the midbrain. The **pineal gland** and related commissures form the posterior wall. The pineal gland is often calcified, and the **habenular commissure** is sometimes calcified, as early as the second decade of life, thereby becoming detectable even on plain radiographs of the skull. The pineal gland is sometimes displaced to one side by a tumor, hematoma, or other space-occupying lesion within the cranial cavity.

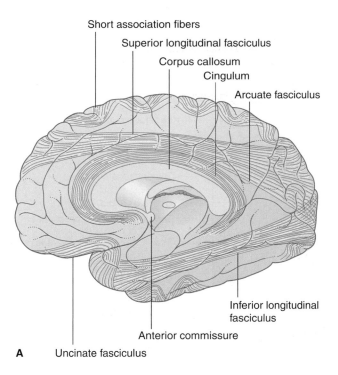

Short association fibers
Superior longitudinal fasciculus
Corpus callosum
Cingulum
Arcuate fasciculus
Inferior longitudinal fasciculus
Anterior commissure
A Uncinate fasciculus

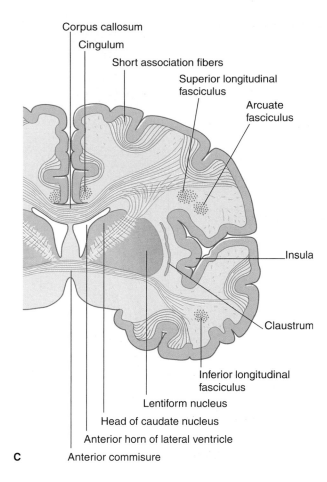

Corpus callosum
Cingulum
Short association fibers
Superior longitudinal fasciculus
Arcuate fasciculus
Insula
Claustrum
Inferior longitudinal fasciculus
Lentiform nucleus
Head of caudate nucleus
Anterior horn of lateral ventricle
C Anterior commisure

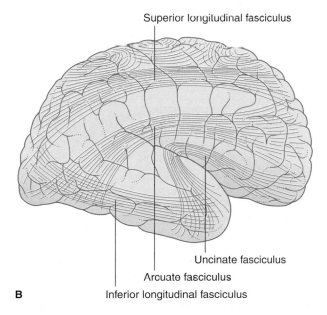

Superior longitudinal fasciculus
Uncinate fasciculus
Arcuate fasciculus
B Inferior longitudinal fasciculus

Figure 2.17 (A) Medial view of 'transparent' right cerebral hemisphere. **(B)** Lateral view of 'transparent' left hemisphere. **(C)** Coronal section, showing position of short and long association fiber bundles.

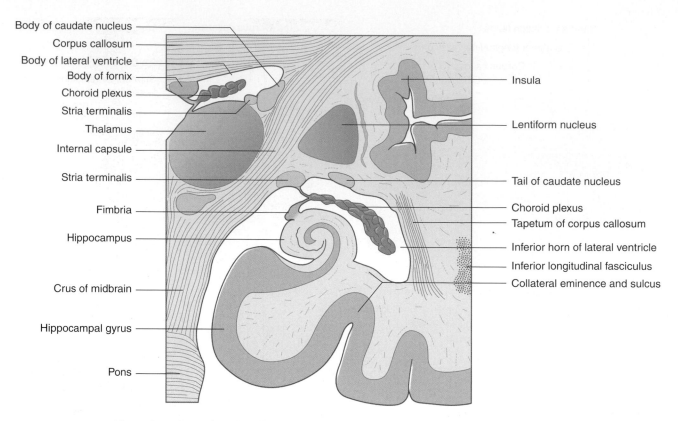

Body of caudate nucleus
Corpus callosum
Body of lateral ventricle
Body of fornix
Choroid plexus
Stria terminalis
Thalamus
Internal capsule
Stria terminalis
Fimbria
Hippocampus
Crus of midbrain
Hippocampal gyrus
Pons

Insula
Lentiform nucleus
Tail of caudate nucleus
Choroid plexus
Tapetum of corpus callosum
Inferior horn of lateral ventricle
Inferior longitudinal fasciculus
Collateral eminence and sulcus

Figure 2.18 Coronal section through the body and inferior horn of the lateral ventricle.

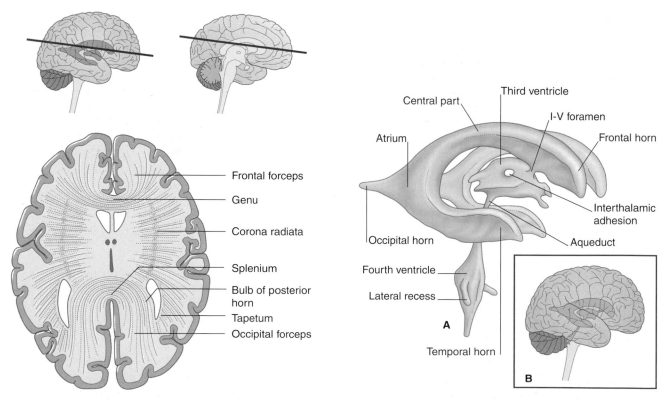

Frontal forceps
Genu
Corona radiata
Splenium
Bulb of posterior horn
Tapetum
Occipital forceps

Central part
Atrium
Occipital horn
Fourth ventricle
Lateral recess
A
Temporal horn

Third ventricle
I-V foramen
Frontal horn
Interthalamic adhesion
Aqueduct

B

Figure 2.19 Horizontal section through genu and splenium of corpus callosum. Fibers passing laterally from the trunk intersect the corona radiata.

Figure 2.20 Ventricular system. **(A)** Isolated cast. **(B)** Ventricular system in situ.

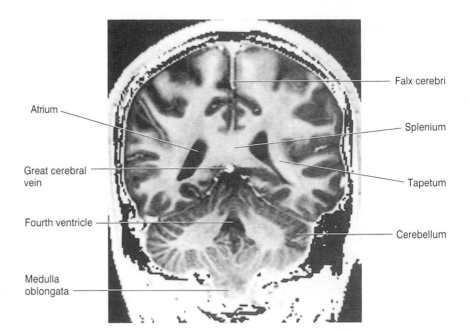

Atrium

Great cerebral vein

Fourth ventricle

Medulla oblongata

Falx cerebri

Splenium

Tapetum

Cerebellum

Figure 2.21 Coronal MRI 'slice' at the level indicated at top. (From a series kindly provided by Professor J. Paul Finn, Director, MRI Facility, Northwestern University Medical School, Chicago.)

Core Information

On the lateral surface of the cerebrum, four lobes are defined by the lateral and central sulci and an imaginary T-shaped line. The frontal lobe has six named gyri, the parietal lobe has seven, the occipital lobe five, and the temporal lobe four. The insula is in the floor of the lateral sulcus.

On the medial surface, the corpus callosum comprises splenium, trunk, genu, and rostrum; the rostrum is attached to the anterior commissure. The septum pellucidum stretches from the corpus callosum to the trunk of the fornix. Separating fornix from thalamus is the choroidal fissure through which the choroid plexus invaginates into the lateral ventricle. The third ventricle has the fornix in its roof; thalamus and hypothalamus in its side wall; infundibulum, tuber cinereum, and mammillary bodies in its floor. Behind it is the pineal gland, often calcified.

The basal ganglia comprise the corpus striatum (caudate and lentiform nuclei), subthalamic nucleus,

and substantia nigra. The lentiform nucleus comprises putamen and globus pallidus. The striatum is made up of caudate and putamen, the pallidum of globus pallidus alone.

The internal capsule is the white matter separating the lentiform nucleus from the thalamus and head of caudate nucleus. The CST descends through the corona radiata, internal capsule, and crus of midbrain.

Association fibers (e.g. longitudinal, arcuate, uncinate fasciculi) link different areas within a hemisphere; commissural fibers (e.g. corpus callosum, anterior and posterior commissures) link matching areas across the midline; projection fibers (e.g. corticothalamic, corticobulbar, corticospinal) pass to thalamus and brainstem. The lateral ventricles have a central part and three horns. Structures determining ventricular shape include corpus callosum, caudate nucleus, thalamus, amygdala, and hippocampus.

REFERENCES

DeArmond, S.J., Fusco, M.M. and Dewey, M.M. (1976) *Structure of the Human Brain: a Photographic Atlas*, 2nd edn. Oxford: Oxford University Press.

England, M.A. and Wakely, J. (1991) *A Colour Atlas of the Brain and Spinal Cord*. London: Wolfe.

Gluhbegovic, N. and Williams, T.H. (1980) *The Human Brain: a Photographic Guide*. New York: Harper & Row.

Kretschmann, H-J. and Weinrich, W. (1998) *Neurofunctional Systems. 3D Reconstructions with Correlated Neuroimaging.*

Stuttgart: Thieme. *Note:* Interactive CD-ROM also available.

Niewenhuys, R., Voogd, J. and van Huijzen, C. (1988) *The Human Central Nervous System: a Synopsis and Atlas*, 3rd edn. New York: Springer-Verlag.

Roberts, M., Hanaway, J. and Morest, D.K. (1987) *Atlas of the Human Brain in Section*, 2nd edn. Philadelphia: Lea & Febiger.

Wicke, L. (1994) *Atlas of Radiologic Anatomy*. Philadelphia: Lea & Febiger.

Midbrain, hindbrain, spinal cord

The midbrain connects the diencephalon to the hindbrain. As explained in Chapter 1, the hindbrain is made up of the pons, medulla oblongata, and cerebellum. The medulla oblongata joins the spinal cord within the foramen magnum of the skull.

In this chapter, the cerebellum (part of the hindbrain) is considered *after* the spinal cord, for the sake of continuity of motor and sensory pathways.

BRAINSTEM

Ventral view   (Figures 3.1, 3.2A)

Midbrain
The ventral surface of the midbrain shows two massive **cerebral peduncles** bordering the **interpeduncular fossa**. The **optic tracts** wind around the midbrain at its junction with the diencephalon. Lateral to the midbrain is the uncus of the temporal lobe. The **oculomotor nerve** (III) emerges from the medial surface of the peduncle. The **trochlear nerve** (IV) passes between the peduncle and the uncus.

Pons
The bulk of the pons is composed of **transverse fibers** which raise numerous surface ridges. On each side, the pons is marked off from the middle cerebellar peduncle by the attachment of the **trigeminal nerve** (V). The **middle cerebellar peduncle** plunges into the hemisphere of the cerebellum.

At the lower border of the pons are the attachments of the **abducens** (VI), **facial** (VII), and **vestibulocochlear** (VIII) nerves (see *Table 3.1*).

Medulla oblongata
The **pyramids** are alongside the anterior median fissure. Just above the spinomedullary junction, the fissure is invaded by the **decussation of the pyramids**, where fibers of the two pyramids intersect while crossing the midline. Lateral to the pyramid is the **olive**, and behind the olive is the **inferior cerebellar peduncle**. Attached between pyramid and olive is the **hypoglossal nerve** (XII). Attached between olive and inferior cerebellar peduncle are the **glossopharyngeal** (IX), **vagus** (X), and **cranial accessory** (XIc) nerves. The **spinal accessory nerve** (XIs) arises from the spinal cord and runs up through the foramen magnum to join the cranial accessory.

Dorsal view   (Figure 3.2B)

The roof or **tectum** of the midbrain is composed of four colliculi. The **superior colliculi** belong to the visual system and the **inferior colliculi** belong to the auditory system. The **trochlear nerve** (IV) emerges below the inferior colliculus on each side.

The diamond-shaped **fourth ventricle** lies behind the pons and upper medulla oblongata, under cover of the cerebellum. The upper half of the diamond is bounded by the **superior cerebellar peduncles** which are attached to the midbrain. The lower half is bounded by the **inferior cerebellar peduncles**, which are attached to the medulla oblongata. The middle cerebellar peduncles enter from the pons and overlap the other two.

Near the midline in the midregion of the ventricle is the **facial colliculus**, which is created by the facial nerve curving around the nucleus of the abducens nerve. The **vestibular area**, and the **vagal** and **hypoglossal trigones** overlie the corresponding cranial nerve nuclei. The **obex** is the posterior apex of the ventricle.

Below the fourth ventricle, the medulla oblongata shows a pair of **gracile tubercles** flanked by a pair of **cuneate tubercles**.

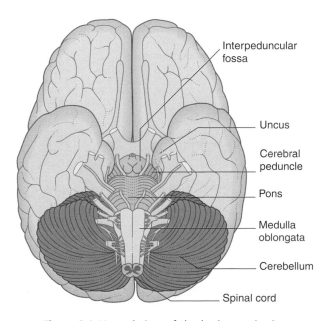

Interpeduncular fossa

Uncus

Cerebral peduncle

Pons

Medulla oblongata

Cerebellum

Spinal cord

Figure 3.1 Ventral view of the brainstem in situ.

Table 3.1 The cranial nerves			
I	Olfactory, enters the olfactory bulb from the nose	VI	Abducens
		VII	Facial
		VIII	Vestibulocochlear
II	Optic	IX	Glossopharyngeal
III	Oculomotor	X	Vagus
IV	Trochlear	XI	Accessory
V	Trigeminal	XII	Hypoglossal

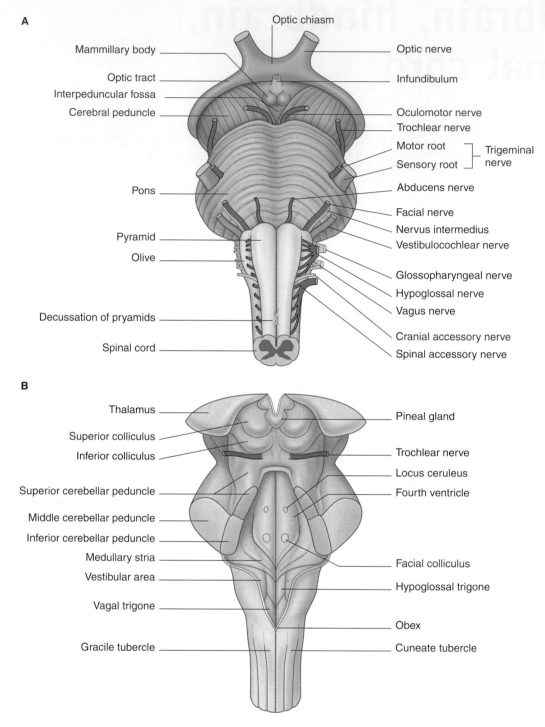

A

Optic chiasm

Mammillary body

Optic nerve

Optic tract

Infundibulum

Interpeduncular fossa

Cerebral peduncle

Oculomotor nerve

Trochlear nerve

Motor root

Trigeminal nerve

Sensory root

Pons

Abducens nerve

Facial nerve

Nervus intermedius

Pyramid

Vestibulocochlear nerve

Olive

Glossopharyngeal nerve

Hypoglossal nerve

Vagus nerve

Decussation of pryamids

Cranial accessory nerve

Spinal cord

Spinal accessory nerve

B

Thalamus

Pineal gland

Superior colliculus

Inferior colliculus

Trochlear nerve

Locus ceruleus

Superior cerebellar peduncle

Fourth ventricle

Middle cerebellar peduncle

Inferior cerebellar peduncle

Medullary stria

Facial colliculus

Vestibular area

Hypoglossal trigone

Vagal trigone

Obex

Gracile tubercle

Cuneate tubercle

Figure 3.2 (A) Anterior and **(B)** posterior view of the brainstem.

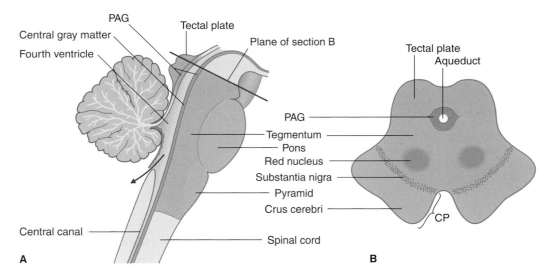

Figure 3.3 Named parts of the midbrain. **(A)** Sagittal section. **(B)** Transverse section. CP, cerebral peduncle; PAG, peri-aqueductal gray matter.

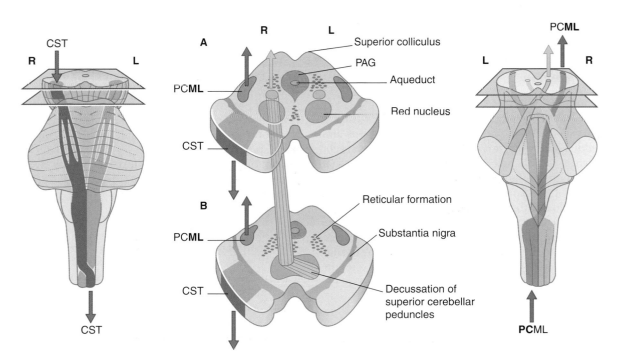

Figure 3.4 Transverse sections of midbrain. **(A)** At level of superior colliculi. **(B)** At level of inferior colliculi. In this and following diagrams, the pathway corticospinal tract (CST) and posterior column–medial lemniscal (PCML) pathways connected to the *right* cerebral hemisphere are highlighted. PAG, peri-aqueductal gray matter.

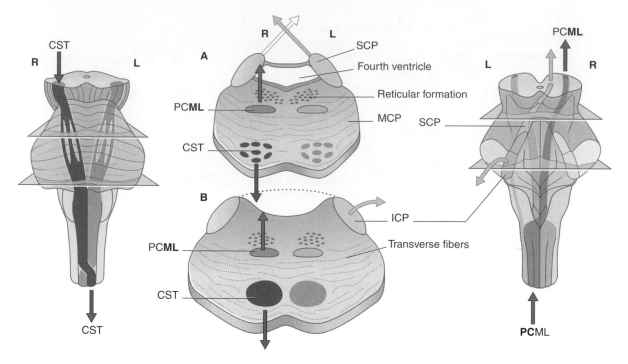

Figure 3.5 Transverse sections of pons. **(A)** Upper pons. **(B)** Lower pons. SCP, MCP, ICP, superior, middle, inferior cerebellar peduncles. CST, corticospinal tract; PCML, posterior column–medial lemniscal pathways.

Sectional views

Sagittal section   (Figure 3.3A)

In the midbrain, the central canal of the embryonic neural tube is represented by the **aqueduct**. Behind the pons and upper medulla oblongata, it is represented by the fourth ventricle, which is tent-shaped in this view. The central canal resumes at midmedullary level; it is continuous with the central canal of the spinal cord, although movement of cerebrospinal fluid into the cord canal is negligible.

The intermediate region of the brainstem is called the **tegmentum** which in the midbrain contains the paired **red nucleus**. Ventral to the tegmentum in the pons is the **basilar region**. Ventral to it in the medulla oblongata are the pyramids.

Transverse sections

The tegmentum of the entire brainstem is permeated by an important network of neurons, the **reticular formation**. The tegmentum also contains *ascending sensory pathways* carrying general sensory information from the trunk and limbs. Illustrated in Figures 3.4–3.7 are the *posterior column–medial lemniscal* (PCML) *pathways*, which inform the brain about the position of the limbs in space. At spinal cord level, the label **PC** ML is used because these pathways occupy the **posterior columns** of white matter in the cord. In the brainstem, the label PCML is used because they continue upward as the **medial lemnisci**.

The most important *motor pathways* from a clinical standpoint are the *corticospinal tracts* (CSTs), the pathways of execution of voluntary movements. The CSTs are placed ven-

trally, occupying the crura of the midbrain, the basilar pons, and the pyramids of the medulla oblongata.

Note that in the medulla oblongata, the PCML and CST *decussate*: one of each pair interesects with the other to gain the contralateral (opposite) side of the neuraxis (brainstem/spinal cord). Crossover of certain pathways is an evolutionary inheritance, as illustrated in *Box 3.1*.

In this introductory account, the positions of the cranial nerve nuclei are not included.

Midbrain   (Figure 3.4)

The main landmarks have already been identified. The medial lemniscal component of PCML occupies the lateral part of the tectum, on its way to a sensory nucleus of the thalamus immediately above this level. The CST has arisen in the cerebral cortex and it is descending in the midregion of the cerebral crus.

The *decussation of the superior cerebellar peduncles* straddles the midline at the level of the inferior colliculi (*Figure 3.4B*). It is the human counterpart of the cerebellothalamic projection shown in *Box 3.1*.

Pons   (Figure 3.5)

In the upper section, the cavity of the fourth ventricle is bordered laterally by the superior cerebellar peduncles which are ascending (arrows) to decussate in the lower midbrain. In the floor of the ventricle is the central gray matter. The medial lemniscus occupies the ventral part of the tegmentum. The basilar region contains millions of *transverse fibers*, some of which separate the CST into bundles of fibers. The

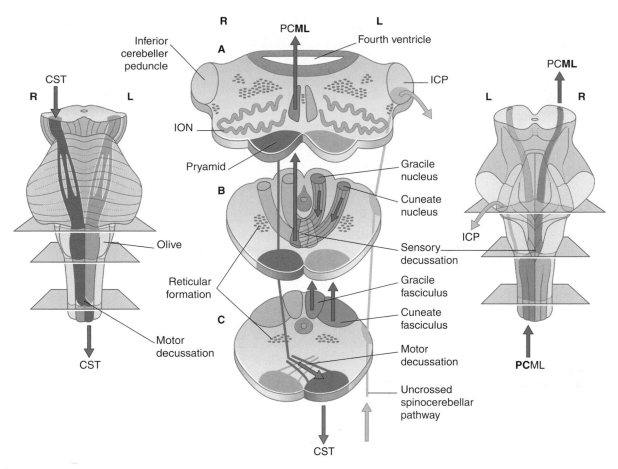

Figure 3.6 Transverse sections of medulla oblongata. **(A)** Level of inferior olivary nucleus (ION). **(B)** Level of sensory decussation. **(C)** Level of motor decussation. ICP, inferior cerebellar peduncle. CST, corticospinal tract; PCML, posterior column–medial lemniscal pathways.

transverse fibers enter the cerebellum via the middle cerebellar peduncles and *appear* to form a bridge (hence, *pons*) connecting the cerebellar hemispheres. But the *individual* transverse fibers arise on one side of the pons and cross to enter the contralateral cerebellar hemisphere. The transverse fibers belong to the pontocerebellar pathway depicted in *Box 3.1*. In mammals, they belong to the giant *corticopontocerebellar pathway* which travels from the cerebral cortex of one side to the contralateral cerebellar hemisphere.

The lower section contains the inferior cerebellar peduncle, about to plunge into the cerebellum. The CST bundles have reunited prior to entering the medulla oblongata.

Medulla oblongata   (Figure 3.6)

Follow the CST from above down. It descends through sections A and B as the **pyramid**. In C, it intersects with its opposite number in the *motor decussation*, prior to entering the contralateral side of the spinal cord.

Follow the PCML pathway from below upward. In section C, it takes the form of the **gracile** and **cuneate fasciculi**, known in the spinal cord as the *posterior columns* of white

matter. In section B, the posterior columns terminate in the **gracile** and **cuneate nuclei**. From these nuclei, fresh sets of fibers swing around the central gray matter and intersect with their opposite numbers in the *sensory decussation*. Having crossed the midline, the fibers turn upward. In section A, they form the medial lemniscal component of PCML.

On the left side of the medulla is shown the *uncrossed, posterior spinocerebellar pathway*. It corresponds to the one depicted in *Box 3.1*, informing the cerebellum of the 'state of play' of ipsilateral (same side) muscles.

The upper third of the medulla shows the wrinkled **inferior olivary nucleus**, which creates the olive of gross anatomy.

SPINAL CORD

General features

The spinal cord occupies the upper half of the vertebral canal. 31 pairs of spinal nerves are attached to it, by means of **anterior** and **posterior nerve roots** (*Figure 3.7A*). The

Box 3.1 Decussations

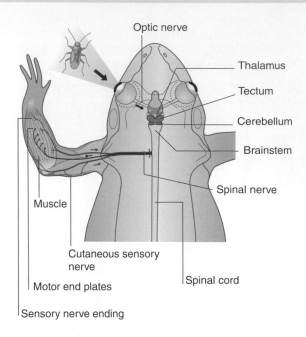

A

Figure Box 3.1.1(A) Monocular view

The evolution of crossed pathways to and from the brain can be traced to the lower vertebrates. During amphibian development, the optic nerves are formed by the growth of bundles of nerve fibers (ensheathed axons) from the retina to reach the brain. The optic nerves meet at a right angle and *decussate* (intersect) and their 'straight ahead' course directs them to the contralateral *tectum*. (In primates, possessing binocular vision, the retinas face forward and the optic nerves intersect obliquely with the result that the fibers in the outer half of each optic nerve remain uncrossed and enter the ipsilateral tectum.) In the diagram, information about an insect is crossing to the tectum on the right side, and the left forelimb will be advanced. Before this can be done, the tectum requires information about the position of the limb and the current state of contraction of the limb muscles. Limb position is signaled by trains of impulses along *afferent* (sensory) nerve fibers supplying the muscles (1M) and skin (1S). The *somas* (cell bodies) of these fibers are *unipolar*, having a single process which divides in the T-shaped manner shown in the second diagram.

The unipolar sensory neurons just described are called *primary* or *first order* afferents in the present context.

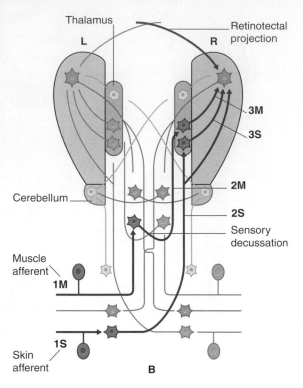

B

Figure Box 3.1.1(B) Higher level afferents

Upon entering the spinal cord, the primary afferents form contacts called *synapses*, upon *secondary* (second-order) sensory neurons. *The secondary neurons project fibers across the midline*. From those receiving cutaneous (skin) primaries, crossover is immediate and the fibers ascend the contralateral cord and brainstem (2S). Some run to the tectum without interruption; others synapse in the thalamus upon *tertiary* afferent neurons (3S) projecting from thalamus to tectum.

With muscle primaries, crossover is delayed. The *centripetal* (Gr. 'center-seeking') processes of these primaries ascend ipsilaterally to the level of the medulla oblongata. There, the second-order muscle afferent neurons, having received inputs from all levels of the cord, send their axons across the midline all at once, in the large *sensory decussation*. The axons ascend (2M) through pons and midbrain before synapsing upon third-order neurons (3M) projecting from thalamus to tectum.

Box 3.1 *Continued*

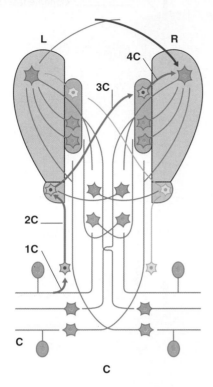 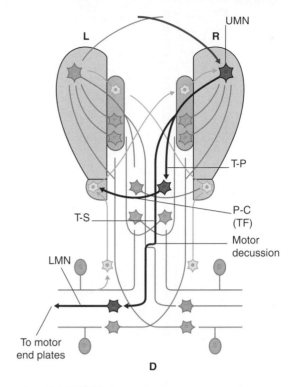

Figure Box 3.1.1(C) Cerebellar control
Before the tectum sends motor instructions, it requires information on the current state of contraction of the limb muscles. This information is stored in the *ipsilateral* hemisphere of the cerebellum.

As indicated in the diagram, neuron 1M is a dual-purpose sensory neuron. It gives off a branch labeled 1C to a *spinocerebellar* neuron which projects (2C) to the ipsilateral cerebellar hemisphere. From here, a *cerebellothalamic* neuron (3C) is shown projecting across the midline to the contralateral thalamus, where a further neuron (4C) relays information to the tectum.

Figure Box 3.1.1(D) Motor output
The tectum now fires impulses along an *upper motor neuron* (UMN) which crosses the midline in the *motor decussation* at the level of the medulla oblongata. This neuron terminates by synapsing upon a *lower motor neuron* (LMN) projecting from the spinal cord to the *motor end plates* on the muscle shown in *Figure 3.1A*.

Note that a copy of the outgoing message is sent to the left cerebellar hemisphere by way of *tectopontine* (T-P) fibers synapsing upon *pontocerebellar* (P-C) neurons sending *transverse fibers* (TF) across the pons.

Sensory and cerebellar neurons are not highlighted here, but both sets do remain active, monitoring the changing position of the limb and the changing state of muscle contraction.

Finally, it may be noted that, at the level of the primates including humans, the emergence of the cerebral cortex results in loss of dominance by the tectum. For example, ascending pathways bypass the tectum and project instead from the thalamus to sensory areas of the cortex; and, although tectopontine and tectospinal neurons persist, they are overshadowed by *corticopontine* and *corticospinal* neurons.

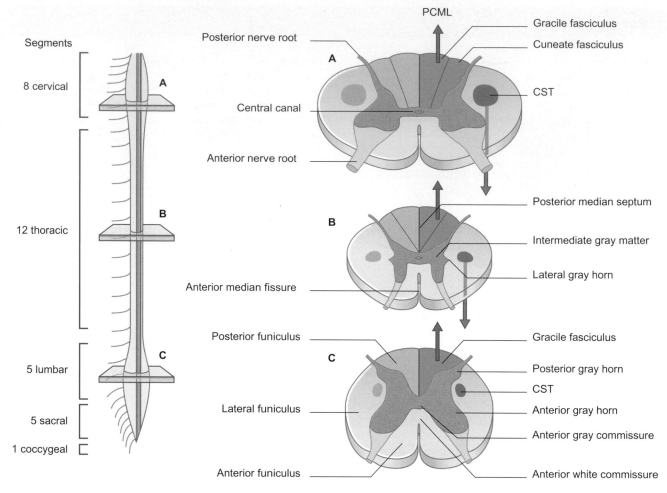

Figure 3.7 Spinal cord. **(A)** Anterior view, with nerve attachments. **(B)** Transverse section at thoracic level. **(C)** General arrangement of pathways in the white matter. CST, corticospinal tract; PCML, posterior column–medial lemniscal pathways.

Core Information

The midbrain comprises tectum, tegmentum, and crus cerebri. The cerebral aqueduct is surrounded by peri-aqueductal gray matter. The tegmentum contains the red nucleus. At all levels of the brainstem, the tegmentum contains elements of the reticular formation. The largest component of the pons is the basilar region containing millions of transverse fibers belonging to the corticopontocerebellar pathways. The most prominent structure in the medulla oblongata is the inferior olivary nucleus.

The CST descends in the crus of midbrain, basilar pons, and medullary pyramid. Its principal component, the lateral CST, passes through the pyramidal decussation and descends the spinal cord in the contralateral lateral funiculus. Most of its fibers terminate in the anterior gray horn.

The posterior columns of the spinal cord comprise the gracile and cuneate fasciculi which terminate in the lower medulla by synapsing upon neurons of the corresponding nuclei. A second set of fibers traverses the sensory decussation before ascending, as the medial lemniscus, to the contralateral sensory thalamus.

The posterior spinocerebellar tract carries information about ipsilateral muscular activity. It enters the inferior cerebellar peduncle. The cerebellum responds by sending signals through the superior cerebellar peduncle of that side to the contralateral motor thalamus via the decussation in the lower midbrain.

Spinal cord
The spinal cord occupies only the upper half of the vertebral canal, the sacral nerve roots being attached to it at the level of the first lumbar vertebra. In all, 31 pairs of roots are attached. The gray matter is most abundant at the levels of attachment of the brachial and lumbosacral plexuses. Anterior and posterior horns are present at all levels, and lateral horns at the

Core Information *Continued*

level of thoracic and upper lumbar root attachments. The white matter comprises anterior, lateral, and posterior funiculi. Axons cross the midline in the gray commissures and in the white commisure. In general, propriospinal pathways are innermost, motor pathways are intermediate, and sensory pathways are outermost.

Cerebellum
The hemispheres are deeply fissured and are linked by the vermis. The oldest part is the flocculonodular lobe. More recent is the anterior lobe. Most recent is the posterior lobe, which includes the tonsils. The white matter contains several nuclei including the dentate nucleus.

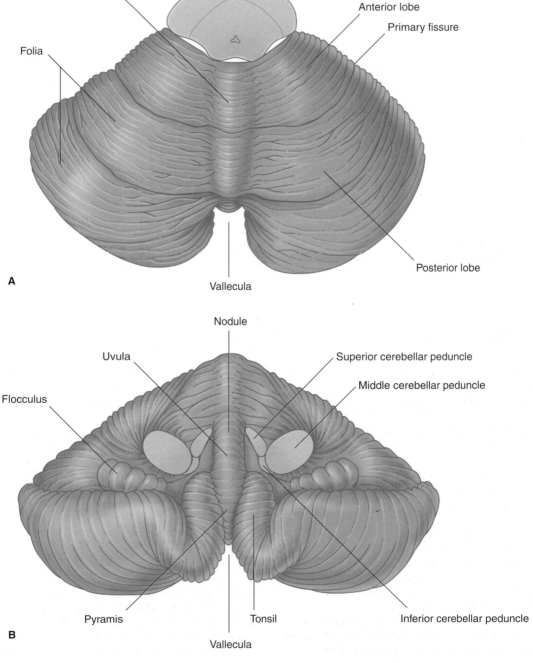

Figure 3.8 Cerebellum. **(A)** Viewed from above. **(B)** Viewed from the position of the pons.

cord shows **cervical** and **lumbar enlargements** which accommodate nerve cells supplying the upper and lower limbs.

Internal anatomy

In transverse sections, the cord shows butterfly-shaped gray matter surrounded by three columns or **funiculi** of white matter (*Figure 3.7B*): an **anterior funiculus** in the interval between the **anterior median fissure** and the emerging **anterior nerve roots**; a **lateral funiculus** between the anterior and **posterior nerve roots**; and a **posterior funiculus** between the posterior roots and the **posterior median septum**.

The gray matter consists of **central gray matter** surrounding a minute central canal, and **anterior and posterior gray horns** on each side. At the levels of attachment of the 12 thoracic and upper two or three lumbar nerve roots, a **lateral gray horn** is present as well. Posterior nerve roots enter the posterior gray horn, and anterior nerve roots emerge from the anterior gray horn.

Axons pass from one side of the spinal cord to the other in the **anterior white** and **gray commissures** deep to the anterior median fissure.

The CST descends the cord within the lateral funiculus. Its principal targets are neurons in the anterior gray horn concerned with activation of skeletal muscles. *Special note*: In Chapter 13, it will be seen that a small, *anterior* CST separates from the main bundle and descends within the anterior funiculus. Accordingly, the full name of the bundle depicted here is the *lateral* CST.

In the cord, the PCML pathway is represented by the **gracile** and **cuneate fasciculi**. The fasciculi are composed of the *central processes of peripheral sensory nerves* supplying muscles, joints, and skin. Processes entering from the lower part of the body form the gracile ('slender') fasciculus; those from the upper part form the cuneate ('wedge-shaped') fasciculus.

CEREBELLUM

The cerebellum is made up of two hemispheres connected by the **vermis** in the midline (*Figure 3.8*). The vermis is distinct only on the under surface, where it occupies the floor of a deep groove, the **vallecula**. The hemispheres show numerous deep **fissures**, with **folia** between. About 80% of the cortex (surface gray matter) is hidden from view on the surfaces of the folia.

The oldest part of the cerebellum (present even in fishes) is the flocculonodular lobe consisting of the **nodule** of the vermis and the **flocculus** in the hemisphere on each side. More recent is the **anterior lobe** which is bounded posteri-

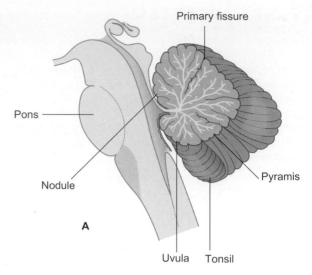

A

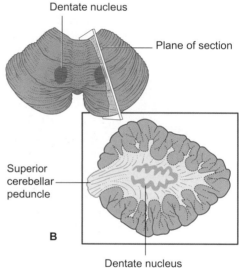

B

Figure 3.9 (A) Sagittal section of hindbrain. **(B)** Oblique section of cerebellum.

orly by the **fissura prima** and contains the **pyramis** and the **uvula**. Most recent is the **posterior lobe**. A prominent feature of the posterior lobe is the **tonsil**. This tonsil lies directly above the foramen magnum of the skull; if the intracranial pressure is raised (e.g. by a brain tumor), one or both tonsils may descend into the foramen and pose a threat to life by compressing the medulla oblongata.

The white matter contains several deep nuclei. The largest of these is the **dentate nucleus** (*Figure 3.9B*).

REFERENCES

See list for Chapter 1.

Meninges

The meninges surround the CNS and suspend it in the protective jacket provided by the CSF. The meninges comprise the tough **dura mater** or **pachymeninx** (*Gr.* thick membrane), and the **leptomeninges** (*Gr.* slender membranes) consisting of the **arachnoid mater** and **pia mater**. Between the arachnoid and the pia is the **subarachnoid space** filled with CSF.

CRANIAL MENINGES

Dura mater

The terminology used to describe the cranial dura mater varies among different authors. It seems best to regard it as a single, tough layer of fibrous tissue which is fused with the inner periosteum of the skull except where it is reflected into the interior of the vault or is stretched across the skull base. Wherever it separates from the periosteum, the intervening space contains venous sinuses (*Figure 4.1*).

Two great dural folds extend into the cranial cavity and help to stabilize the brain. These are the **falx cerebri** and the **tentorium cerebelli**.

The falx cerebri occupies the longitudinal fissure between the cerebral hemispheres. Its attached border extends from the crista galli of the ethmoid bone to the upper surface of the tentorium cerebelli. Along the vault of the skull it encloses the **superior sagittal sinus**. Its free border contains the **inferior sagittal sinus** which unites with the **great cerebral vein** to form the **straight sinus**. The straight sinus travels along the line of attachment of falx cerebri to tento-

rium cerebelli and meets the superior sagittal sinus at the **confluence of the sinuses**.

The crescentic **tentorium cerebelli** arches like a tent above the posterior cranial fossa, being lifted up by the falx cerebri in the midline. The attached margin of the tentorium encloses the **transverse sinuses** on the inner surface of the occipital bone and the **superior petrosal sinuses** along the upper border of the petrous temporal bone. The attached margin reaches to the posterior clinoid processes of the sphenoid bone. Most of the blood from the superior sagittal sinus enters the right transverse sinus (*Figure 4.2*).

The free margin of the tentorium is U-shaped. The tips of the U are attached to the anterior clinoid processes. Just behind this, the two limbs of the U are linked by a sheet of dura, the **diaphragma sellae**, which is pierced by the pituitary stalk. Laterally, the dura falls away into the middle cranial fossae from the limbs of the U, creating the **cavernous sinus** on each side (*Figure 4.3*). Behind the sphenoid bone, the concavity of the U encloses the midbrain.

The cavernous sinus receives blood from the orbit via the ophthalmic veins. The superior petrosal sinus joins the transverse sinus at its junction with the **sigmoid sinus**. The sigmoid sinus descends along the occipital bone and discharges into the bulb of the internal jugular vein. The bulb receives the inferior petrosal sinus which descends along the edge of the occipital bone.

The tentorium cerebelli divides the cranial cavity into a **supratentorial compartment** containing the forebrain and an **infratentorial compartment** containing the hindbrain. A small **falx cerebelli** is attached to the under surface of the

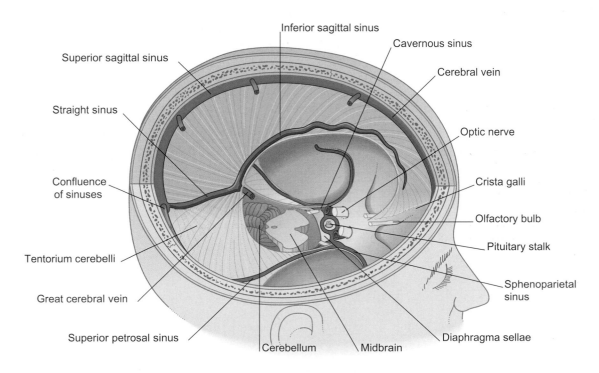

Figure 4.1 Dural reflections and venous sinuses. The midbrain occupies the tentorial notch.

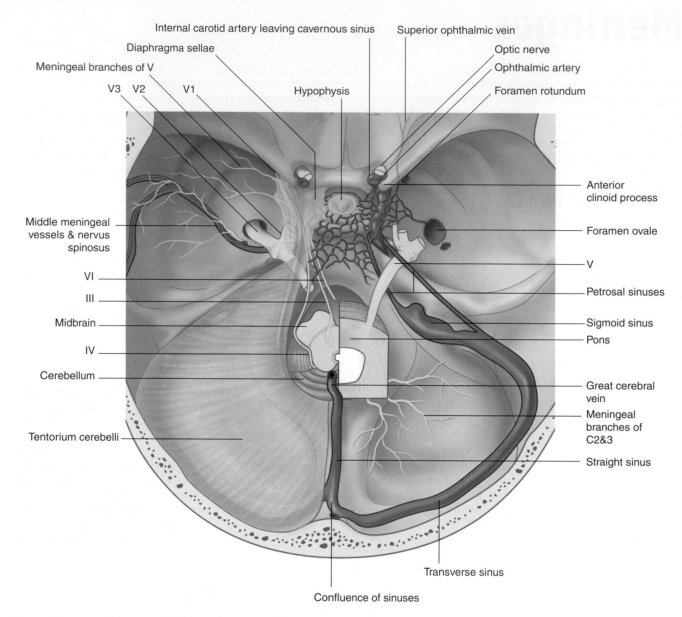

Internal carotid artery leaving cavernous sinus

Superior ophthalmic vein

Diaphragma sellae

Optic nerve

Meningeal branches of V

Ophthalmic artery

V3 V2 V1

Hypophysis

Foramen rotundum

Middle meningeal vessels & nervus spinosus

Anterior clinoid process

Foramen ovale

VI

V

III

Petrosal sinuses

Midbrain

Sigmoid sinus

IV

Pons

Cerebellum

Great cerebral vein

Tentorium cerebelli

Meningeal branches of C2&3

Straight sinus

Transverse sinus

Confluence of sinuses

Figure 4.2 Venous sinuses on the base of the skull. The dura mater has been removed on the right side. The inset indicates where grooves for sinuses are seen on the dry skull. *Note:* On the left, the midbrain is seen at the level of the tentorial notch. On the right, a lower level section shows the trigeminal nerve attached to the pons.

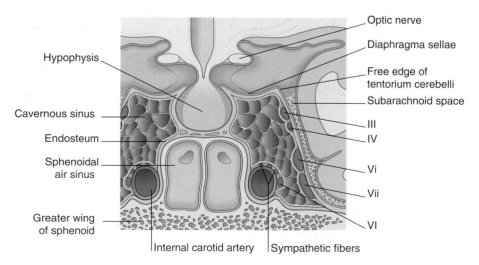

Optic nerve

Diaphragma sellae

Hypophysis

Free edge of tentorium cerebelli

Cavernous sinus

Subarachnoid space

III

Endosteum

IV

Sphenoidal air sinus

Vi

Vii

Greater wing of sphenoid

VI

Internal carotid artery

Sympathetic fibers

Figure 4.3 Coronal section of the cavernous sinus.

tentorium cerebelli and to the internal occipital crest of the occipital bone.

Innervation of the cranial dura mater

The dura mater lining the supratentorial compartment of the cranial cavity receives sensory innervation from the trigeminal nerve. That lining the anterior cranial fossa and anterior part of the skull vault is supplied by the ophthalmic nerve; that lining the middle cranial fossa and midregion of the vault is mainly supplied by the **nervus spinosus** (*Figure 4.2*). This nerve leaves the mandibular outside the foramen ovale, to return via the foramen spinosum and accompany the **middle meningeal artery** and its branches. Stretching or inflammation of the supratentorial dura gives rise to frontal or parietal headache.

The dura mater lining the infratentorial compartment is supplied by branches of the upper cervical spinal nerves entering the foramen magnum (*Figure 4.2*). Occipital and posterior neck pains accompany disturbance of the infratentorial dura. Acute meningitis involving the posterior cranial fossa is associated with *neck rigidity* and often with *head retraction* brought about by reflex contraction of the posterior nuchal muscles, which are supplied by cervical nerves. Violent occipital headache also follows *subarachnoid hemorrhage*, (Ch. 27) where free blood swirls around the hindbrain.

Meningeal arteries

Embedded in the inner periosteum of the skull are several **meningeal arteries** whose main function is to supply the diploë (bone marrow). Much the largest is the middle meningeal artery, which ramifies over the inner surface of the temporal and parietal bones. Tearing of this artery, with its accompanying vein, is the usual source of an *extradural hematoma* (*Clinical Panel 4.1*).

Arachnoid mater

The arachnoid (*Gr.* spidery) is a thin, fibrocellular layer in direct contact with the dura mater (*Figure 4.4*). The outermost cells of the arachnoid are bonded to one another by tight junctions which seal the **subarachnoid space**. Innumerable **arachnoid trabeculae** cross the space to reach the pia mater.

Pia mater

The pia mater invests the brain closely, following its contours and lining the various sulci (*Figure 4.4*). Like the arachnoid,

it is fibrocellular. The cellular component of the pia is external and is permeable to CSF. The fibrous component occupies a narrow **subpial space** which is continuous with **perivascular spaces** around cerebral blood vessels penetrating the brain surface.

Note: Although the subarachnoid and subpial spaces are proven, there is no sign of any 'subdural space' in properly fixed material. Such a space can be created, however, by leakage of blood into the cellular layer of the dura mater following a tear of a cerebral vein at its point of anchorage to the fibrous layer. (See *subdural hematoma* in *Clinical Panel 4.1*.)

Subarachnoid cisterns

Along the base of the brain and the sides of the brainstem, pools of CSF occupy subarachnoid cisterns (*Figures 4.5 and 4.6*). The largest of these is the **cisterna magna**, in the interval between the cerebellum and the medulla oblongata. More rostrally are the **cisterna pontis** ventral to the pons, the **interpeduncular cistern** between the cerebral peduncles, and the **cisterna ambiens** at the side of the midbrain. The complete list of cisterns is in *Table 4.1*.

Sheath of the optic nerve

The optic nerve is composed of CNS white matter, and it has a complete meningeal investment. The dura mater fuses with the scleral shell of the eyeball; the subarachnoid space is a tubular *cul de sac* (dead end). The central vessels of the retina pierce the meninges to enter it (*Figure 4.7*). Any sustained elevation of intracranial pressure will be transmitted to the subarachnoid sleeve surrounding the nerve. The **central vein** will be compressed, resulting in swelling of the retinal tributaries of the vein and edema of the optic papilla, where the optic nerve begins. The condition is known as *papilledema* (*Figure 4.8*). It can be recognized on inspection of the retina with an ophthalmoscope.

SPINAL MENINGES   (Figure 4.9)

The spinal dural sac is like a test tube, attached to the rim of the foramen magnum and reaching down to the level of the second sacral vertebra. The outer surface of the tube is adherent to the posterior longitudinal ligament of the vertebrae in the midline; elsewhere it is surrounded by fat containing the **epidural**, **internal vertebral venous plexus** (Ch. 11).

Table 4.1 Subarachnoid cisterns

Cistern	Location
Posterior cerebellomedullary (cisterna magna)	Between cerebellum and dorsal surface of medulla oblongata
Lateral cerebellomedullary	Along each side of the medulla
Cistern of lateral cerebral fossa	Along the lateral sulcus (Sylvian fissure)
Chiasmatic	Behind and above the optic chiasm
Interpeduncular	Interpeduncular fossa
Ambient (cisterna ambiens)	On each side of the midbrain
Quadrigeminal	Surrounding the great cerebral vein dorsal to the midbrain colliculi (quadrigeminal bodies)

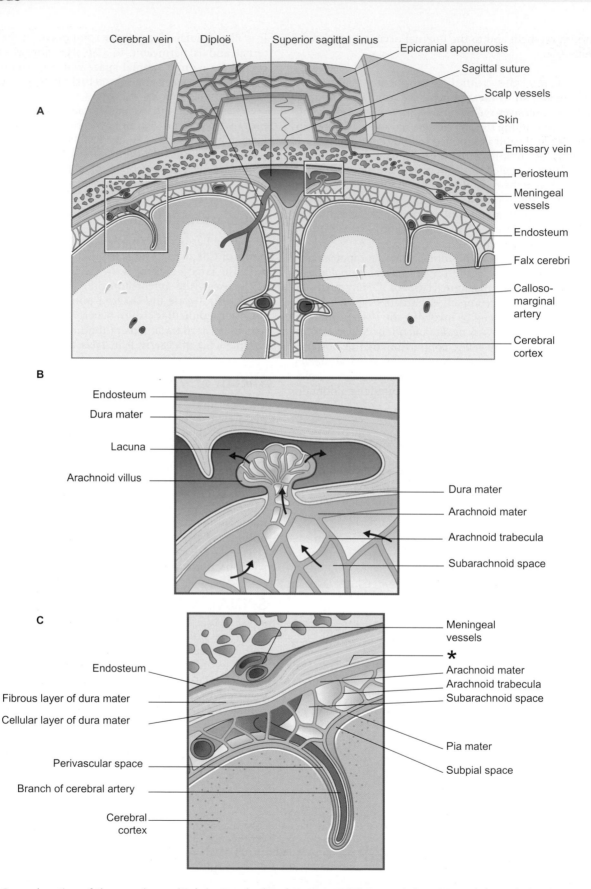

Figure 4.4 Coronal section of the superior sagittal sinus and related structures. **(A)** General view. Most of the scalp has been removed, to show two emissary veins transferring blood from the diploë into scalp veins on the surface of the epicranial aponeurosis. On the right, the diploë is being fed and drained by meningeal vessels. Also seen is a cerebral vein draining into the superior sagittal sinus. **(B)** Enlargement from (A) showing an arachnoid granulation transferring cerebrospinal fluid from the subarachnoid space to a lacuna connected to the superior sagittal sinus. **(C)** Enlargement from (A) showing an artery sequentially surrounded by subarachnoid, subpial, and perivascular space extracellular fluid. *Marks the potential space between dura and arachnoid, for spread of subdural blood from a torn cerebral vein. Note the extradural position of the meningeal vessels.

Clinical Panel 4.1 Extradural/subdural hematomas

An *extradural (epidural) hematoma* is typically caused by a blow to the side of the head severe enough to cause a fracture with associated tearing of the anterior or posterior branch of the middle meningeal artery. Following the initial *concussion* of the brain, with loss of consciousness, there may be a *lucid interval* of several hours. Onset of increasing headache and drowsiness signals *cerebral compression* produced by expansion of the hematoma. Coma and death will supervene unless the hematoma is drained though a burr-hole. The favored site of access is the H-shaped suture complex known as the *pterion*, which overlies the anterior branch of the middle meningeal artery (*Figure CP 4.1.1*).

Subdural hematomas are caused by rupture of superficial cerebral veins in transit from the brain to an intracranial venous sinus.

An *acute subdural hematoma* most often follows severe head injury in children. It must always be suspected where a child remains unconscious after a head injury. Child battering is a possible explanation if this situation arises in the home.

A *subacute subdural hematoma* may follow head injury at any age. Symptoms and signs of raised intracranial pressure (described in Ch. 6) develop up to 3 weeks after the injury.

Chronic subdural hematomas occur in older people, where the transit veins have become brittle and made taut by shrinkage of the aging brain. Head injury may be mild or even absent. A significant number of these patients are alcoholics with reduced blood clotting. Presenting symptoms are variable and include personality changes, headaches, and epileptic seizures.

Figure CP 4.1.1 The circle encloses the pterion.

Clinical Panel 4.2 Hydrocephalus

Hydrocephalus (*Gr.* water in the head) denotes accumulation of CSF in the ventricular system. With the exception of overproduction of CSF by a rare papilloma of the choroid plexus, hydrocephalus results from obstruction of the normal CSF circulation, with consequent dilatation of the ventricles. (The term is not used to describe the accumulation of fluid in the ventricles and subarachnoid space in association with senile atrophy of the brain.)

In the great majority of cases, hydrocephalus is caused by obstruction of the foramina opening the fourth ventricle to the subarachnoid space. A major cause of outlet obstruction in *infancy* is the *Arnold–Chiari malformation*, in which the cerebellum is partly extruded into the vertebral canal during fetal life because the posterior cranial fossa is underdeveloped. In untreated cases, the child's head may become as large as a football and the cerebral hemispheres paper thin. The condition is nearly always associated with spina bifida (Ch. 11). Early treatment is essential to prevent severe brain damage. The obstruction can be bypassed by means of a catheter having one end inserted into a lateral ventricle and the other inserted into the internal jugular vein.

A major cause of outlet obstruction in *adults* is displacement of the cerebellum into the foramen magnum by a space-occupying lesion such as a tumor or hematoma (see Ch. 6).

Meningitis can cause hydrocephalus at any age. The development of leptomeningeal adhesions may compromise CSF circulation at the level of the ventricular outlets, the tentorial notch, and/or the arachnoid granulations.

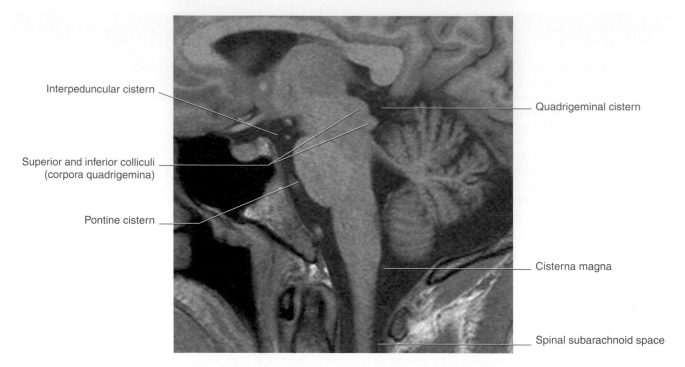

Interpeduncular cistern

Superior and inferior colliculi
(corpora quadrigemina)

Pontine cistern

Quadrigeminal cistern

Cisterna magna

Spinal subarachnoid space

Figure 4.5 Portion of Figure 2.7 showing subarachnoid cisterns.

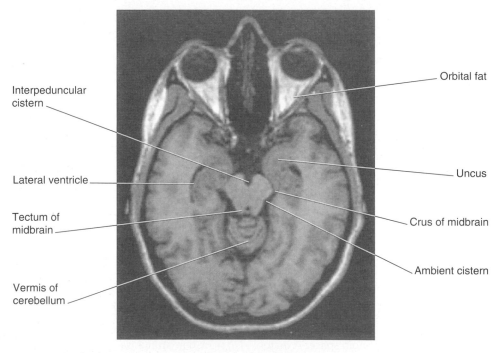

Interpeduncular
cistern

Lateral ventricle

Tectum of
midbrain

Vermis of
cerebellum

Orbital fat

Uncus

Crus of midbrain

Ambient cistern

Figure 4.6 Horizontal MRI 'slice' at the level indicated at top. Note the proximity of the uncus to the crus of the midbrain (cf. uncal herniation *Clinical Panel 6.2* in Ch. 6). (From a series kindly provided by Professor J. Paul Finn, Director, MRI Facility, Northwestern University School of Medicine, Chicago.)

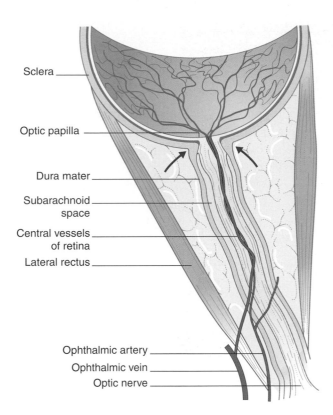

Sclera

Optic papilla

Dura mater

Subarachnoid space

Central vessels of retina

Lateral rectus

Ophthalmic artery

Ophthalmic vein

Optic nerve

Figure 4.7 Horizontal section of the left orbit. The subarachnoid space extends forward to the level of fusion of dura mater with the scleral coat of the eyeball (arrows).

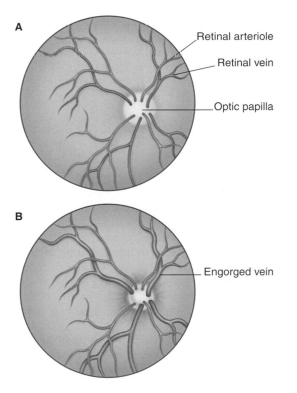

A

Retinal arteriole

Retinal vein

Optic papilla

B

Engorged vein

Figure 4.8 Fundus oculi as seen with an ophthalmoscope. **(A)** Normal. **(B)** Papilledema resulting from raised intracranial pressure.

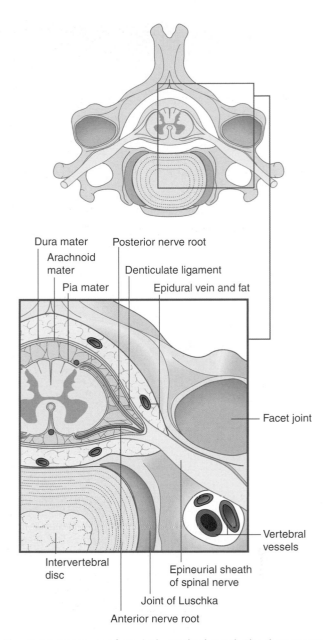

Dura mater   Posterior nerve root
Arachnoid mater
Pia mater   Denticulate ligament
Epidural vein and fat

Facet joint

Vertebral vessels

Intervertebral disc

Epineurial sheath of spinal nerve

Joint of Luschka

Anterior nerve root

Figure 4.9 Contents of cervical vertebral canal. The dura mater blends with the epineurium of the spinal nerve trunk.

The internal surface of the dura is lined with arachnoid mater. The pia mater lines the surface of the spinal cord and is attached to the dura mater at regular intervals by the serrated **denticulate ligament**.

Because the spinal cord reaches only to first or second lumbar vertebral level, a large **lumbar cistern** is created, containing the free-floating roots of the sacral and lower lumbar spinal nerves (Ch. 11). The lumbar cistern may be tapped to procure samples of CSF for analysis (*Clinical Panel 4.3*), or to deliver a spinal anesthetic (Ch. 11).

CIRCULATION OF CEREBROSPINAL FLUID   (Figure 4.10)

The principal source of the CSF is the secretion of the choroid plexuses into the ventricles of the brain. From the

Clinical Panel 4.3   Lumbar puncture

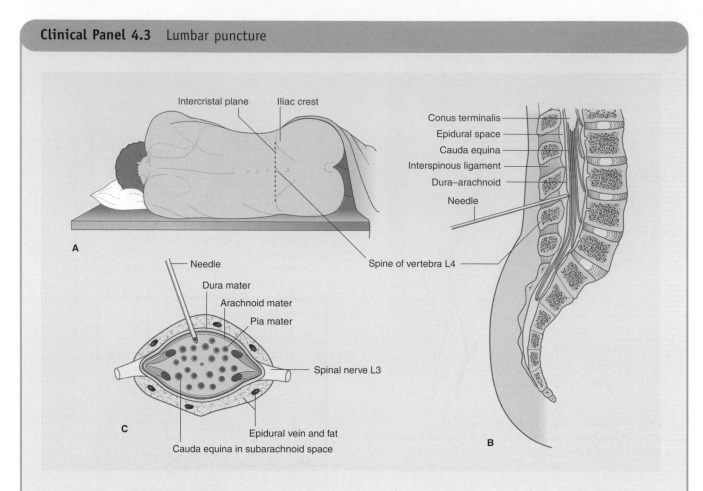

Figure CP 4.3.1 Lumbar puncture (spinal tap). **(A)** The patient lies on one side, curled forwards to open the interspinous spaces of the lumbar region. The spine of vertebra L4 is identified in the intercristal (supracristal) plane at the level of the tops of the iliac crests. **(B)** Under aseptic conditions, a lumbar puncture needle is introduced obliquely above the spine of vertebra L4, parallel to the plane of the spine. The needle is passed through the interspinous ligament. A slight 'give' is perceived when the needle pierces the dura–arachnoid mater and enters the subarachnoid space. **(C)** Transverse section showing the cauda equina floating in the subarachnoid space. The anterior and posterior roots of spinal nerve L3 are coming together as they leave the lumbar cistern.

lateral ventricles, the CSF enters the third through the interventricular foramen. It descends to the fourth ventricle through the aqueduct and squirts into the subarachnoid space through the median and lateral apertures. (Flow within the central canal of the spinal cord is negligible.)

Within the subarachnoid space, some of the CSF descends through the foramen magnum, reaching the lumbar cistern in about 12 hours. From the subarachnoid space at the base of the brain, the CSF ascends through the tentorial notch and bathes the surface of the cerebral hemispheres before being returned to the blood through the **arachnoid granulations** (*Figure 4.4*). The arachnoid granulations are pinhead pouches of arachnoid mater projecting through the dural wall of the major venous sinuses – especially the superior sagittal sinus and the small venous **lacunae** that open into it. CSF is transported across the arachnoid epithelium in giant vacuoles.

As much as a quarter of the circulating CSF may not reach the superior sagittal sinus. Some enters small arachnoid villi projecting into spinal veins exiting intervertebral foramina; and some drains into lymphatics in the adventitia of arteries at the base of the brain and in the epineurium of cranial nerves. These lymphatics drain into cervical lymph nodes. Bimanual downward massage of the sides of the neck is sometimes used to enhance this drainage in patients suffering from cerebral edema.

About 300 ml of CSF are secreted by the choroid plexuses every 24 hours. Another 200 ml are produced from other sources, as described in Chapter 5. Blockage of flow through the ventricular system or cranial subarachnoid space will cause back-up within the ventricular system: a state of *hydrocephalus* (*Clinical Panel 4.2*).

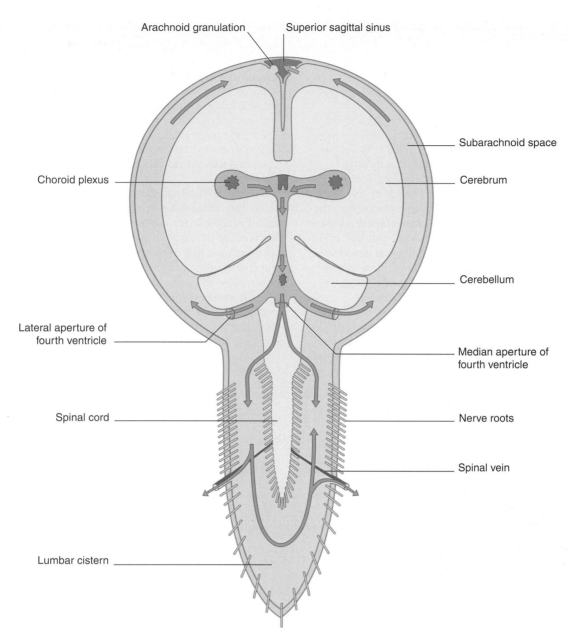

Arachnoid granulation

Superior sagittal sinus

Subarachnoid space

Choroid plexus

Cerebrum

Cerebellum

Lateral aperture of
fourth ventricle

Median aperture of
fourth ventricle

Spinal cord

Nerve roots

Spinal vein

Lumbar cistern

Figure 4.10 Circulation of cerebrospinal fluid.

Core Information

Meninges

The meninges comprise dura, arachnoid, and pia mater. The subarachnoid space contains CSF.

The cranial dura mater shows two large folds: the falx cerebri encloses the superior sagittal sinus, which usually enters the right of the two transverse sinuses enclosed by the tentorium cerebelli. The inferior sagittal sinus joins the great cerebral vein, forming the straight sinus which joins the confluence of the sagittal and transverse sinuses. The transverse sinus enters the sigmoid sinus which empties into the internal jugular vein. The midbrain is partly enclosed by the free edge of the tentorium, which is attached to the anterior clinoid processes of the sphenoid bone; dura drapes from the free edge into the middle cranial fossa, creating the cavernous sinus on each side. The supratentorial dura mater is innervated by the trigeminal nerve, the infratentorial dura by upper cervical nerves. The meningeal vessels run extradurally to supply the diploë; if torn by skull fracture, they may form an extradural hematoma compressing the brain.

Cerebrospinal fluid

Pools of CSF at the base of the brain include the cisterna magna, the cisterna pontis, the interpeduncular cistern, and the cisterna ambiens. CSF also extends along the meningeal sheath of the optic nerve, and raised intracranial pressure may compress the central vein of the retina, causing papilledema.

The spinal dural sac extends down to S2 vertebral level. The lumbar cistern contains spinal nerve roots and is accessible for lumbar puncture (spinal tap). CSF secreted by the choroid plexuses escapes into the subarachnoid space through the three apertures of the fourth ventricle. Some descends to the lumbar cistern. The CSF ascends through the tentorial notch and the cerebral subarachnoid space to reach the superior sagittal sinus and its lacunae via the arachnoid granulations. Blockage of CSF flow anywhere along its course leads to hydrocephalus.

REFERENCES

Brinker, T., Ludemann, W., Berens von Rautenfeld, D. and Samii, M. (1997) Dynamic properties of lymphatic pathways for the absorption of cerebrospinal fluid. *Acta Neuropathol. (Berlin)* **94**: 493–498.

Hutchings, M. and Weller, R.O. (1986) Anatomical relationships of the pia mater to cerebral blood vessels in man. *J. Neurosurg.* **65**: 316–325.

Nicholas, D.S. and Weller, R.O. (1988) The fine anatomy of the human spinal meninges. *J. Neurosurg.* **69**: 276–282.

Prockop, L.D. and Shah, C.P. (1989) Hydrocephalus. In *Merritt's Textbook of Neurology*, 8th edn (Rowland, L.P., ed.). Philadelphia: Lea & Febiger.

Vandenabeele, L., Creemers, J. and Lambrichts, I. (1996) Ultrastructure of the human spinal arachnoid mater and dura mater. *J. Anat.* **189**: 417–430.

Blood supply of the brain

INTRODUCTORY NOTE

Cerebrovascular disease is so prevalent as to be the leading cause of neurological disability. Its diverse manifestations are largely accounted for by the anatomical distribution of the stems and branches of the cerebral and brainstem vessels. Because interpretation of the symptoms produced by cerebrovascular accidents requires prior knowledge of brain function, Clinical Panels on this subject are placed in the final chapter. On the other hand, a Clinical Panel on blood–brain barrier pathology is placed in this chapter because the symptoms are of a general nature.

The brain is absolutely dependent on a continuous supply of oxygenated blood. It controls the delivery of blood by sensing the momentary pressure changes in its main arteries of supply, the internal carotids. It controls the arterial oxygen tension by monitoring respiratory gas levels in the internal carotid artery and in the CSF beside the medulla oblongata (Ch. 19). The control systems used by the brain are exquisitely sophisticated but they can be brought to nothing if a distributing artery ruptures spontaneously or is rammed shut by an embolus.

ARTERIAL SUPPLY OF THE FOREBRAIN

The blood supply to the forebrain is derived from the two **internal carotid arteries** and from the **basilar artery** (*Figure 5.1*).

Each internal carotid artery enters the subarachnoid space by piercing the roof of the cavernous sinus. In the subarachnoid space, it gives off **ophthalmic, posterior communicating**, and **anterior choroidal arteries** before dividing into the **anterior** and **middle cerebral arteries**.

The basilar artery divides at the upper border of the pons into the two **posterior cerebral arteries**. The **cerebral arterial circle** (*circle of Willis*) is completed by a linkage of the posterior communicating artery with the posterior cerebral on each side, and by linkage of the two anterior cerebrals by the **anterior communicating artery**.

The choroid plexus of the lateral ventricle is supplied from the **anterior choroidal** branch of the internal carotid artery and by the **posterior choroidal** branch from the posterior cerebral artery.

Dozens of fine **central (perforating) branches** are given off by the constituent arteries of the circle of Willis. They enter the brain through the **anterior perforated substance** beside the optic chiasm and through the **posterior perforated substance** behind the mammillary bodies. They have been classified in various ways but can be conveniently grouped into short and long branches. **Short central branches** arise from all of the constituent arteries and from the two choroidal arteries. They supply the optic nerve, chiasm, and tract, and the hypothalamus. **Long central branches** arise from the three cerebral arteries. They supply the thalamus, corpus striatum, and internal capsule. They include the **striate branches** of the anterior and middle cerebral arteries.

Anterior cerebral artery   (Figure 5.2)

The anterior cerebral artery passes above the optic chiasm to gain the medial surface of the cerebral hemisphere. It forms an arch around the genu of the corpus callosum. making it easy to identify in a carotid angiogram (see later). Close to the anterior communicating artery, it gives off the **medial striate artery**, also known as the *recurrent artery of Heubner* (*pron.* 'Hoibner') which contributes to the blood supply of the internal capsule. Cortical branches of the anterior cerebral artery supply the medial surface of the hemisphere as far back as the parieto-occipital sulcus (*Table 5.1*). The branches overlap onto the orbital and lateral surfaces of the hemisphere.

Middle cerebral artery   (Figure 5.3)

The middle cerebral artery is the main continuation of the internal carotid, receiving 60–80% of the carotid blood flow. It immediately gives off important central branches, then passes along the depth of the lateral fissure to reach the surface of the insula. There it usually breaks into upper and lower divisions. The upper division supplies the frontal lobe, the lower division supplies the parietal temporal lobes, and the midregion of the optic radiation. Named branches and their territories are listed in Table 5.2. Overall, the middle cerebral supplies two-thirds of the lateral surface of the brain.

The **central branches** of the middle cerebral include the **lateral striate** arteries (*Figure 5.4*). These arteries supply the corpus striatum, internal capsule, and thalamus. Occlusion of one of the lateral striate arteries is the chief cause of classic *stroke*, where damage to the pyramidal tract in the posterior limb of the internal capsule causes *hemiplegia*, a term denoting paralysis of the contralateral arm, leg, and lower part of face.

Note: Additional information on the blood supply of the internal capsule is provided in Chapter 30.

Table 5.1 Named cortical* branches of the anterior cerebral artery

Branch	Territory
Orbitofrontal	Orbital surface of frontal lobe
Polar frontal	Frontal pole
Callosomarginal	Cingulate and superior frontal gyri; paracentral lobule
Pericallosal	Corpus callosum

*The term 'cortical' is conventional. 'Terminal' is better because these arteries also supply the underlying white matter.

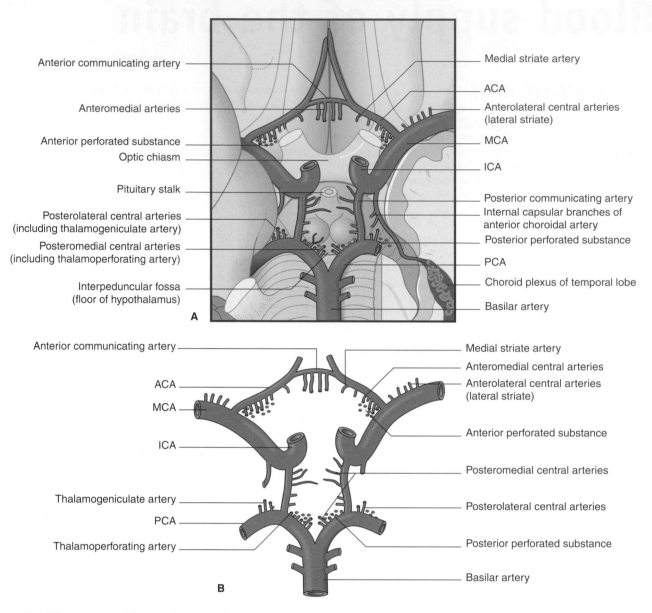

Figure 5.1 (A) Brain viewed from below, showing background structures related to the circle of Willis. Part of the left temporal lobe (to right of picture) has been removed to show the choroid plexus in the inferior horn of the lateral ventricle. **(B)** The arteries comprising the circle of Willis. The four groups of central branches are shown; the thalamoperforating artery belongs to the posteromedial group and the thalamogeniculate artery belongs to the posterolateral group. ACA, MCA, PCA, anterior, middle, posterior cerebral arteries; ICA, internal carotid artery.

Posterior cerebral artery (Figures 5.2, 5.5)

The two posterior cerebral arteries are the terminal branches of the basilar. However, in embryonic life they originated from the internal carotid, and in about 25% of individuals the internal carotid persists as the primary source of blood on one or both sides, by way of a large posterior communicating artery.

Close to its origin, each posterior cerebral artery gives branches to the midbrain and a **posterior choroidal artery** to the choroid plexus of the lateral ventricle. Additional, **central branches** are sent into the posterior perforated substance (*Figure 5.1*). The main artery winds around the midbrain in company with the optic tract. It supplies the splenium of the corpus callosum and the cortex of the occip-

ital and temporal lobes. Named cortical branches and their territories are given in *Table 5.3*.

The central branches, called **thalamoperforating** and **thalamogeniculate**, supply the thalamus, subthalamic nucleus, and optic radiation.

Note: Additional information on the central branches is provided in Chapter 30.

Neuroangiography

The cerebral arteries and veins can be diplayed under general anesthesia by rapid injection of a radiopaque dye into the internal carotid or vertebral artery followed by serial radiography every 2 seconds. The dye completes its journey through the arteries, brain capillaries, and veins in about 10

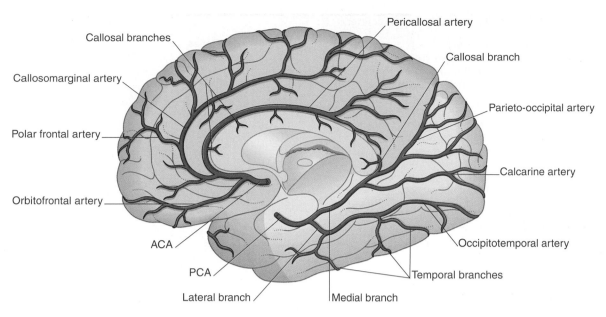

Figure 5.2 Medial view of the right hemisphere showing the cortical branches and territories of the three cerebral arteries. ACA, PCA, anterior, posterior cerebral arteries.

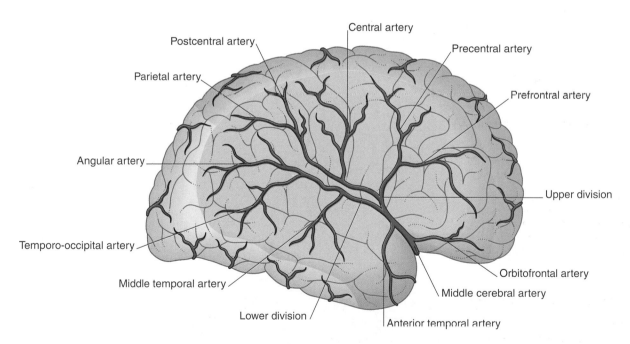

Figure 5.3 Lateral view of right cerebral hemisphere showing the cortical branches and territories of the three cerebral arteries.

Table 5.2 Cortical branches of the middle cerebral artery

Origin	Branch(es)	Territory
Stem	Frontobasal	Orbital surface of frontal lobe
	Anterior temporal	Anterior temporal cortex
Upper division	Prefrontal	Prefrontal cortex
	Precentral	Premotor areas
	Central	Pre- and postcentral gyri
	Postcentral	Postcentral and anterior parietal cortex
	Parietal	Posterior parietal cortex
Lower division	Middle temporal	Midtemporal cortex
	Temporo-occipital	Temporal and occipital cortex
	Angular	Angular and neighboring gyri

Table 5.3 Named cortical branches of the posterior cerebral artery

Branch	Artery	Territory
Lateral	Anterior temporal	Anterior temporal cortex
	Posterior temporal	Posterior temporal cortex
	Occipitotemporal	Posterior temporal and occipital cortex
Medial	Calcarine	Calcarine cortex
	Parieto-occipital	Cuneus and precuneus
	Callosal	Splenium of corpus callosum

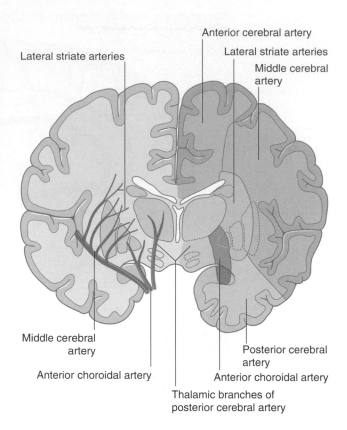

Figure 5.4 Distribution of perforating branches of the middle cerebral, anterior choroidal, and posterior cerebral arteries (schematic). The anterior choroidal artery arises from the internal carotid.

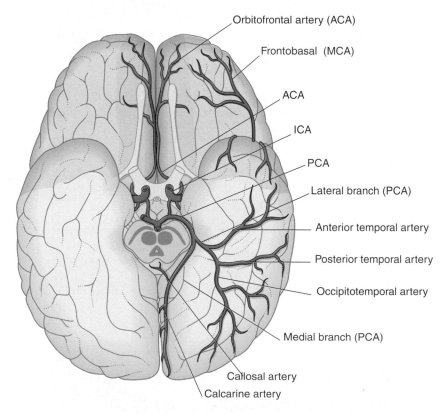

Figure 5.5 View from below of the cerebral hemispheres showing the cortical branches and territories of the three cerebral arteries.

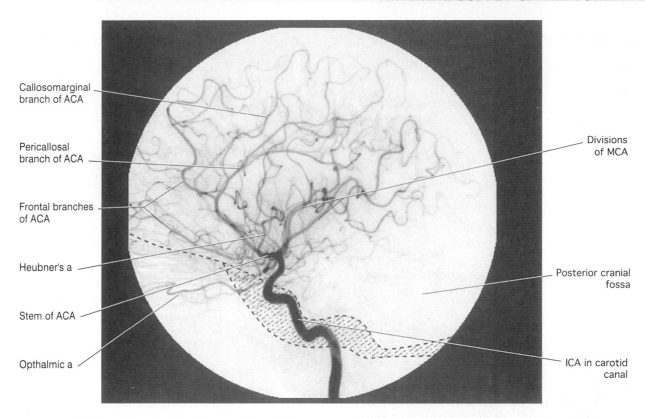

Callosomarginal branch of ACA

Pericallosal branch of ACA

Frontal branches of ACA

Heubner's a

Stem of ACA

Opthalmic a

Divisions of MCA

Posterior cranial fossa

ICA in carotid canal

Figure 5.6 Arterial phase of a carotid angiogram, lateral view. Contrast medium injected into the left internal carotid artery is passing through the anterior and middle cerebral arteries (ACA, MCA). The base of the skull is shown in hatched outline. ICA, internal carotid artery. (From an original series kindly provided by Dr. Michael Modic, Dept of Radiology, The Cleveland Clinic Foundation.)

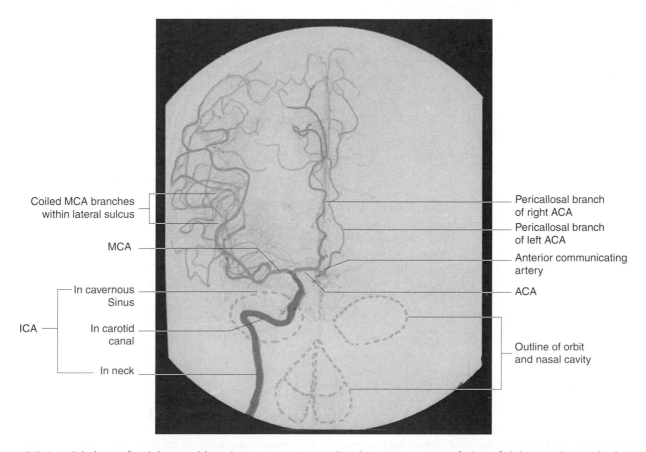

Coiled MCA branches within lateral sulcus

MCA

ICA — In cavernous Sinus

In carotid canal

In neck

Pericallosal branch of right ACA

Pericallosal branch of left ACA

Anterior communicating artery

ACA

Outline of orbit and nasal cavity

Figure 5.7 Arterial phase of a right carotid angiogram, anteroposterior view. Note some perfusion of right anterior cerebral artery (ACA) territory (via the anterior communicating artery. ICA), internal carotid artery; MCA, middle cerebral artery. (Angiogram kindly provided by Dr Pearse Morris, Director, Interventional Neuroradiology, Wake Forest University School of Medicine, Winston-Salem, N. Carolina, USA.)

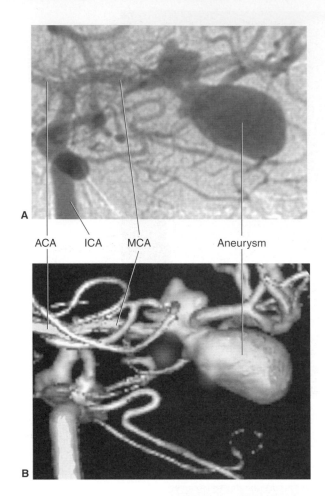

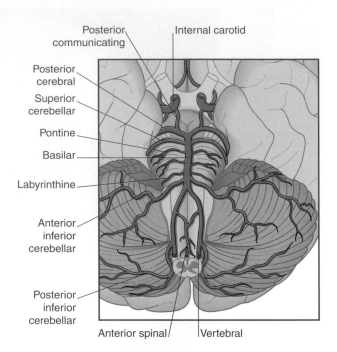

Figure 5.9 Arterial supply of hindbrain.

Figure 5.8 (A) Excerpt from a conventional carotid angiogram, anteroposterior view, showing an aneurysm attached to the middle cerebral artery. **(B)** Excerpt from a 3D image of the same area. ACA, MCA, anterior and middle cerebral arteries; ICA, internal carotid artery. (Originals kindly provided by Dr Pearse Morris, Director, Interventional Neuroradiology, Wake Forest University School of Medicine, Winston-Salem, N. Carolina, USA.)

seconds. The *arterial phase* of the journey yields either a *carotid angiogram* or a *vertebrobasilar angiogram*. Improved vascular definition in radiographs of the arterial phase or of the *venous phase* can be procured by a process of *subtraction* whereby positive and negative images of the overlying skull are superimposed on one another, thereby virtually deleting the skull image.

A recent development, *three-dimensional* angiography, is based upon simultaneous angiography from two slightly separate perspectives.

Arterial phases of carotid angiograms are shown in *Figures 5.6–5.8*.

ARTERIAL SUPPLY TO HINDBRAIN

The brainstem and cerebellum are supplied by the vertebral and basilar arteries and their branches (*Figure 5.9*).

The two **vertebral arteries** arise from the subclavian arter-

ies and ascend the neck in the foramina transversaria of the upper six cervical vertebrae. They enter the skull through the foramen magnum and unite at the lower border of the pons to form the **basilar artery**. The basilar artery ascends to the upper border of the pons and divides into two posterior cerebral arteries (*Figures 5.10, 5.11*).

All of the primary branches of the vertebral and basilar arteries give branches to the brainstem.

Vertebral branches

The **posterior inferior cerebellar artery** supplies the side of the medulla before giving branches to the cerebellum. **Anterior** and **posterior spinal arteries** supply the ventral and dorsal medulla, respectively, before descending through the foramen magnum.

Basilar branches

The **anterior inferior cerebellar** and **superior cerebellar arteries** supply the side of the pons before giving branches to the cerebellum. The anterior inferior cerebellar usually gives off the **labyrinthine artery** to the inner ear.

About a dozen **pontine arteries** supply the full thickness of the medial part of the pons.

The midbrain is supplied by the **posterior cerebral artery**, and by the **posterior communicating artery** linking the posterior cerebral to the internal carotid.

VENOUS DRAINAGE OF THE BRAIN

The venous drainage of the brain is of great importance in relation to neurosurgical procedures. It is also important to

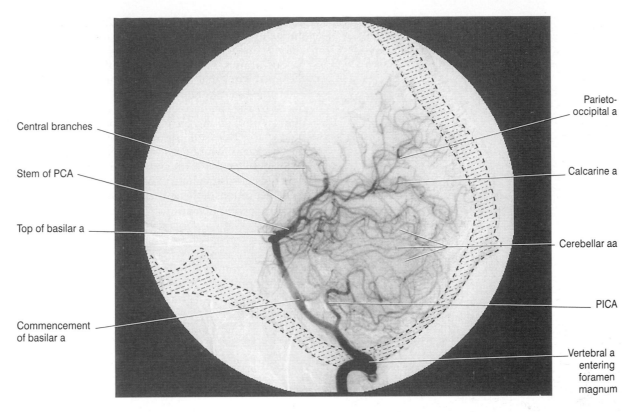

Central branches

Stem of PCA

Top of basilar a

Commencement
of basilar a

Parieto-
occipital a

Calcarine a

Cerebellar aa

PICA

Vertebral a
entering
foramen
magnum

Figure 5.10 Vertebrobasilar angiogram, lateral view. Contrast medium was injected into the left vertebral artery. PCA, posterior cerebral artery; PICA, posterior inferior cerebellar artery. Basilar supply to the upper half of the cerebellum is somewhat obscured by overlying posterior parietal branches of the PCA. (From an original series kindly provided by Dr Michael Modic, Dept of Radiology, The Cleveland Clinic Foundation.)

the professional neurologist because a variety of clinical syndromes can be produced by venous obstruction, venous thrombosis, and congenital arteriovenous communications. In general medical practice, however, problems caused by cerebral veins are rare in comparison with arterial disease.

The cerebral hemispheres are drained by superficial and deep cerebral veins. Like the intracranial venous sinuses, they are devoid of valves.

Superficial veins

The **superficial cerebral veins** lie in the subarachnoid space overlying the hemispheres. They drain the cerebral cortex and underlying white matter and empty into intracranial venous sinuses (*Figures 5.12A, 5.13, 5.14*).

The upper part of each hemisphere drains into the superior sagittal sinus. The middle part drains into the cavernous sinus (as a rule) by way of the **superficial middle cerebral vein**. The lower part drains into the transverse sinus.

Deep veins   (Figure 5.12B)

The deep cerebral veins drain the corpus striatum, thalamus, and choroid plexuses.

A **thalamostriate vein** drains the thalamus and caudate nucleus. Together with a **choroidal vein**, it forms the **internal cerebral vein**. The two internal cerebral veins unite

beneath the corpus callosum to form the **great cerebral vein** (of Galen).

A **basal vein** is formed beneath the anterior perforated substance by the union of **anterior** and **deep middle cerebral veins**. The basal vein runs around the crus cerebri and empties into the great cerebral vein.

Finally, the great cerebral vein enters the midpoint of the tentorium cerebelli. As it does so, it unites with the **inferior sagittal sinus** to form the **straight sinus**. The straight sinus empties in turn into the **left transverse sinus**.

REGULATION OF BLOOD FLOW

Blood flow in the cerebral vessels is primarily controlled by *autoregulation,* which is defined as the capacity of a tissue to regulate its own blood supply.

The most powerful source of autoregulation in the CNS is the *H+ ion concentration* in the extracellular fluid surrounding the arterioles within the brain parenchyma. Generalized relaxation of arteriolar smooth muscle tone is produced by hypercapnia (excess plasma $P\text{CO}_2$). On the other hand, hypocapnia causes arteriolar vasoconstriction.

A second powerful source of autoregulation is the *intraluminal pressure* within the arterioles. Any increase in pressure elicits a direct, myogenic response. When other factors are controlled (in animal experiments), the myogenic response is sufficient to maintain steady-state perfusion of

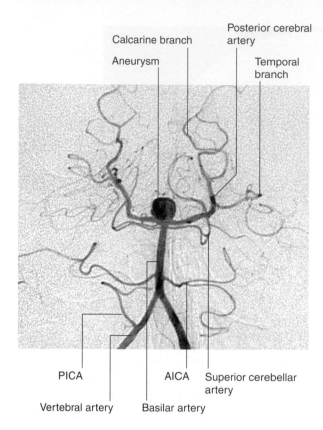

Calcarine branch
Posterior cerebral artery
Aneurysm
Temporal branch

PICA
AICA
Superior cerebellar artery

Vertebral artery
Basilar artery

Figure 5.11 Vertebrobasilar angiogram, Townes' view, (from above and in front) showing the vertebrobasilar arterial system. Note the large aneurysm arising from the bifurcation point of the basilar artery and accounting for the patient's persistent headache. AICA, anterior inferior cerebellar artery; PICA, posterior inferior cerebellar artery. (Kindly provided by Dr Pearse Morris, Director, Interventional Neuroradiology, Wake Forest University School of Medicine, Winston-Salem, N. Carolina, USA.)

the brain within a systemic blood pressure range of 80–180 mmHg (11–24 kPa).

Local blood flow increases within cortical areas and deep nuclei involved in particular motor, sensory, or cognitive tasks. The local arteriolar relaxation can be accounted for by a rise in K^+ levels caused by propagation of action potentials, and by a rise in H^+ caused by increased cell metabolism.

A large number of vasoactive substances have been identified in neural networks surrounding the cerebral conducting arteries and the arterioles. A specific role is difficult to assign to any of them, within the physiological range of blood flow.

THE BLOOD–BRAIN BARRIER

The nervous system is isolated from the blood by a barrier system that provides a stable and chemically optimal environment for neuronal function. The neurons and neuroglia are bathed in *brain extracellular fluid* (ECF) which accounts for 15% of total brain volume.

The extracellular compartments of the CNS are shown diagrammatically in *Figure 5.15*. As previously described

(Ch. 4), CSF secreted by the choroid plexuses circulates through the ventricular system and the subarachnoid space before passing through the arachnoid villi into the dural venous sinuses. In addition, CSF diffuses passively through the ependyma–glial membrane lining the ventricles and enters the brain extracellular spaces. It adds to the ECF produced by the capillary bed and by cell metabolism, and it diffuses through the pia-glial membrane into the subarachnoid space. This 'sink' movement of fluid compensates for the absence of lymphatics in the CNS.

Metabolic water is the only component of the CSF which does not pass through the blood–brain barrier. It carries with it any neurotransmitter substances that have not been recaptured following liberation by neurons, and it accounts for the presence in the subarachnoid space of transmitters and transmitter metabolites that could not penetrate the blood–brain barrier.

Relative contributions to the CSF obtained from a spinal tap are approximately as follows:

Choroid plexuses	60%
Capillary bed	30%
Metabolic water	10%

The blood–brain barrier has two components. One is at the level of the choroid plexus, the other resides in the CNS capillary bed.

Blood–CSF barrier (Figure 5.16A)

The blood–CSF barrier resides in the specialized ependymal lining of the choroid plexuses. This choroidal epithelium differs from the general ependymal epithelium in three ways:

1 Cilia are almost completely replaced by microvilli.
2 The cells are bonded by tight junctions. These pericellular belts of membrane fusion are the actual site of the blood–CSF barrier.
3 The epithelium contains numerous enzymes specifically involved in transport of ions and metabolites.

Blood–ECF barrier (Figure 5.16B)

The blood–ECF barrier resides in the CNS capillary bed, which differs from that of other capillary beds in three ways:

- The endothelial cells are bonded by tight junctions.
- Pinocytotic vesicles are rare, and fenestrations are absent.
- The cells contain the same transport systems as those of the choroidal epithelium.

Roles of microvascular pericytes
Pericytes are in cytoplasmic continuity with the endothelial cells, by way of gap junctions. Tissue culture studies have provided strong evidence for their primary roles in capillary angiogenesis during development and in the production and maintenance of the tight junctions.

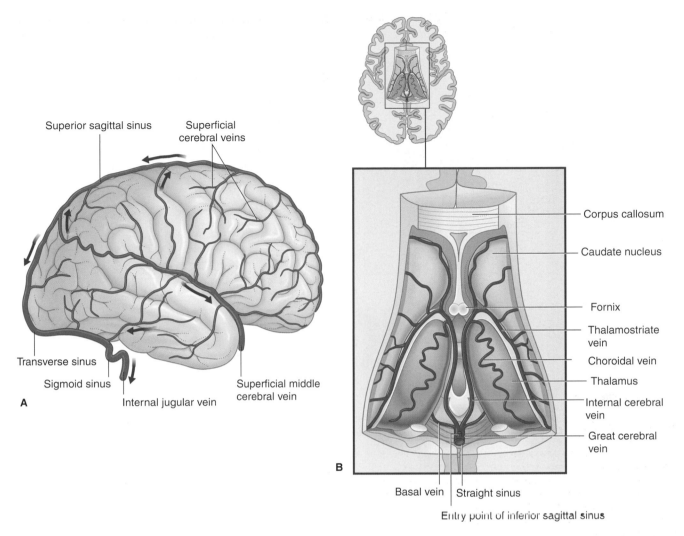

Superior sagittal sinus

Superficial cerebral veins

Transverse sinus

Sigmoid sinus

Internal jugular vein

Superficial middle cerebral vein

A

Corpus callosum

Caudate nucleus

Fornix

Thalamostriate vein

Choroidal vein

Thalamus

Internal cerebral vein

Great cerebral vein

B

Basal vein   Straight sinus

Entry point of inferior sagittal sinus

Figure 5.12 Cerebral veins. **(A)** Superficial veins viewed from the right side; arrows indicate direction of blood flow. **(B)** Deep veins viewed from above.

Pericytes express receptors for vasoactive mediators including norepinephrine, vasopressin, and angiotensin II, all indicative of a role in cerebrovascular autoregulation. In the presence of chronic hypertension, they strengthen the capillary bed by undergoing hypertrophy, hyperplasia, and internal production of cytoplasmic contractile protein filaments.

Pericytes are equipped for a hemostatic function, having an appropriate membrane surface for assembly of the prothrombin complex.

Pericytes are also phagocytic, and possess immunoregulatory cytokines.

The surface area of the brain capillary bed is about the size of a tennis court! This huge area accounts for the brain's consumption of 20% of basal oxygen intake by the lungs. The density of the cortical capillary bed is demonstrated in the latex cast shown in *Figure 5.17*.

Functions of the blood–brain barrier

- Modulation of the entry of metabolic substrates. Glucose, in particular, is a fundamental source of energy for neurons. The level of glucose in the brain ECF is more stable than that of the blood because the specific carrier becomes saturated when blood glucose rises and becomes hyperactive when it falls.

- Control of ion movements. Na^+-K^+ ATPase in the barrier cells pumps sodium into the CSF and pumps potassium out of the CSF into the blood.

- Prevention of access to the CNS by toxins and by peripheral neurotransmitters escaping into the bloodstream from autonomic nerve endings.

For some clinical notes concerning the blood–brain barrier, see *Clinical Panel 5.1*.

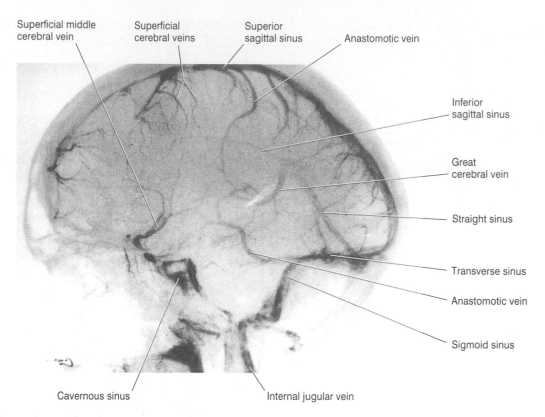

Superficial middle cerebral vein

Superficial cerebral veins

Superior sagittal sinus

Anastomotic vein

Inferior sagittal sinus

Great cerebral vein

Straight sinus

Transverse sinus

Anastomotic vein

Sigmoid sinus

Cavernous sinus

Internal jugular vein

Figure 5.13 Internal carotid angiogram, venous phase, lateral view. The dye is draining into the dural venous sinuses. (Photograph kindly provided by Dr James Toland, Dept of Radiology, Beaumont Hospital, Dublin.)

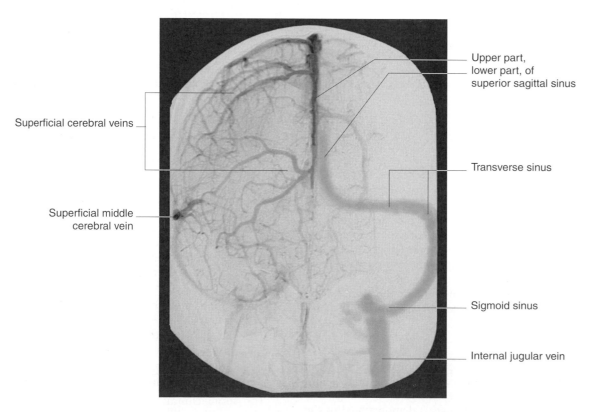

Upper part, lower part, of superior sagittal sinus

Superficial cerebral veins

Superficial middle cerebral vein

Transverse sinus

Sigmoid sinus

Internal jugular vein

Figure 5.14 Internal carotid angiogram, venous phase, anteroposterior view. Same patient as in *Figure 5.6*, this picture taken circa 8 seconds later. The vascular pattern is unusual in that the left rather than the right transverse sinus is dominant. (Angiogram kindly provided by Dr Pearse Morris, Director, Interventional Neuroradiology, Wake Forest University School of Medicine, Winston-Salem, N. Carolina, USA.)

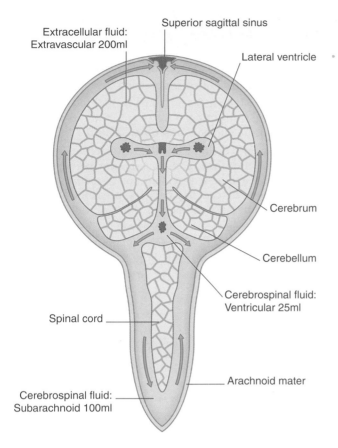

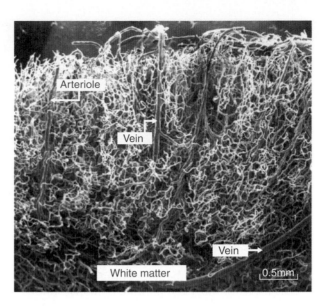

Figure 5.17 Latex-injection cast of the blood vessels in human postmortem brain. The convoluted whitish threads represent cortical capillaries. (Reprinted from Duvernoy, H.M., Delon, S., and Vannson, J.L. (1981) *Brain Res. Bull.* **7**: 519, with permission.)

Figure 5.15 Extracellular compartments of the brain. Arrows indicate circulation of cerebrospinal fluid.

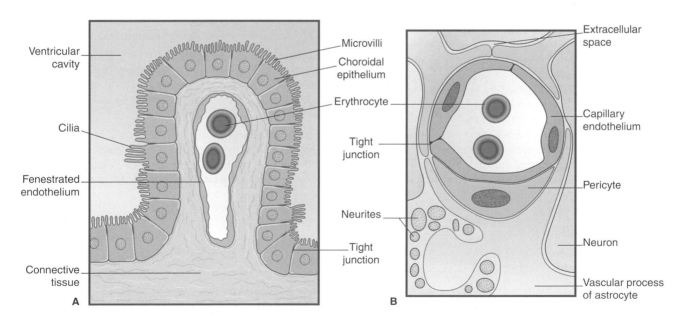

Figure 5.16 (A) Structure of blood–cerebrospinal fluid barrier. **(B)** Structure of blood–extracellular fluid barrier. Astrocytes are described in Chapter 6.

Clinical Panel 5.1   Blood–brain barrier pathology

The following five conditions are associated with breakdown of the blood–brain barrier:

1 Patients suffering from hypertension are liable to attacks of *hypertensive encephalopathy* should the blood pressure exceed the power of the arterioles to control it. The pressure may then open the tight junctions of the brain capillary endothelium. Rapid exudation of plasma causes *cerebral edema* with severe headache and vomiting, sometimes progressing to convulsions and coma.

2 In patients with severe *hypercapnia* brought about by reduced ventilation of the lungs (as in pulmonary or heart disease, or after surgery), relaxation of arteriolar muscle may be sufficient to induce cerebral edema even if the blood pressure is normal. In this case, the edema may be expressed by mental confusion and drowsiness progressing to coma.

3 *Brain injury*, whether from trauma or spontaneous hemorrhage, leads to edema owing to the osmotic effects of tissue damage (and other factors).

4 *Infections* of the brain or meninges are accompanied by breakdown of the blood–brain barrier, perhaps because of the large-scale emigration of leukocytes through the brain capillary bed. The breakdown can be exploited because the porous capillary walls will permit the passage of non-lipid-soluble antibiotics.

5 The capillary bed of *brain tumors* is fenestrated. As a result, radioactive tracers too large to penetrate healthy brain capillaries can be detected within tumors.

Core Information

Arteries
The circle of Willis comprises the anterior communicating artery and two anterior cerebral arteries, the internal carotids, two posterior communicating arteries, and the two posterior cerebral arteries.

The anterior cerebral artery gives off Heubner's artery to the antero-inferior internal capsule, then arches around the corpus callosum and supplies the medial surface of the hemisphere as far back as the parieto-occipital sulcus, with overlap on to the lateral surface.

The middle cerebral artery enters the lateral sulcus and supplies two-thirds of the lateral surface of the hemisphere. Its central branches include the leak-prone lateral striate supplying the upper part of the internal capsule.

The posterior cerebral artery arises from the basilar artery; it supplies the splenium of corpus callosum and the occipital and temporal cortex.

The vertebral arteries enter the foramen magnum. They supply spinal cord, posterior–inferior cerebellum and medulla oblongata before uniting to form the basilar artery.

The basilar artery supplies the anterior–inferior and superior cerebellum, the pons and inner ear, before dividing into posterior cerebral arteries.

Veins
Superficial cerebral veins drain the cerebral cortex and empty into dural venous sinuses. The internal cerebral veins drain the thalami and unite as the great cerebral vein. The great veins drain the corpus striatum via the basal vein before entering the straight sinus.

Autoregulation
Hypercapnia causes arteriolar dilatation; hypocapnia causes constriction. A rise of intraluminal pressure produces a direct, myogenic response by arteriolar walls.

Blood–brain barrier
A blood–CSF barrier resides in the choroidal epithelium (modified ependyma) of the ventricles. A blood–ECF barrier resides in the endothelium of the brain capillary bed.

REFERENCES

Balabanonov, B. and Dore-Duffy, P. (1998) Role of the microvascular pericyte in the blood–brain barrier. *J. Neurosci. Res.* **53**: 637–644.

Duvernoy, H.M. (1978) *Human Brainstem Vessels.* New York: Springer-Verlag.

Duvernoy, H.M., Delon, S. and Vannson, J.L. (1981) Cortical blood vessels of the human brain. *Brain Res. Bull.* **7**: 519–530.

Gloger, S., Gloger, A., Vogt. H. and Kretschmann, H-J. (1994) Computer-assisted 3D reconstruction of the terminal branches of the cerebral arteries. *Neuroradiol.* **36**: 173–180; 181–187; 251–257.

Kapp, J.P. (1984) *The Cerebral Venous System and its Disorders.* Orlando: Grune & Stratton.

Sage, M.R. and Wilson, A.J. (1994) The blood–brain barrier: an important concept in neuroimaging. *Am. J. Neuroradiol.* **94**: 601–622.

Wahl, M. and Schilling, L. (1993) Regulation of cerebral blood flow – a brief review. *Acta Neurochir.* **59**: 3–10.

Neurons and neuroglia

Nerve cells, or **neurons**, are the structural and functional units of the nervous system. They generate and conduct electrical changes in the form of nerve impulses. They communicate chemically with other neurons at points of contact called **synapses**. **Neuroglia** (literally, 'nerve glue') is the connective tissue of the nervous system.

Neuroglial cells outnumber neurons by about five to one. They have important nutritive and supportive functions.

NEURONS

Billions of neurons form a shell, or **cortex**, on the surface of the cerebral and cerebellar hemispheres. **Nuclei** are aggregates of neurons buried within the white matter.

In the CNS, almost all neurons are multipolar, their cell bodies or **somas** having multiple poles or angles. At every pole but one, a **dendrite** emerges and divides repeatedly (*Figure 6.1*). On some neurons, the shafts of the dendrites are smooth. On others, the shafts show numerous short **spines**. The dendrites receive synaptic contacts from other neurons, both on the spines and on the shaft surface.

The remaining pole of the soma gives rise to the **axon**, which conducts nerve impulses. Most axons give off *collateral* branches (*Figure 6.2*). *Terminal* branches synapse upon target neurons.

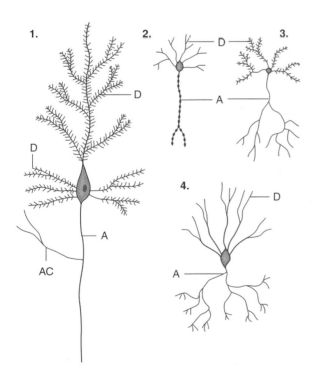

Figure 6.1 Profiles of neurons from the brain. **1**, Pyramidal cell, cerebral cortex. **2**, Neuroendocrine cell, hypothalamus. **3**, Spiny neuron, corpus striatum. **4**, Basket cell, cerebellum. Neurons **1** and **3** show dendritic spines. A, axon; AC, axon collateral; D, dendrites.

Most synaptic contacts between neurons are either **axodendritic** or **axosomatic**. Axodendritic synapses are usually excitatory in their effect upon target neurons, whereas most axosomatic synapses have an inhibitory effect.

Internal structure of neurons

All parts of neurons are permeated by **microtubules** and **neurofilaments** (*Figure 6.3*). The soma contains the nucleus and the cytoplasm or **perikaryon** (*Gr.* around the nucleus). The perikaryon contains clumps of granular endoplasmic reticulum known as *Nissl bodies*; also Golgi complexes, free ribosomes, mitochondria, and smooth endoplasmic reticulum (SER).

Intracellular transport

Turnover of membranous and skeletal material takes place in all cells. In neurons, fresh components are continuously synthesized in the soma and moved into the axon and dendrites by a process of *anterograde transport*. At the same time, worn-out materials are returned to the soma by *retrograde transport*, for degradation in lysosomes (see also *target recognition*, later).

Anterograde transport is of two kinds, rapid and slow. Included in *rapid* transport (at a speed of 300–400 mm per day) are free elements such as synaptic vesicles, transmitter substances (or their precursor molecules), and mitochondria. Also included are lipid and protein molecules (including receptor proteins) for insertion into the plasma membrane. Included in *slow* transport (at 5–10 mm per day) are the skeletal elements, and soluble proteins including some of those involved in transmitter release at nerve endings. Microtubules seem to be largely constructed within the axon. They are exported from the soma in pre-assembled short sheaves which propel one another along the initial segment of the axon; further progress is mainly by a process of elongation (up to 1 mm apiece) performed by the addition of tubulin polymers at their distal ends, with some disassembly at their proximal ends. The bulk movement of neurofilaments slows down to almost zero distally; there, the filaments are refreshed by the insertion of filament polymers moving from the soma by slow transport.

Retrograde transport of worn-out mitochondria, SER, and plasma membrane (including receptors therein) is fairly rapid (150–200 mm per day). In addition to its function in waste disposal, retrograde transport is involved in *target cell recognition*. At synaptic contacts, axons constantly 'nibble' the plasma membrane of target neurons by means of endocytotic vesicular uptake, the vesicles being brought to the soma and incorporated into Golgi complexes there. Uptake of target cell 'marker' molecules is important for cell recognition during development. It may also be necessary for viability later on because adult neurons shrink and may even die if their axons are severed proximal to their first branches.

Survival of neurons depends upon *neurotrophins*. Longest known is NGF (nerve growth factor), on which the developing peripheral sensory and autonomic systems are

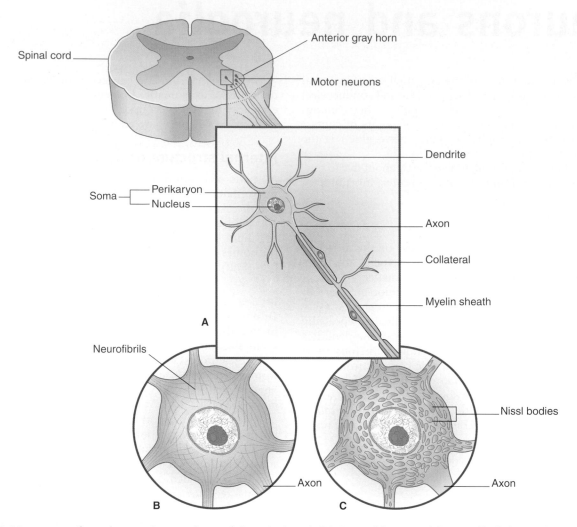

Figure 6.2 Motoneuron from the anterior gray horn of the spinal cord. **(A)** General features. **(B)** Neurofibrils (matted neurofilaments) seen after staining with silver salts. **(C)** Nissl bodies (clumps of granular endoplasmic reticulum) seen after staining with a cationic dye such as thionin.

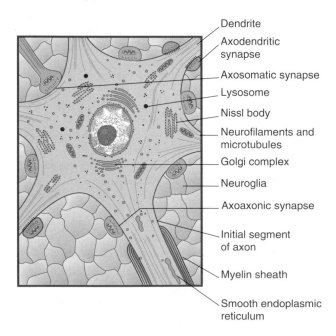

Figure 6.3 Ultrastructure of a motoneuron. Stems of five dendrites are included; also three excitatory synapses (red) and five inhibitory synapses.

especially dependent. NGF is taken up from target tissues and taken to the soma by retrograde transport. Adult brain neurons synthesize brain-derived neurotrophic factor (BDNF) in the soma and send it to their nerve endings by anterograde transport. Animal studies have shown that BDNF maintains the general health of neurons in terms of metabolic activity, impulse propagation, and synaptic transmission.

Transport mechanisms

Microtubules are the supporting structures for neuronal transport. Microtubule-binding proteins, in the form of ATPases, propel organelles and molecules along the outer surface of the microtubules. Distinct ATPases are used for anterograde and retrograde work.

Neurofilaments do not seem to be involved in the transport mechanism. They are rather evenly spaced, having side-arms that keep them apart and provide skeletal stability by attachment to proteins beneath the axolemmal membrane. Neurofilament numbers are in direct proportion to axonal diameter and the filaments may in truth *determine* axonal diameter.

Some points of clinical relevance are highlighted in *Clinical Panel 6.1.*

Clinical Panel 6.1 Clinical relevance of neuronal transport

Tetanus

Wounds contaminated by soil or street dust may contain *Clostridium tetani*. The toxin produced by this organism binds to the plasma membrane of nerve endings, is taken up by endocytosis, and is carried to the spinal cord by retrograde transport. Other neurons upstream take in the toxin by endocytosis – notably Renshaw cells (Ch. 12) which normally exert a braking action upon motor neurons through the release of an inhibitory transmitter substance, glycine. Tetanus toxin prevents the release of glycine. As a result, motor neurons go out of control, particularly those supplying the muscles of the face, jaws, and spine. These muscles exhibit prolonged, agonizing spasms. About half of the patients who show these classic signs of tetanus die of exhaustion within a few days. Tetanus is entirely preventable by appropriate and timely immunization.

Viruses and toxic metals

Retrograde axonal transport has been blamed for the passage of viruses from the nasopharynx to the CNS; also for the uptake of toxic metals such as lead and aluminum. Viruses, in particular, may be spread widely through the brain by means of retrograde transneuronal uptake.

Peripheral neuropathies

Defective anterograde transport seems to be involved in certain 'dying back' neuropathies in which the distal parts of the longer peripheral nerves undergo progressive atrophy (see Clinical Panel 7.1).

SYNAPSES

Chemical synapses

Synapses are the points of contact between neurons. Conventional synapses are *chemical*, depending for their effect on the release of a *transmitter substance*. The typical chemical synapse comprises a **presynaptic membrane**, a **synaptic cleft**, and a **postsynaptic membrane** (*Figure 6.4*). The presynaptic membrane belongs to the terminal bouton, the **postsynaptic** membrane to the target neuron. Transmitter substance is released from the bouton by exocytosis, traverses the narrow synaptic cleft, and activates receptors in the postsynaptic membrane. Underlying the postsynaptic membrane is a **subsynaptic web**, in which numerous biochemical changes are initiated by receptor activation.

The bouton contains **synaptic vesicles** loaded with transmitter substance, together with numerous mitochondria and sacs of SER. Following conventional methods of fixation, *presynaptic dense projections* are visible (*Figure 6.4*), and microtubules seem to guide the synaptic vesicles to active zones in the intervals between the projections.

Receptor activation

Transmitter molecules cross the synaptic cleft and activate receptor proteins which straddle the postsynaptic membrane (*Figure 6.5*). The activated receptors initiate ionic events that either depolarize the postsynaptic membrane (excitatory postsynaptic effect) or hyperpolarize it (inhibitory postsynaptic effect). The voltage change passes over the soma in a decremental wave called *electrotonus*, and alters the resting potential of the first part or **initial segment** of the axon. (See physiology texts for details of the ionic events.) If excitatory postsynaptic potentials are dominant, the initial segment

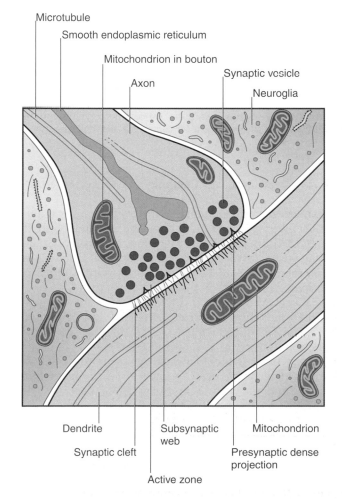

Figure 6.4 Ultrastructure of an axodendritic synapse following conventional tissue fixation.

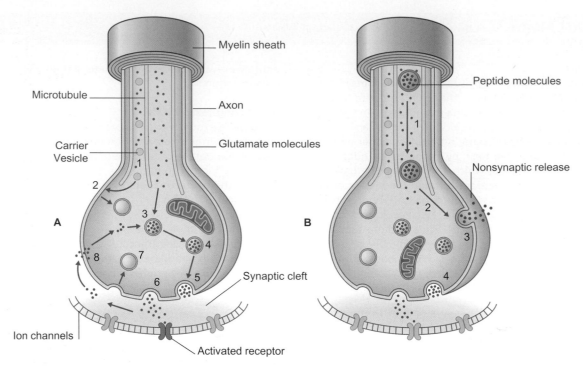

Figure 6.5 Dynamic events at two types of nerve terminals. **(A)** Small molecule transmitter, exemplified by a glutamatergic nerve ending. **(1)** Carrier vesicles containing synaptic vesicle membrane proteins are rapidly transported along microtubules and stored in the plasma membrane of the terminal bouton. At the same time, enzymes and glutamate molecules are conveyed by slow transport. **(2)** Vesicle membrane proteins are retrieved from the plasma membrane and form synaptic vesicles. **(3)** Glutamate is taken into the vesicles where it is stored and concentrated. **(4)** Loaded vesicles approach the presynaptic membrane. **(5)** Following depolarization, the 'docked' vesicles undergo exocytosis. **(6)** Released transmitter diffuses across the synaptic cleft and activates specific receptors in the postsynaptic membrane. **(7)** Vesicular membranes are retrieved by means of endocytosis. **(8)** Some glutamate is actively transported back into the bouton for recycling. **(B)** Neuropeptide cotransmission. The example here is peptide *substance P* contransmission with glutamate, a combination found at the central end of unipolar neurons serving pain sensation. **(1)** The vesicles and peptide precursors (propeptides) are synthesized in Golgi complexes in the perikaryon and taken to the terminal bouton by rapid transport. **(2)** As they enter the bouton, peptide formation is being completed, whereupon the vesicle approaches the plasma membrane. **(3)** Following membrane depolarization, the vesicular contents are sent into the intercellular space by means of exocytosis. **(4)** Glutamate is simultaneously released into the synaptic cleft.

will be depolarized to threshold and generate action potentials.

In the CNS, the commonest excitatory transmitter is glutamate; the commonest inhibitory one is γ-aminobutyric acid (GABA). In the peripheral nervous system (PNS), the transmitter for motor neurons supplying striated muscle is *acetylcholine*; the main transmitter for sensory neurons is *glutamate*.

The sequence of events involved in *glutamatergic* synaptic transmission is shown in *Figure 6.5A*. In the case of peptide *co-transmission* with glutamate, release of (one or more) peptides is *nonsynaptic*, as shown in *Figure 6.5B*.

Many sensory neurons liberate one or more *peptides* as well as glutamate; the peptides may be shed from any part of the neuron, but their usual role is to modulate (raise or lower) the effectiveness of the transmitter.

A further kind of transmission is known as *volume* transmission. This kind is typical of *monoamine (biogenic amine)* neurons, which fall into two categories. One category synthesizes a *catecholamine*, namely *norepinephrine* or *dopamine*, both synthesized from the amino-acid tyrosine. The other synthesizes *serotonin*, derived from tryptophane. As illustrated in *Figure 6.6 for dopamine*, the transmitter is liberated

from *varicosities* (where they are also synthesized) as well as from synaptic contacts. The transmitter enters the ECF of the CNS and activates specific receptors up to 100μm away before being degraded. The monoamine neurons have enormous territorial distribution, and deviation from normal function is implicated in a variety of ailments including Parkinson's disease, schizophrenia, and major depression.

Nitric oxide within glutamatergic neurons is also associated with volume transmission. Excess nitric oxide liberation is *cytotoxic*, notably in areas rendered avascular by cerebral arterial thrombosis. Glutamate itself is also potentially cytotoxic.

In the context of volume transmission, the conventional kind is called 'wiring' to indicate its relatively fixed nature.

Lock and key analogy for drug therapy

The receptor may be likened to a lock, the transmitter being the key that operates it. The transmitter output of certain neurons may falter as a consequence of age or disease, and a duplicate key can often be provided in the form of a drug which mimics the action of the transmitter. Such a drug is

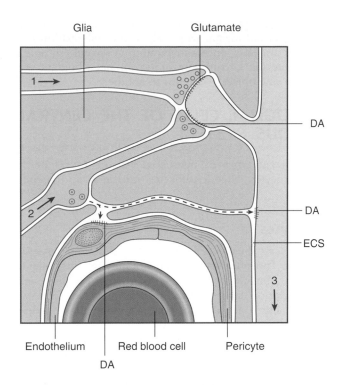

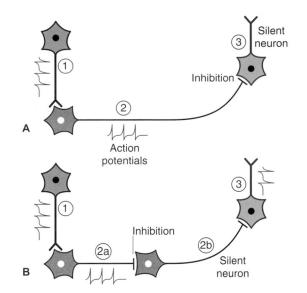

Figure 6.7 (A) Excitatory neuron 1 is activating inhibitory neuron 2 with consequent silencing of neuron 3 by neuron 2. **(B)** Interpolation of a second inhibitory neuron (2b) has the opposite effect on neuron 3 because 2b is silenced. Neuron 3 (spontaneously active unless inhibited) is released.

Figure 6.6 Volume transmission in the brain. The axon of a glutamatergic neuron (1) and of a dopaminergic neuron (2) are making conventional synaptic contacts on the spine of a spiny stellate cell (3) in the striatum. Dopamine (DA) is also escaping from a varicosity and diffusing through the extracellular space (ECS) to activate dopamine receptors on the dendritic shaft and on the wall of a capillary pericyte (see Ch. 5).

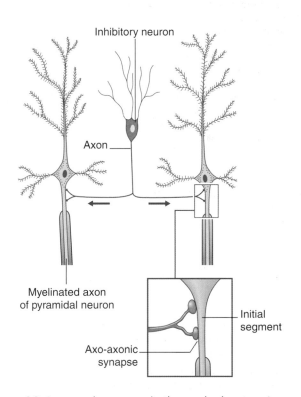

Figure 6.8 Axo-axonic synapses in the cerebral cortex. Arrows indicate direction of impulse conduction.

called an *agonist*. On the other hand, excessive production of a transmitter may be countered by a *receptor blocker* – the equivalent of a dummy key which will occupy the lock without activating it.

Inhibition versus disinhibition

Spontaneously active neurons are often held in check by inhibitory neurons (usually GABAergic) as shown in *Figure 6.7A*. The inhibitory neurons may be silenced by others of the same kind, leading to *disinhibition* of the target cell (*Figure 6.7B*). Disinhibition is a major feature of neuronal activity on the basal ganglia (Ch. 28).

Less common chemical synapses

Two varieties of **axo-axonic** synapses are recognized. In both cases, the boutons belong to inhibitory neurons. One variety occurs on the initial segment of the axon, where it exercises a powerful veto on impulse generation (*Figure 6.8*). In the second kind, the boutons are applied to excitatory boutons of other neurons, and they inhibit transmitter release. The effect is called *presynaptic inhibition*, any conventional contact being *postsynaptic* in this context (*Figure 6.9*).

Dendrodendritic (D-D) synapses occur between dendritic spines of contiguous spiny neurons and alter the electrotonus of the target neuron rather than generating nerve impulses. In *one-way* D-D synapses, one of the two spines contains synaptic vesicles. In *reciprocal* synapses, both do. Excitatory D-D synapses are shown in *Figure 6.10*. Inhibitory D-D synapses are numerous in relay nuclei of the thalamus (Ch. 22).

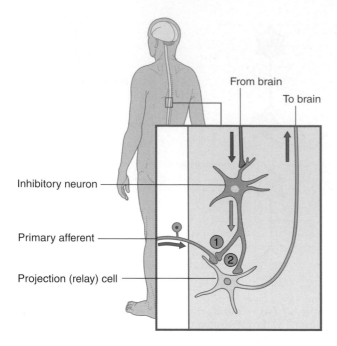

Figure 6.9 **(1)** Presynaptic and **(2)** postsynaptic inhibition of a spinal neuron projecting to the brain. Arrows indicate directions of impulse conduction (relay cell may be silenced by inhibitory cell activity).

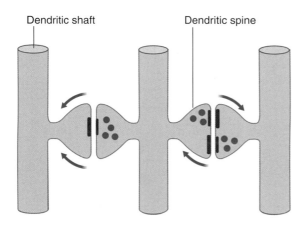

Figure 6.10 Dendrodendritic excitation. The dendrites belong to three separate neurons. On the right is a reciprocal synapse. Arrows indicate direction of electrotonic waves.

Somatodendritic and **somatosomatic** synapses have also been identified, but they are scarce.

Electrical synapses

Electrical synapses are scarce in the mammalian nervous system. They consist of gap junctions (nexuses) between dendrites or somas of contiguous neurons, where there is cytoplasmic continuity through 1.5 nm channels. No transmitter is involved and there is no synaptic delay. They permit electrotonic changes to pass from one neuron to another. Being tightly coupled, modulation is not possible. Their function is to ensure synchronous activity of neurons having a common action. An example is the inspiratory center in the medulla oblongata, where all of the cells exhibit synchronous discharge during inspiration. A second example is among neuronal circuits controlling *saccades*, where the eyes dart from one object of interest to another.

NEUROGLIAL CELLS OF THE CENTRAL NERVOUS SYSTEM

Four different types of neuroglial cell are found in the CNS: astrocytes, oligodendrocytes, microglia, and ependymal cells.

Astrocytes

Astrocytes are bushy cells with dozens of fine radiating processes. The cytoplasm contains abundant intermediate filaments. This confers a degree of rigidity on these cells which helps to support the brain as a whole. Glycogen granules, which are also abundant, provide an immediate source of glucose for the neurons.

Some astrocyte processes from **glial-limiting membranes** on the inner (ventricular) and outer (pial) surfaces of the brain. Other processes invest synaptic contacts between neurons (*Figure 6.11*). In addition, *vascular processes* invest brain capillaries.

Astrocytes are engaged in mopping up K$^+$ ions during periods of intense neuronal activity. They participate in recycling certain neurotransmitter substances following release, notably the chief excitatory CNS transmitter, *glutamate* and the chief inhibitory transmitter, *GABA*.

Unlike neurons, whose multiplication has ceased around the time of birth, astrocytes can multiply at any time. As part of the healing process following CNS injury, proliferation of astrocytes and their processes results in dense glial scar tissue (*gliosis*). More importantly, spontaneous local proliferation of astrocytes may give rise to a brain tumor (*Clinical Panel 6.2*).

Oligodendrocytes

Oligodendrocytes are responsible for wrapping myelin sheaths around axons in the white matter. In the gray matter, they form **satellite cells** which seem to participate in ion exchange with neurons.

Myelination

Myelination commences during the middle period of gestation, and continues well into the second decade. A single oligodendrocyte lays myelin on upwards of three dozen axons by means of a spiraling process whereby the inner and outer faces of the plasma membrane form the alternating **major** and **minor dense lines** seen in transverse sections of the myelin sheath (*Figure 6.12*). Some cytoplasm remains in **paranodal pockets** at the ends of each myelin segment. In the intervals between the glial wrappings, the axon is relatively exposed, at nodes.

Myelination greatly increases the speed of impulse conduction because the depolarization process jumps from node to node (see Ch. 7). During myelination, K$^+$ ion channels are deleted from the underlying axolemma. For this

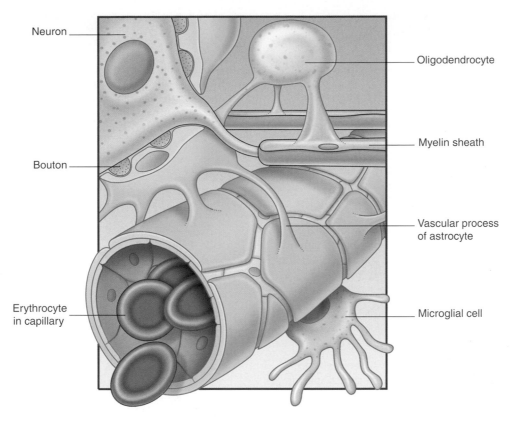

Neuron

Bouton

Erythrocyte
in capillary

Oligodendrocyte

Myelin sheath

Vascular process
of astrocyte

Microglial cell

Figure 6.11 Three neuroglial cell types.

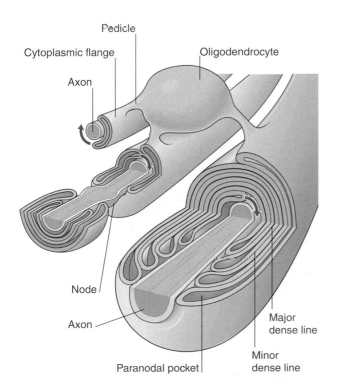

Pedicle

Cytoplasmic flange

Axon

Oligodendrocyte

Node

Axon

Paranodal pocket

Major
dense line

Minor
dense line

Figure 6.12 Myelination in the CNS. Arrows indicate movement
of the growing edge of the cytoplasmic flange of the
oligodendrocyte.

reason, demyelinating diseases such as multiple sclerosis
(*Clinical Panel 6.3*) are accompanied by failure of impulse
conduction.

Unmyelinated axons abound in the gray matter. They
are fine (0.2 μm in diameter or less) and not individually
ensheathed.

Microglia (Figure 6.11)

The weight of evidence indicates that both embryonic and
post traumatic microglial cells are of mesodermal origin.
Resting microglial cells are minute (hence the name), but
when *activated* by inflammation or by myelin sheath breakdown, they enlarge and become motile phagocytes.

Ependyma

Ependymal cells line the ventricular system of the brain.
Cilia on their free surface help the propulsion of CSF
through the ventricles.

Clinical Panel 6.2   Gliomas

Brain tumors most commonly originate from neuroglial cells, especially astrocytes.

General symptoms produced by expanding brain tumors are those of *raised intracranial pressure*. They include headache, drowsiness, and vomiting. Radiological investigation may reveal displacement of midline structures to the opposite side. Tumors below the tentorium (usually cerebellar) are likely to block the exit of CSF from the fourth ventricle, in which case ballooning of the ventricular system will add to the intracranial pressure.

Local symptoms depend upon the position of the tumor. For example, clumsiness of an arm or leg may be caused by a cerebellar tumor on the same side; and motor weakness of an arm or leg may be caused by a cerebral tumor on the opposite side.

Progression

Expansion of a tumor may cause one or more brain hernias to develop, as shown in *Figure CP 6.2.1*:

1 *Subfalcal herniation* (in the interval between falx cerebri and corpus callosum) seldom causes specific symptoms.

2 *Uncal herniation* is the term used to denote displacement of the uncus of the temporal lobe into the tentorial notch. Compression of the ipsilateral crus cerebri by the uncus may give rise to *contralateral* motor weakness. Alternatively, compression of the contralateral crus against the sharp edge of the tentorium cerebelli may cause *ipsilateral* motor weakness.

3 *Pressure coning:* a cone of cerebellar tissue (the tonsil) may descend into the foramen magnum, squeezing the medulla oblongata and causing death from respiratory/cardiovascular failure by inactivation of *vital centers* in the reticular formation (Ch. 19).

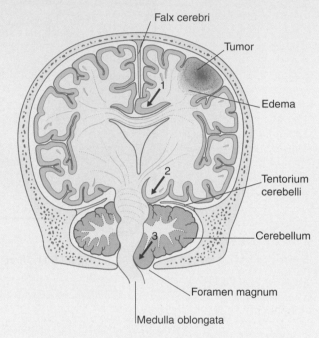

Figure CP 6.2.1 Brain herniations. For numbers, see text.

Core Information

Neurons

The multipolar neuron of the CNS comprises soma, dendrites, and axon; the axon gives off collateral and terminal branches. The soma contains rough and smooth endoplasmic reticulum, Golgi complexes, neurofilaments, and microtubules. Microtubules pervade the entire neuron; they are involved in anterograde transport of synaptic vesicles, mitochondria, and membranous replacement material; and in retrograde transport of marker molecules and degraded organelles.

The three kinds of chemical neuronal interaction are synaptic (e.g., glutamatergic), nonsynaptic (e.g., peptidergic), and volume (e.g., monoaminergic, serotonergic).

Anatomical varieties of chemical synapse include axodendritic, axosomatic, axo-axonic, and dendrodendritic. Structure includes pre- and postsynaptic membranes, synaptic cleft, and subsynaptic web.

Electrical synapses via gap junctions render some neuronal groups electrically coupled, for synchronous activation.

Neuroglia

Astrocytes have supportive, nutritive, and retrieval functions. They are the main source of brain tumors. Oligodendrocytes form CNS myelin sheaths, which are subject to destruction in demyelinating diseases. Microglia are potential phagocytes.

Clinical Panel 6.3   Multiple sclerosis

Multiple sclerosis (MS) is the commonest neurological disorder of young adults in the temperate latitudes north and south of the equator. It is more prevalent in women, with a female : male ratio of 3 : 2. The peak age of onset is around 30 years, the range being 15 to 45.

MS is a *primary demyelinating disease*: the initial feature is the development of plaques (patches) of demyelination in the white matter while the axons remain intact. The denuded axons are unable to conduct impulses because K+ channels are normally deleted from the axolemmal membrane when myelin sheaths are initially laid down. Impulse conduction in neighboring myelinated fibers is also compromised by edema (inflammatory exudate). Over time, the plaques are progressively replaced by glial scar tissue and the trapped axons degenerate as well. Old plaques feel firm (sclerotic) in postmortem slices of the brain.

Common locations of early plaques are the cervical spinal cord, upper brainstem, optic nerve, and periventricular white matter including that of the cerebellum. MS is not a systems disease: it is not anatomically selective, and a plaque may involve parts of adjacent motor and sensory pathways.

Presenting symptoms can be correlated with lesion sites, as follows:

- *Motor weakness*, usually in one or both legs, signifies a lesion involving the CST.

- *Clumsiness* in reaching and grasping usually accompanies a lesion in the cerebellar white matter.

- *Numbness/tingling*, often spreading up from the legs to the trunk, may be caused by a lesion in the posterior white matter of the spinal cord. Tingling ('pins and needles') is attributed to spontaneous firing of partially demyelinated sensory fibers.

- *Diplopia* (double vision) may be produced by a plaque within the pons or midbrain affecting the function of one of the ocular motor nerves.

- A *scotoma* (patch of blindness in the visual field of one eye) is produced by a plaque within the optic nerve.

- *Urinary retention* (failure of the bladder to empty) can be caused by interruption of the central autonomic pathway descending from the brainstem to the lower part of the cord.

The usual course of the disease is one of remissions and relapses, with an overall slow progression and development of multiple disabilities.

REFERENCES

Alter, C.A., Cal, N., Bliven, T., Juhasz, M., Conner, J.M., Acheson, A.L., Lindsay, R.M. and Weigand, S.J. (1997) Anterograde transport of brain-derived neurotrophic factor and its role in the brain. *Nature* **389**: 856–859.

Calakos, N. and Scheller, R.H. (1996) Synaptic vesicle biogenesis, docking, and fusion: a molecular description. *Physiol. Rev.* **76**: 1–29.

Federoff, S. (1995) Development of microglia. In *Neuroglia* (Kettenmann, H. and Ransom, B.R., eds), pp. 163–184. New York: Oxford University Press.

Gehrmann, J., Matsumoto, Y. and Kreutzberg, D.W. (1995) Microglia: intrinsic immunoeffector cells of the brain. *Brain Res. Rev.* **20**: 269–287.

Golding, D.W. (1994) Synaptic, non-synaptic and parasynaptic exocytosis. *BioEssays* **16**: 503–508.

Grafstein, B. (1995) Axonal transport: function and mechanisms. In *The Axon* (Waxman, S., Kocsis, J.D. and Stys, P.K., eds), pp. 185–199. New York: Oxford University Press.

Grafstein, B. (1999) Intracellular traffic in nerve cells. *Brain Res. Bull.* **50**: 311–322.

Kaur, C. et al. (2001) Origin of microglia. *Microsc. RW. Tech* **54**: 2–9

Lee, R.M.K.W. (1995) Morphology of cerebral arteries. *Pharmacol. Therap.* **66**: 149–173.

Mercer, J.A., Albanesci, J.P. and Brady, S.T. (1994) Molecular motors and cell motility in the brain. *Brain Pathol.* **4**: 167–179.

Morell, P. and Quarles, R.H. (1989) Formation, structure, and biochemistry of myelin. In *Basic Neurochemistry: Molecular, Cellular, and Medical Aspects*, 4th edn (Siegel, G.J., et al., eds), pp. 109–138. New York: Raven Press.

Norenberg, M.D. (1994) Astrocyte responses to injury. *J. Neuropath. Exp. Neurol.* **53**: 213–220.

Privat, A., Giminez-Robotta, M. and Ridet, J-L. (1995) Morphology of astrocytes. In *Neuroglia* (Kettenmann, H. and Ransom, B.R., eds), pp. 3–22. New York: Oxford University Press.

Raine, C.S. (1989) Neurocellular anatomy. In *Basic Neurochemistry: Molecular, Cellular, and Medical Aspects*, 4th edn (Siegel, G.J., et al., eds), pp. 3–33. New York: Raven Press.

Sano, Y. (1989) Morphological aspects of neurons as secretory cells. *Arch. Histol. Cytol.* **52**: 107–112.

Volknandt, W. (1995) The synaptic vesicle and its targets. *Neurosci.* **64**: 277–300.

Zoli, M., Torri, C., Ferrari, R., Jansson, A., Zinni, I., Fuxe, K. and Agnati, L.F. (1998) The emergence of the volume transmission concept. *Brain Res. Rev.* **26**: 136–147.

Peripheral nerves

7

GENERAL FEATURES

The peripheral nerves comprise the cranial and spinal nerves linking the brain and spinal cord to the peripheral tissues. The spinal nerves are formed by the union of **anterior** and **posterior nerve roots** at their points of exit from the vertebral canal (*Figure 7.1*). The swelling on each posterior root is a **spinal** or **posterior root ganglion**. The **spinal nerve** is only 1 cm long and occupies an intervertebral foramen. Upon emerging from the foramen, it divides into **anterior** and **posterior rami**.

The posterior rami supply the erector spinae muscles and the overlying skin of the trunk. The anterior rami supply the muscles and skin of the side and front of the trunk, including the muscles and skin of the limbs; they also supply sensory fibers to the parietal pleura and parietal peritoneum.

The cervical, brachial and lumbosacral plexuses are derived from anterior rami, which form the *roots* of the plexuses. The term 'root' therefore has two different meanings, depending on the context. (Details of the plexi are in standard anatomy texts.)

The neurons contributing to peripheral nerves are partly contained within the CNS (*Figure 7.2*). The cells giving rise to the motor (*efferent*) nerves to skeletal muscles are **multipolar** *alpha* and *gamma* **neurons** of similar configuration to the one depicted in *Figure 6.3*; in the spinal cord, they occupy the anterior horn of gray matter. Further details are in Chapter 8. Those giving rise to posterior nerve roots are **unipolar neurons** whose cell bodies lie in posterior root ganglia and whose sensory (*afferent*) central processes enter the posterior horn of gray matter.

The spinal nerves supply *somatic efferent fibers* to the skeletal muscles of the trunk and limbs, and *somatic afferent fibers* to the skin, muscles, and joints. They all carry *visceral effer-*

ent, autonomic fibers and some spinal nerves contain visceral afferent fibers as well.

MICROSCOPIC STRUCTURE OF PERIPHERAL NERVES

Figure 7.3 illustrates the structure of a typical peripheral nerve. It is not possible to designate individual nerve fibers as motor or sensory on the basis of structural features alone.

Peripheral nerves are invested with **epineurium**, a loose, vascular connective tissue sheath surrounding the fascicles (bundles of fibers) that make up the nerve. Never fibers are exchanged between fascicles along the course of the nerve.

Each fascicle is covered by **perineurium**, composed of several layers of pavement epithelium bonded by tight junctions. Surrounding the individual Schwann cells is a network of reticular collagenous fibers, the **endoneurium**.

Less than half of the nerve fibers are enclosed in myelin sheaths. The remaining, unmyelinated fibers travel in deep gutters along the surface of Schwann cells.

The term 'nerve fiber' is usually used in the context of nerve impulse conduction, where it is equivalent to 'axon'. An anatomical definition is possible for a myelinated fiber: it comprises axon, myelin, and neurolemmal sheaths, and endoneurium. A definition is not possible for unmyelinated axons because they share *neurolemmal* (Schwann cell) and endoneurial sheaths.

Myelin formation

The **Schwann cell** is the representative neuroglial cell of the PNS. It forms chains of neurolemmal cells along the nerves. Modified Schwann cells form **satellite cells** in posterior root ganglia and in autonomic ganglia, and **teloglia** at encapsulated sensory nerve endings (Ch. 9).

If an axon is to be myelinated, it receives the simultaneous attention of a sequence of Schwann cells along its length. Each one encloses the axon completely, creating a 'mesentery' of plasma membrane, the **mesaxon** (*Figure 7.4*). The mesaxon is displaced progressively, being rotated around the axon. Successive layers of plasma membrane come into apposition to form the **major** and **minor dense lines** (*Figure 7.4*). (See histology texts for details of myelin ultrastructure.)

Paranodal pockets of cytoplasm persist at the ends of the myelin segments, on each side of the nodes of Ranvier. (Louis Ranvier identified them 80 years before CNS nodes were demonstrated with the electron microscope in the early 1960s.) The paranodal pockets may be responsible for maintaining the dense population (about 10^5) of Na$^+$ channels in the nodal plasma membrane.

Myelin expedites conduction

Along unmyelinated fibers, impulse conduction is *continuous* (uninterrupted). Its maximum speed is 15 m/s (meters per

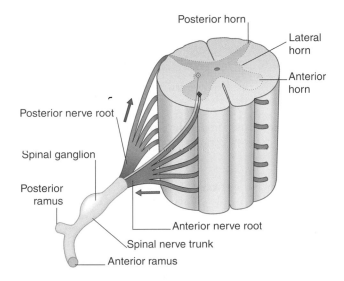

Figure 7.1 Segment of thoracic spinal cord with attached nerve roots. Arrows indicate directions of impulse conduction. *Green* indicates sympathetic outflow.

Posterior horn

Lateral horn

Anterior horn

Posterior nerve root

Spinal ganglion

Posterior ramus

Anterior nerve root

Spinal nerve trunk

Anterior ramus

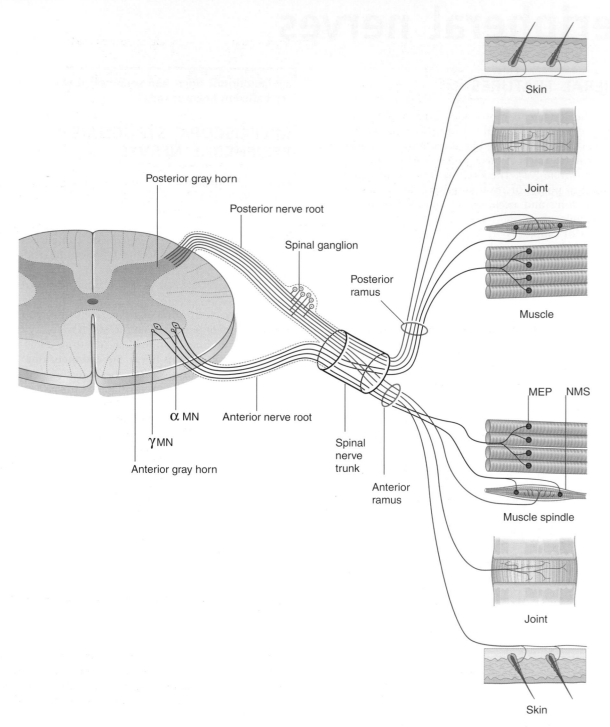

Figure 7.2 Composition and distribution of a cervical spinal nerve. *Note:* The sympathetic component is not shown. MEP, motor end plate; MN, multipolar neurons; NMS, neuromuscular spindle.

second). Along myelinated fibers, excitable membrane is confined to the nodes of Ranvier because myelin is an electrical insulator. Impulse conduction is called *saltatory* ('jumping') because it jumps from node to node. Speed of conduction is much greater along myelinated fibers, with a maximum of 120 m/s. The number of impulses that can be conducted by myelinated fibers is also much greater than by unmyelinated ones.

The larger the myelinated fiber, the more rapid the conduction, because larger fibers have longer internodal segments and the nerve impulses take longer 'strides' between nodes. A 'rule of six' can be used to express the ratio between size and speed: a fiber of 10 μm external diameter will conduct at 60 m/s, one of 15 μm at 90 m/s, and so on.

In physiological recordings, peripheral nerve fibers are classified in accordance with conduction velocities and other criteria. Motor fibers are classified into Groups A, B, and C in descending order. Sensory fibers are classified into Types I–IV. In practice, there is some interchange of usage: e.g.

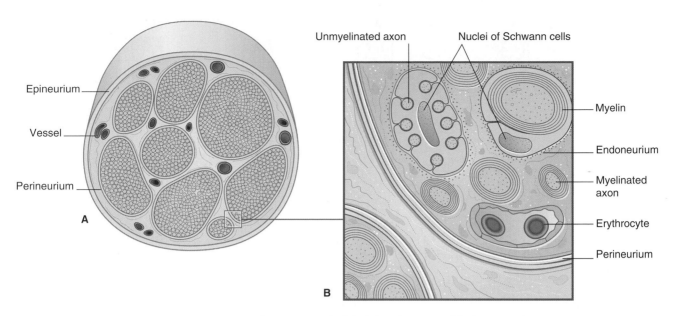

Figure 7.3 Transverse section of a nerve trunk. **(A)** Light microscopy. **(B)** Electron microscopy.

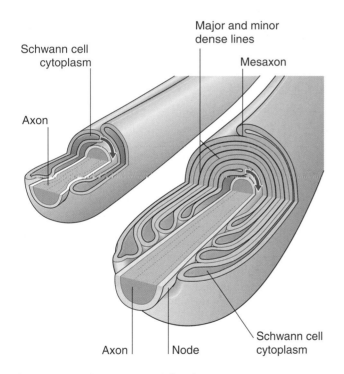

Figure 7.4 Myelination in peripheral nervous system. Arrows indicate movement of flange of Schwann cell cytoplasm.

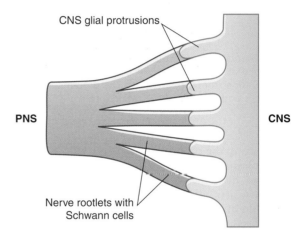

Figure 7.5 Central nervous system–peripheral nervous system transitional zone.

unmyelinated sensory fibers are usually called C fibers rather than Type IV.

Central nervous system–peripheral nervous system transitional region

Close to the brainstem and spinal cord, peripheral nerves enter the *CNS–PNS transitional region* (*Figure 7.5*). Astrocyte processes reach out of the CNS into the endoneurial compartments of peripheral nerve rootlets and interdigitate with the Schwann cells. In unmyelinated fibers, the astrocytes

burrow into the space between axons and Schwann cells. In myelinated fibers, nodes are bounded by Schwann cell myelin (showing some transitional features) on the peripheral side and by oligodendrocytic myelin centrally.

DEGENERATION AND REGENERATION

When nerves are cut or crushed, their axons degenerate distal to the lesion, because axons are pseudopodial outgrowths and depend on their parent cells for survival. In the PNS regeneration is vigorous and it is often complete. In the CNS, on the other hand, it is neither vigorous nor complete.

Wallerian degeneration of peripheral nerves

The principal events in peripheral nerve degeneration are represented in *Figure 7.6* and described in the caption. Following a crush or cut injury to a nerve, the axons and myelin

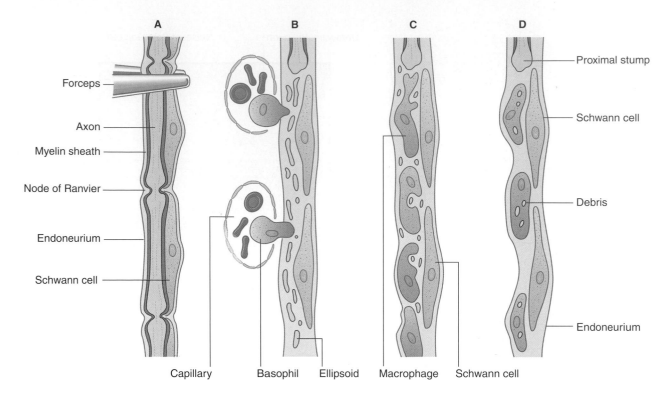

Figure 7.6 Events in degeneration of a single myelinated nerve fiber. **(A)** Intact fiber, showing its four components. The fiber is being pinched at its upper end. **(B)** The myelin and axon have broken up into 'ellipsoids' and droplets. Monocytes are entering the endoneurial tube from the blood. **(C)** The droplets are being engulfed by monocytes. **(D)** Clearance of debris is almost complete. Schwann cells and endoneurium remain intact.

sheaths distal to the cut break up to form 'ellipsoids' during the first 48 hours – mainly because of Ca^{2+} activated release of proteases by Schwann cells. The debris is cleared by monocytes which enter the damaged endoneurial sheaths from the blood and become macrophages. In addition to their phagocytic function, the macrophages are mitogenic to Schwann cells and participate with Schwann cells in provision of trophic (feeding) and tropic (guidance) factors for regenerating axons.

The end result of degeneration is a shrunken nerve skeleton with intact connective tissue and perineurial sheaths, and a core of intact, multiplying Schwann cells.

Regeneration of peripheral nerves

The principal events in regeneration of a peripheral nerve are summarized in *Figure 7.7*. Following a clean cut, axons begin to sprout from the face of the proximal stump within a few hours, but in the more common crush or tear injuries seen clinically, the axons die back for 1 cm or more and sprouting may be delayed for a week. Successful regeneration requires that the axons make contact with Schwann cells of the distal stump. Failure to make contact leads to production of a *neuroma* consisting of whorls of regenerating axons trapped in scar tissue at the site of the initial injury. Following amputation of a limb, an *amputation neuroma* can be a source of severe pain.

Two reparative events are in simultaneous progress within hours of the injury. In the proximal stump, multiple branchlets begin to extend distally, their tips exhibiting swellings called **growth cones**; and in the distal stump, Schwann cells send processes in the direction of the growth cones. The cones are surmounted by antenna-like **filopodia**, and these develop surface receptors which become anchored temporarily to complementary *cell surface adhesion molecules* in Schwann cell basement membranes. Filaments of actin within the filopodia become attached to the surface receptors; from these points of anchorage, they are able to exert onward traction on the growth cones.

Growth cones are mitogenic to Schwann cells, which divide further before wrapping the larger axons with myelin lamellae.

Regeneration proceeds at about 5 mm per day in the larger nerve trunks, slowing down to 2 mm per day in the finer branches. Not surprisingly, the functional outlook is better after a crush injury (endoneurium preserved) than after complete severance. At the same time, filopodia of motor and sensory axons 'recognize' Schwann cell basement membranes previously occupied by axons of similar kind.

When nerve trunks have been completely severed, it is common practice to wait about 3 weeks before attempting repair. By that time, the connective tissue sheaths will have thickened a little and will be better able to hold suture material than freshly injured, edematous sheaths. Moreover, the trimming of the nerves required before insertion of sutures creates a second axotomy, on the axons emerging from the proximal stump. In animal experiments, a second axotomy induces a more vigorous and sustained regenerative response.

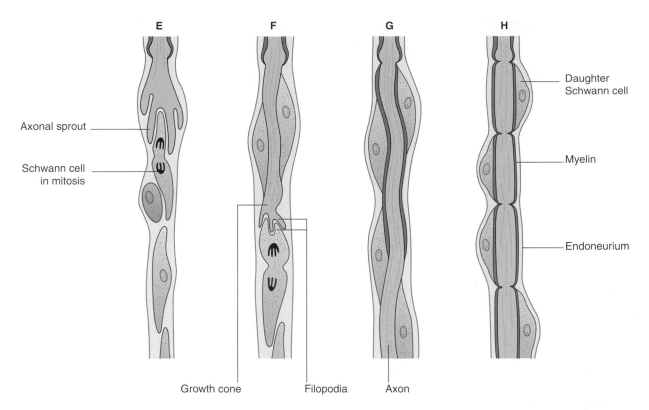

Figure 7.7 Events in regeneration. **(E)** An axonal sprout has entered the distal stump. The sprout is mitogenetic to each Schwann cell it encounters. **(F)** The growth cone is extending distally along the surface of Schwann cells. **(G)** Myelination is commencing along the proximal part of the regenerating axon. **(H)** When regeneration is complete, the fiber has a normal appearance but the myelin segments are shorter than the originals.

Upstream effects of nerve section

- Within a few days of axotomy, Nissl bodies can no longer be identified by cationic dyes in parent cells in the dorsal root ganglia and spinal gray matter (*Figure 7.8*). The phenomenon is known as *chromatolysis* ('loss of color'). Electron microscopy reveals that the granular endoplasmic reticulum is in fact increased in amount. Instead of being in clumps, it is dispersed throughout the perikaryon, with accumulations located deep to the plasma membrane.

- The nucleus becomes eccentric because of osmotic changes in the perikaryon.

- Parent motor neurons become isolated from synaptic contacts in the gray matter by the intrusion of neuroglial cells into all of the synaptic clefts.

- In monkeys, it has been demonstrated that, following transection of sensory nerves, 30–40% of their posterior nerve root terminals undergo Wallerian degeneration. Because their terminals are in central gray matter, they do not regenerate; however, some of their synaptic sites are taken over by *collateral sprouts* given off by healthy neighbors. Overall, this observation may account for the usually incomplete recovery of sensory function in patients.

Degeneration in the central nervous system

Following injury to the white matter, distal degeneration occurs after the manner of peripheral nerves. However, clearance of debris by microglial cells and fresh monocytes is much slower. Debris can still be identified after 6 months in the CNS, whereas in peripheral nerves it is virtually cleared in 6 days.

Chromatolysis is unusual in the CNS. Instead, large-scale necrosis (death) of injured neurons is the rule. Neurons that survive may appear wasted, with permanent isolation from synaptic contacts.

Transneuronal atrophy

CNS neurons have a trophic (sustaining) effect upon one another. If the main input to a group of neurons is destroyed, the group is likely to waste away and die. This is known as *orthograde transneuronal atrophy*. It is comparable to the atrophy that occurs in skeletal muscle when its motor nerve is cut. In some situations, *retrograde transneuronal degeneration* takes place in neurons upstream to those destroyed by a lesion.

End result of central nervous system injury

If the lesion has been small, the neuronal debris is ultimately replaced by a glial scar composed of astrocyte processes. A large lesion may result in cystic cavities walled by scar tissue, containing CSF and hemolyzed blood.

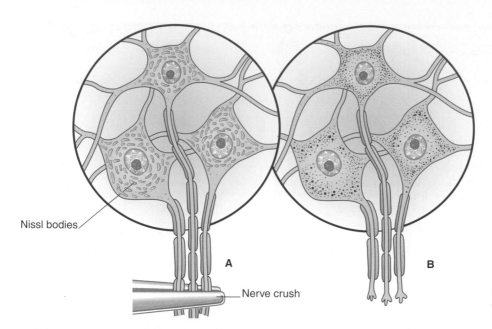

Nissl bodies

A

B

Nerve crush

Figure 7.8 Dispersal of granular endoplasmic reticulum in motor neurons in response to axonal injury.

Clinical Panel 7.1   Peripheral polyneuropathies

The term 'polyneuropathy' refers to a generalized pathology of sensory and motor (and sometimes, autonomic) nerves. Possible causes include chronic vitamin deficiency (especially one or more of the B complex), chronic diabetes, chronic hypothyroidism, and an acute, postviral polyneuropathy called *Guillain–Barré syndrome* which will not be considered here.

In the chronic neuropathies listed, the primary pathology affects the myelin sheaths while axons remain relatively intact. Myelin degeneration occurs initially in the longest and largest sensory fibers, and is expressed clinically as 'glove and stocking' paresthesia (*Figure CP 7.1.1*). The term *paresthesia* refers to sensations of numbness and/or tingling. After several months, motor weakness and wasting may become evident in the muscles of the hands and feet. With further progression, *joint sense* and *vibration* sense may be lost in the hands and feet. (Joint sense refers to the ability to detect passive movement at a joint performed by a clinician; vibration sense refers to the ability to feel the buzz of a tuning fork applied to bone (see Ch. 12).

The most prevalent form of chronic polyneuropathy occurs in late middle age and is of unknown causation; hence the terms *idiopathic* ('private pathology') and *cryptogenic* ('hidden origin') applied to this condition. Biopsy studies have demonstrated that the initial pathology is *axonal*, in the form of a distal-to-proximal *dying back* process. In contrast to demyelinating neuropathies, the leading symptom is *chronic pain* in the feet, sometimes later in the hands also. The pain is attributed to abnormal firing patterns in axons during the breakdown period and is associated with reduced conduction rates and smaller spike amplitudes. At the same time, there is reduced sensitivity to pinprick. Peripheral motor weakness sets in gradually but is seldom debilitating.

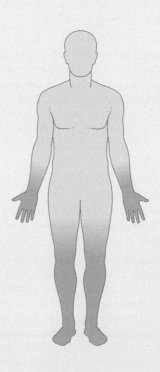

Figure CP 7.1.1 'Glove and stocking' paresthesia.

Core Information

Structure

Spinal nerve trunks occupy intervertebral foramina. They are formed by the union of anterior (motor) and posterior (sensory) nerve roots and they divide into (mixed) anterior and posterior rami. The roots of the limb plexuses are in fact anterior rami. Peripheral nerves have an outer, epineurial connective tissue sheath, a fascicular perineurial sheath, and an endoneurial collagenous sheath investing Schwann cells. A myelinated fiber comprises axon, myelin sheath, Schwann cytoplasm (neurolemma), and endoneurium. Myelin sheaths are derived from chains of Schwann cells; they give rise to saltatory conduction of nerve impulses, at a rate proportionate to fiber diameter.

Degeneration and regeneration

Separation of fibers from parent somas causes axons and myelin sheaths to break down, the debris being removed by phagocytes. Neurolemmal and connective tissue sheaths survive. Axons regenerate by sprouting along vacated neurolemmal sheaths while exhibiting growth cones with filopodia. Motor and sensory end organs may be successfully re-innervated, and fresh myelin sheaths formed. Regeneration in the CNS is very limited, but the use of grafts of embryonic neurons has yielded some encouraging results.

Regeneration in the central nervous system

Remarkable degrees of functional recovery are often observed after CNS lesions. However, injured motor and sensory pathways do not re-establish their original connections. They regenerate for a few millimeters at most, and such synapses as develop are upon other neurons close to the site of injury. Adult CNS neurons (in laboratory animals at least) do have regenerative capacity, as witnessed by their liberal sprouting and invasion of the endoneurial tubes of implanted peripheral nerves. The principal deterrents to spontaneous regeneration following CNS injury are obstruction by developing glial scar tissue, and growth inhibition by oligodendrocyte breakdown products.

One of the most active areas in neurobiological research is the use of embryonic nervous tissue to replace neurons that have been lost owing to injury or disease. The mammalian CNS in general seems to be lacking in *trophic factors* required for successful regeneration.

Trophic factors are also abundant in *embryonic* central neurons because when these are transplanted (with immunological precautions) into adult brain they grow well. This approach is under investigation in animal models of Parkinson's disease, Alzheimer's disease, and spinal cord injury, with limited benefits in all three. In Parkinson's disease, loss of dopaminergic function in the striatum is a key factor in pathogenesis. Implantation of human fetal dopaminergic neurons into the caudate nucleus has led to sufficient improvement sufficient in many cases to warrant reduction in the amount of ongoing drug therapy.

REFERENCES

Berthold, C.H. and Rydmark, M. (1995) Morphology of normal peripheral axons. In *The Axon* (Waxman, S. Kocsis, J.D. and Stys, P.K., eds), pp. 13–48. New York: Oxford University Press.

Bisby, M.A. (1995) Regeneration of peripheral nervous system axons. In *The Axon* (Waxman, S., Kocsis, J.D. and Stys, P.K., eds), pp. 355–374. New York: Oxford University Press.

Boyer, K.L. and Bakay, R.A.E. (1995) The history, theory and present status of brain transplantation. *Neurosurg. Clin. N. Am.* **6**: 113–125.

Gag, F.H. and Fisher, L.J. (1991) Intracerebral grafting: a tool for the neurobiologist. *Neuron* **6**: 1–12.

Fraher, J.P. (1999) The transitional zone and CNS regeneration. *J. Anat.* **194**: 161–182.

Liss, A.G. and Wiberg, M. (1997) Loss of nerve endings in the spinal dorsal horn after a peripheral nerve injury. An anatomical study in *Macaca fascicularis* monkeys. *Eur. J. Neurosci.* **9**: 2187–2192.

Koutouzis, T.K., Emerich, D.F., Bourlongan, C.V., Freeman, T.B., Cahill, D.W. and Sanberg, P.R. (1994) Cell transplantation for central nervous disorders. *Crit. Rev. Neurobiol.* **8**: 125–162.

McQuarry, I.G. (1988) Cytoskeleton of the regenerating axon. In *Current Issues in Neural Regeneration Research*, pp. 23–32. New York: Alan R. Liss.

O'Reilly, P.M.R. and FitzGerald, M.J.T. (1985) Internodal segments in human laryngeal nerves. *J. Anat.* **140**: 645–650.

Stoll, G., Griffin, J.W., Li, C.Y. and Trapp, R.D. (1989) Wallerian degeneration in the peripheral nervous system: participation of both Schwann cells and macrophages in myelin degradation. *J. Neurocytol.* **18**: 671–683.

Terenghi, G. (1999) Peripheral nerve regeneration and neurotrophic factors. *J. Anat.* **194**: 1–14.

Tetzlaff, W., Graeber, M.B. and Kreutzberg, G.W. (1986) Reaction of motoneurons and their microenvironment to axotomy. *Exp. Brain Res. Suppl.* **13**: S3–S8.

Wolfe G.I., Baker, N.S., Amato, A.A., Jackson, C.E., Nations, S.P., Saperstein, D.S., Cha, C.H., Katz, J.S., Bryan, W.W. and Barohn, R.J. (1999) Chronic cryptogenic sensory polyneuropathy. *Arch. Neurol.* **56**: 540–548.

Innervation of muscles and joints

In gross anatomy, the nerves to skeletal muscles are branches of mixed peripheral nerves. The branches enter the muscles about one-third of the way along their length, at *motor points* (*Figure 8.1*). Motor points have been identified for all major muscle groups, for the purpose of *functional electrical stimulation* by physical therapists, in order to increase muscle power.

Only 60% of the axons in the nerve to a given muscle are motor to the muscle fibers that make up the bulk of the muscle. The rest are sensory in nature although the largest sensory receptors – the neuromuscular spindles – have a motor supply of their own.

MOTOR INNERVATION OF SKELETAL MUSCLE

The nerve of supply branches within the muscle belly, forming a plexus from which groups of axons emerge to supply the muscle fibers (*Figure 8.1*). The axons supply single motor end plates placed about half way along the muscle fibers (*Figure 8.2A*).

A *motor unit* comprises a motor neuron in the spinal cord or brainstem together with the *squad* of muscle fibers it innervates. In large muscles (e.g. the flexors of the hip or knee), each motor unit contains 1000 muscle fibers or more. In small muscles (e.g. the intrinsic muscles of the hand), each unit contains 10 muscle fibers or less. Small units contribute to the finely graded contractions used for delicate manipulations.

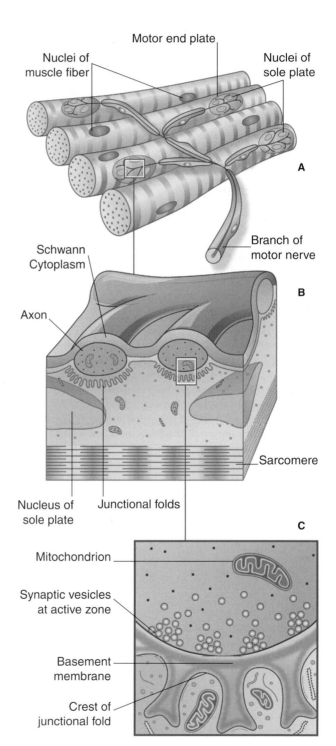

Figure 8.2 Motor nerve supply to skeletal muscle. **(A)** Four motor end plates supplied from a single axon. **(B)** Enlargement from **(A)**. **(C)** Enlargement from **(B)** showing active zones.

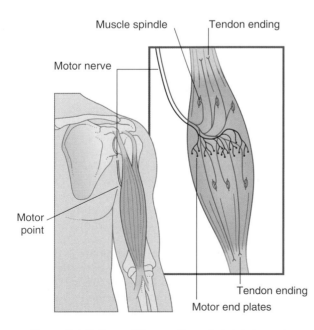

Figure 8.1 Pattern of innervation of skeletal muscle.

There are three different types of skeletal muscle fiber:

1 *Slow-twitch, oxidative (SO) fibers* are small, rich in mitochondria and blood capillaries (hence, they are red). They exert small forces and are fatigue resistant. They are deeply placed and suited to sustained postural activities, including standing.

2 *Fast, glycolytic (FG) fibers* are large, mitochondria poor, and capillary poor (hence, white). They produce brief, powerful contractions. They predominate in superficial muscles.

3 *Intermediate (fast, oxidative-glycolytic, FOG)* fibers have properties intermediate between the other two. Every muscle contains all three kinds of fiber, but a given motor unit contains only one kind. The fibers of each unit interdigitate with those of other units.

Motor end plates

At the **myoneural junction**, the axon forms a handful of branchlets which groove the surface of the muscle fiber (*Figure 8.2B*). The underlying sarcolemma is thrown into **junctional folds**. The basement membrane of the muscle fiber traverses the synaptic cleft and lines the folds. The underlying sacroplasm shows an accumulation of nuclei, mitochondria, and ribosomes known as a sole plate.

Each axonal branchlet forms an elongated terminal bouton, containing thousands of synaptic vesicles loaded with acetylcholine (ACh). Synaptic transmission takes place at **active zones** facing the crests of the junctional folds (*Figure 8.2C*). ACh is extruded by exocytosis into the synaptic cleft. It diffuses through the basement membrane to reach ACh receptors in the sarcolemma. Activation of the receptors leads to depolarization of the sarcolemma. The depolarization is led into the interior of the muscle fiber by T-tubules. The sarcoplasmic reticulum liberates Ca^{2+} ions which initiate contraction of the sarcomeres (see biochemistry texts for details).

Cholinesterase enzyme is concentrated in the basement membrane, and about 30% of released ACh is hydrolyzed

without reaching the postsynaptic membrane. After hydrolysis, the choline moiety is returned to the axoplasm.

Also found within terminal boutons are *dense-cored vesicles* containing one or more peptides (*Figure 8.2C*). Best known is *CGRP (calcitonin-gene-related peptide)* which, upon extrasynaptic release (Ch. 6), is a potent vasodilator.

Motor units in the elderly

The progressive wasting of muscles seen in the elderly is due to loss of motor neurons from the spinal cord and brainstem, and to low-grade peripheral neuropathy arising from vascular disease and often from nutritional deficiency. Electromyographic (EMG) records taken from contracting muscles show *giant motor unit potentials* during the seventh and eighth decades. The extra-large potentials result from takeover of vacated motor end plates of lost motor neurons by collateral sprouts from the axons of adjacent healthy motor units.

The commonest disorder of the myoneural junction is *myasthenia gravis (Clinical Panel 8.1)*.

SENSORY INNERVATION OF SKELETAL MUSCLE

Neuromuscular spindles

Muscle spindles are up to 1 cm in length and vary in number from a dozen to several hundred in different muscles. They are abundant (a) in the antigravity muscles along the vertebral column, femur, and tibia; (b) in the muscles of the neck; and (c) in the intrinsic muscles of the hand. All of these muscles are rich in slow, oxidative muscle fibers. Spindles are scarce where FG or FOG fibers predominate.

Muscle spindles contain up to a dozen **intrafusal muscle fibers** (*Figure 8.3*). (Ordinary muscle fibers are extrafusal in this context.) The larger intrafusal fibers emerge from the **poles** (ends) of the spindle and are anchored to connective tissue (perimysium). The smaller ones are anchored to the

---

Clinical Panel 8.1   Myasthenia gravis

The ACh receptors of skeletal muscle normally undergo turnover with a half-life (i.e. a 50% loss) of 10 days. New receptors are constantly synthesized in Golgi complexes located around the nuclei of the sole plate and inserted into the sarcolemma of the junctional folds. Old receptors are removed by endocytosis and degraded by lysosomes.

In myasthenia gravis, the immune system produces antibodies to the ACh receptor. The antigen–antibody complex has a half-life of only 2 days, leading to a progressive loss of receptors and of junctional folds. Muscles most affected are those supplied by cranial nerves.

Clinically, myasthenia gravis is characterized by

weakness and easy fatigue of the muscles of the orbit, face, and mouth. The limbs are sometimes affected as well. In severe cases, weakness of the muscles of swallowing and respiration may be life-threatening.

Administration of an anticholinesterase drug such as neostigmine can be both diagnostic and therapeutic. By prolonging the binding time of ACh with the remaining receptors, it usually causes prompt improvement in muscle power.

The abnormal antibodies seem to originate in the thymus gland, which is usually hyperplastic in these cases and contains a lymphoid tumor in 10% of patients. Removal of the thymus may be beneficial if symptoms cannot be otherwise controlled.

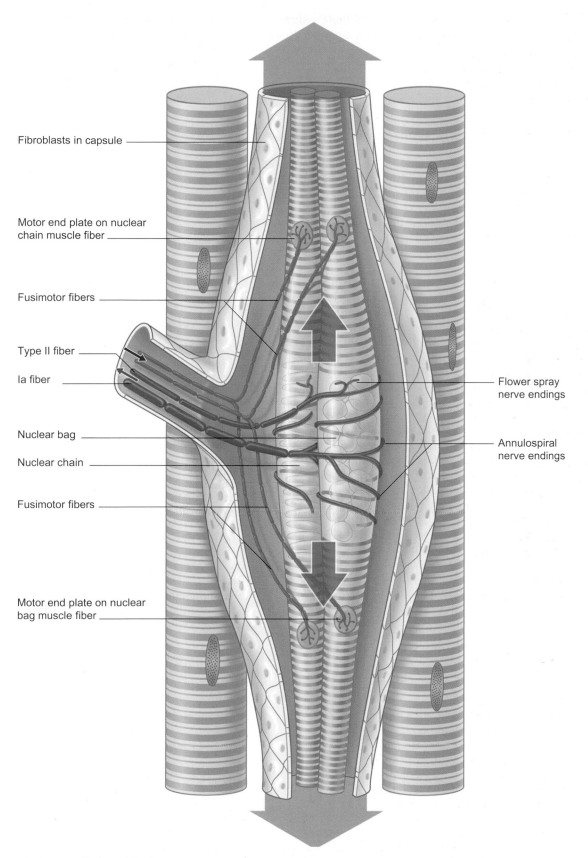

Fibroblasts in capsule

Motor end plate on nuclear chain muscle fiber

Fusimotor fibers

Type II fiber

Ia fiber

Nuclear bag

Nuclear chain

Fusimotor fibers

Motor end plate on nuclear bag muscle fiber

Flower spray nerve endings

Annulospiral nerve endings

Figure 8.3 Neuromuscular spindle (simplified). *Large arrows* indicate passive stretch of the annulospiral endings produced by lengthening of the relaxed muscle as a whole. *Medium arrows* indicate active stretch of annulospiral endings produced by activity of fusimotor nerve fibers. Active stretch more than compensates for the unloading effect of simultaneous extrafusal muscle fiber contraction. *Small arrows* indicate directions of impulse conduction to and from the spindle when the parent muscle is in use.

collagenous spindle capsule. At the spindle **equator** (middle), the sarcomeres are replaced almost entirely by nuclei, in the form of 'bags' (in large fibers) or 'chains' (in small fibers).

Innervation

Spindles have a motor as well as a sensory nerve supply. The motor fibers, called *fusimotor*, are in the Aγ size range, in contrast to the Aα fibers supplying extrafusal muscle. The fusimotor axons divide to supply the striated segments at both ends of the intrafusal muscles (*Figure 8.3*). A single *primary* sensory fiber of Type Ia caliber forms *annulospiral* wrappings around the bag/chain segments of the intrafusal muscle fibers. *Secondary* 'flower spray' sensory endings are found on one or both sides of the primary; they are supplied by Type II fibers.

Activation

Muscle spindles are *stretch receptors*. Ion channels in the surface membrane of the sensory terminals are opened by stretch, creating positive electronic waves which summate close to the final heminode of the parent sensory fiber. Summation produces a *receptor potential* which will fire off nerve impulses when it reaches threshold.

Muscle spindles may be stretched either *passively* or *actively*.

Passive stretch

Passive stretch of muscle spindles occurs when an entire muscle belly is passively lengthened. For example, in eliciting a tendon reflex such as the *knee jerk*, the spindles in the belly of the muscle are passively stretched when the tendon is struck. The Type Ia and Type II fibers discharge to the spinal cord, where they synapse upon the dendrites of α motor neurons (*Figure 8.4*). (α Motor neurons are so called because they give rise to axons of Aα diameter.) The response to the *positive feedback* from spindles is a twitch of contraction in the extrafusal muscle fibers. The spindles, because they lie in parallel with the extrafusal muscle, are passively shortened; they are described as being *unloaded*.

Tendon reflexes are monosynaptic reflexes. They have a *latency* (stimulus–response interval) of about 15–25 msec.

In addition to exciting homonymous motor neurons (i.e. motor neurons supplying the same muscles), the spindle afferents *inhibit* the α motor neurons supplying the antagonist muscles, through the medium of inhibitory internuncial (interposed) neurons (*Figure 8.4*). This effect is called *reciprocal inhibition*. The inhibitory neurons involved are called *Ia internuncials*.

Information coding

Spindle primary afferents are most active *during* the stretching process. The more rapid the stretch, the more impulses they fire off. They therefore encode the *rate of stretch*.

Spindle secondary afferents are more active than the primaries when a given position is held. The greater the degree of *maintained* stretch, the more impulses they fire off. They therefore encode the *degree* of muscle stretch.

Active stretch

Active stretch is produced by the fusimotor neurons, which elicit contraction of the striated segments of the intrafusal

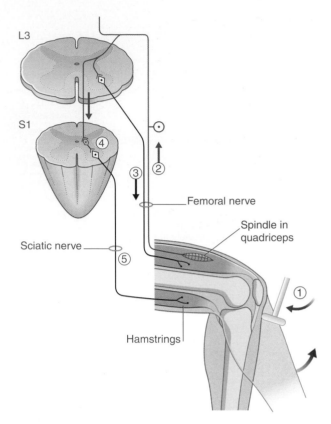

Figure 8.4 Patellar reflex, including reciprocal inhibition. Arrows indicate nerve impulses. **(1)** A tap to the patellar ligament stretches the spindles in quadriceps femoris. **(2)** Spindles discharge excitatory impulses to the spinal cord. **(3)** α Motor neurons respond by eliciting a twitch in quadriceps, with extension of the knee. **(4,5)** Ia inhibitory internuncials respond by suppressing any activity in the hamstrings.

muscle fibers. As the connective tissue attachments are relatively fixed, the intrafusal fibers stretch the spindle equators by pulling them in the direction of the spindle poles. (This could be called a 'Christmas-cracker' effect.)

During voluntary movements, α and γ motor neurons are *coactivated* by the corticospinal (pyramidal) tract. As a result, the spindles are *not* unloaded by extrafusal muscle contraction. Through ascending connections, the spindle afferents on both sides of the relevant joints are able to keep the brain informed about contractions and relaxations during any given movement.

Tendon endings

Golgi tendon organs are found at muscle–tendon junctions (*Figure 8.5*). A single Ib caliber nerve fiber forms elaborate sprays which intertwine with tendon fiber bundles enclosed within a connective tissue capsule.

A dozen or more muscle fibers insert into the intracapsular tendon fibers, which are *in series* with the muscle fibers. The bulbous nerve endings are activated by the tension that develops during muscle contraction. Because the rate of impulse discharge along the parent fiber is related to the applied tension, tendon endings signal the *force* of muscle contraction.

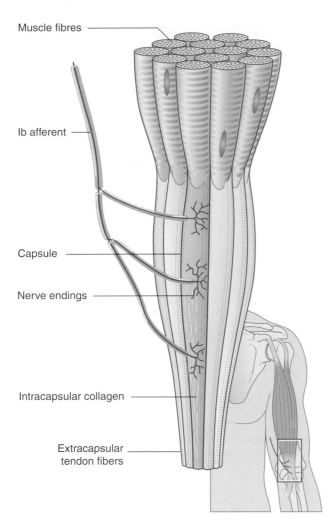

Muscle fibres

Ib afferent

Capsule

Nerve endings

Intracapsular collagen

Extracapsular
tendon fibers

Figure 8.5 Golgi tendon organ.

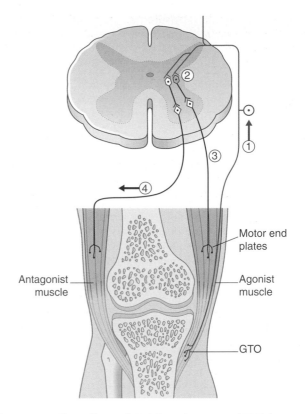

Motor end
plates

Antagonist
muscle

Agonist
muscle

GTO

Figure 8.6 Reflex effects of Golgi tendon organ (GTO) stimulation. **(1)** Agonist contraction excites GTO afferent which **(2)** excites inhibitory internuncial synapsing on **(3)** homonymous motoneuron and excites excitatory internuncial synapsing on **(4)** motoneuron supplying antagonist.

The Ib afferents exert *negative feedback* on to the homonymous motor neurons, in contrast to the positive feedback exerted by muscle spindle afferents. The effect is called *autogenetic inhibition*, and the reflex arc is disynaptic because of the interpolation of an inhibitory neuron (*Figure 8.6*). If need be, there follows *reciprocal excitation* of motor neurons supplying antagonist muscles. An important function of tendon organ afferents is to dampen (restrict) the inherent tendency of moving limb segments to oscillate (sway to and fro). Dampening introduces an element known to physiologists as *joint stiffness*. Paradoxically, when 1b afferents are allowed too much freedom, as in *Parkinson's disease* (Ch. 25), they reinforce the inherent tendency to oscillate, and contribute to the characteristic *resting tremor* which is most obvious in the forearm (pronation–supination) and in the fingers ('pill-rolling' of the thumb pad by adjacent fingers).

Free nerve endings

Muscles are rich in freely ending nerve fibers, distributed to the intramuscular connective tissue and investing fascial envelopes. They are responsible for pain sensation caused by direct injury or by accumulation of metabolites including lactic acid.

INNERVATION OF JOINTS

Freely ending unmyelinated nerve fibers are abundant in joint ligaments and capsules, and in the outer parts of intra-articular menisci. They mediate pain when a joint is strained, and they operate an excitatory reflex to protect the capsule. For example, the anterior wrist capsule is supplied by the median and ulnar nerves; if it is suddenly stretched by forced extension, motor fibers in these nerves are reflexly activated and cause wrist flexion.

Animal experiments have shown that when a joint is inflamed, more freely ending nerve fibers are excited than is the case when a healthy joint capsule is stretched. It seems that some nerve endings are *only* stimulated by inflammation.

Encapsulated nerve endings in and around joint capsules include Ruffini endings which signal tension, lamellated endings responsive to pressure, and Pacinian corpuscles responsive to vibration (see Ch. 9).

Core Information

Muscle

A motor unit comprises a motor neuron and the group of muscle fibers it supplies. Each unit contains only one histochemical type of muscle fiber. At the myoneural synapse, the terminal bouton (containing vesicular ACh quanta) is separated from sarcolemmal junctional folds (containing ACh receptors) by basement membrane containing acetylcholinesterase.

Muscle spindles contain intrafusal muscle fibers supplied at each end by γ fusimotor neurons. Sensory fibers of Type Ia diameter provide primary annulospiral endings at the equator and fibers of Type II diameter provide secondary endings nearby; both kinds are stretch receptors. Stretch may be passive, e.g. by a tendon reflex, or active during fusimotor activity. Homonymous motor neurons are monosynaptically excited; antagonists are reciprocally inhibited via Ia internuncials. Spindle primaries signal the rate of muscle stretch; secondaries signal the degree. During voluntary movements, α and γ motor neurons are coactivated.

Golgi tendon organs signal the force of muscle contraction. They comprise encapsulated tendon tissue innervated by Type 1b diameter afferents, which exert disynaptic inhibition on homonymous motor neurons and reciprocal excitation of antagonists.

Free intramuscular nerve endings subserve pain sensation.

Joints

Free nerve endings abound in ligaments and capsules and in the outer part of menisci. They mediate pain, and operate an articular protective reflex. Encapsulated endings signal joint movement.

REFERENCES

Arvidsson, U., Piehl, F., Johnson, H., Ulfhake, B., Cullheim, S. and Hokfelt, T. (1993) The peptidergic motoneurone. *Neuroreport* **4**: 849–856.

Burke, D. and Gandevia, S.C. (1990) Peripheral motor system. In *The Human Nervous System* (Paxinos, G., ed.), pp. 125–148. San Diego: Academic Press.

McCloskey, D.I. (1994) Human proprioceptive sensation. *J. Clin. Neurosci.* **1**: 173–177.

McCloskey, D.I. and Gandevia, S.C. (1993) Aspects of proprioception. In *Science and Practice in Clinical Neurology* (Gandevia, S.C., Burke, D. and Anthony, M., eds), pp. 3–19. Cambridge: Cambridge University Press.

Salpeter, M.M. (1987) Vertebrate neuromuscular junctions: general morphology, molecular organization, and functional consequences. In *The Vertebrate Neuromuscular Junction* (Salpeter, M.M., ed.), pp. 55–116. New York: Alan R. Liss.

Innervation of skin

From the cutaneous branches of the spinal nerves, innumerable fine twigs enter a **dermal nerve plexus** located in the base of the dermis. Within the plexus, individual nerve fibers divide and overlap extensively with others before terminating at higher levels of the skin. Because of overlap, the area of anesthesia resulting from injury to a cutaneous nerve (e.g. superficial radial, saphenous) is smaller than its anatomical territory.

SENSORY UNITS

A given stem fiber forms the same kind of nerve ending at all of its terminals. In physiological recordings, the stem fiber and its family of endings constitute a *sensory unit*. Together with its parent unipolar nerve cell, the sensory unit is analogous to the motor unit described in Chapter 8.

The territory from which a sensory unit can be excited is its *receptive field*. There is an inverse relationship between the size of receptive fields and sensory acuity, e.g. fields measure about $2\,cm^2$ on the arm, $1\,cm^2$ at the wrist, and $5\,mm^2$ on the finger pads.

Sensory units interdigitate so that different *modalities* of sensation can be perceived from a given patch of skin.

NERVE ENDINGS

Free nerve endings   (Figure 9.1A, B)

As they run toward the skin surface, many sensory fibers shed their perineural sheaths and then their myelin sheaths (if any) before branching further in a subepidermal network. The Schwann cell sheaths open to permit naked axons to terminate between collagen bundles (**dermal nerve endings**) or within the epidermis (**epidermal nerve endings**).

Functions
Some sensory units with free nerve endings are *thermoreceptors*. They supply either 'warm spots' or 'cold spots' scattered over the skin. Two kinds of *nociceptors* (pain transducing) units with free endings are also found. One kind responds to severe mechanical deformation of the skin, e.g. pinching with a forceps. The parent fibers are finely myelinated ($A\delta$). The other kind comprises *polymodal nociceptors*; these are C fiber units able to transduce mechanical deformation, intense heat (some also intense cold), and irritant chemicals.

C fiber units are responsible for the axon reflex (*Clinical Panel 9.1*).

Follicular nerve endings   (Figure 9.1A, D)

Just below the level of the sebaceous glands, myelinated fibers apply a *palisade* of naked terminals along the outer root sheath epithelium of the hair follicles. Outside this is a *circumferential* set of terminals.

Each follicular unit supplies many follicles and there is much territorial overlap. Follicular units are *rapidly adapting*: they fire when the hairs are being bent, but not when the

bent position is held. Rapid adaptation accounts for our being largely unaware of our clothing except when donning or offing.

Merkel cell–neurite complexes   (Figure 9.1A, C)

Expanded nerve terminals are applied to **Merkel cells** (*tactile menisci*) in the basal epithelium of epidermal pegs and ridges. These *Merkel cell–neurite complexes* are *slowly adapting*. They discharge continuously in response to sustained pressure, e.g. while we hold a pen or wear spectacles), and they are markedly sensitive to the *edges* of objects held in the hand.

Encapsulated nerve endings

The *capsules* of the three nerve endings to be described comprise an outer coat of connective tissue, a middle coat of perineural epithelium, and an inner coat of modified Schwann cells (**teloglia**). All three are *mechanoreceptors*, transducing mechanical stimuli.

- **Meissner's corpuscles** are most numerous in the finger pads, where they lie beside the intermediate ridges of the epidermis (*Figure 9.2A–C*). In these ovoid receptors, several axons zigzag among stacks of teloglial lamellae. Meissner's corpuscles are rapidly adapting. Together with the slowly adapting Merkel cell–neurite complexes, they provide the tools for delicate detective work on textured surfaces such as cloth or wood, or on embossed surfaces such as Braille text. Elevations as little as $5\,\mu m$ in height can be detected!

- **Ruffini endings** are found in both hairy and glabrous skin (*Figures 9.1A, 9.2D*). They respond to *drag* (shearing stress) and are slowly adapting. Their structure resembles that of Golgi tendon organs, having a collagenous core in which several axons branch liberally.

- **Pacinian corpuscles** (*Figure 9.2B, E*) are the size of rice grains. They number about 300 in the hand. They are subcutaneous, close to the underlying periosteum, and numerous along the sides of the fingers and in the palm. Inside a thin connective sheath are onion-like layers of perineural epithelium containing some blood capillaries. Innermost are several teloglial lamellae surrounding a single central axon which has shed its myelin sheath at point of entry. Pacinian corpuscles are rapidly adapting and are especially responsive to *vibration* – particularly to bone vibration. In the limbs, many corpuscles are embedded in the periosteum of the long bones.

Pacinian corpuscles discharge one or two impulses when compressed, and again when released. In the hands, they seem to function in group mode: when an object such as an orange is picked up, as many as 100 or more corpuscles are activated momentarily, with a momentary repetition when the object is released. For this reason they have been called 'event detectors' during object manipulation.

The digital receptors are classified as follows by sensory physiologists:

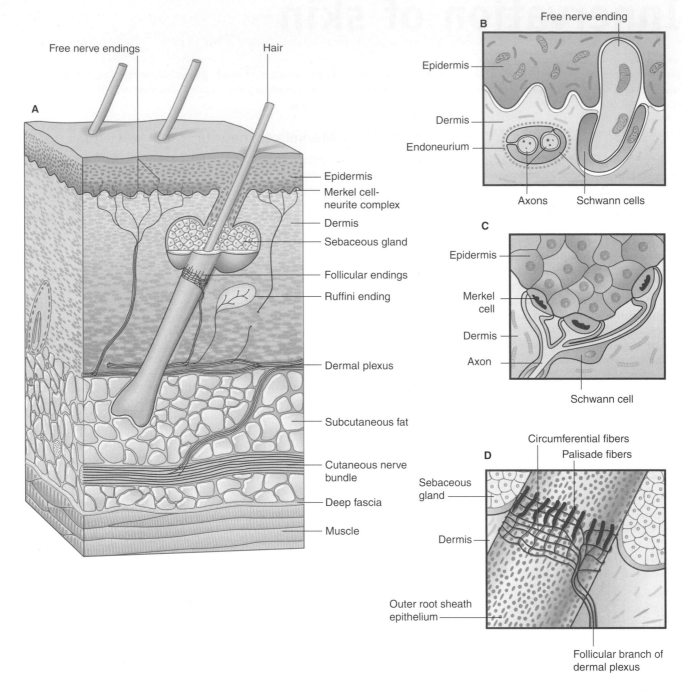

Figure 9.1 Innervation of hairy skin. **(A)** Three morphological types of sensory nerve endings in hairy skin. **(B)** Free nerve ending in the basal layer of the epidermis. **(C)** Merkel cell–neurite complex. **(D)** Palisade and circumferential nerve endings on the surface of the outer root sheath of a hair follicle.

- Merkel cell–neurite complexes = SA I
- Meissner's corpuscles = RA I
- Ruffini endings = SA II
- Pacinian corpuscles = RA II

When three-dimensional objects are being manipulated out of sight, significant contributions to perceptual evaluation are made by muscle afferents (especially from muscle spindles) and articular afferents from joint capsules. The cutaneous, muscular, and articular afferents relay informa-tion independently to the contralateral somatic sensory cortex. The three kinds of information serve the function of *tactile discrimination*. They are integrated (brought together at cellular level) in the posterior part of the contralateral pari-etal lobe, which is specialized for *spatial sense*, both tactile and visual. Spatial tactile sense is called *stereognosis*. In the clinic, stereognosis is tested by asking the patient to identify an object such as a key without looking at it.

Clinical Panel 9.2 gives a short account of *peripheral neuropathies*, with special reference to leprosy.

Clinical Panel 9.1   Neurogenic inflammation: the axon reflex

When sensitive skin is stroked with a sharp object, a red line appears in seconds owing to capillary dilatation in direct response to the injury. A few minutes later, a red *flare* spreads into the surrounding skin, owing to arteriolar dilatation, followed by a white *wheal* owing to exudation of plasma from the capillaries. These phenomena constitute the *triple response*. The wheal and flare responses are produced by *axon reflexes* in the local sensory cutaneous nerves. The sequence of events follows the numbers in Figure CP 9.1.1.

1 The noxious stimulus is transduced (converted to nerve impulses) by polymodal nociceptors.

2 As well as transmitting impulses to the CNS in the normal, orthodromic direction, the axons send impulses in an *antidromic* direction from points of bifurcation into the neighboring skin. The nociceptive endings respond to antidromic stimulation by releasing one or more peptide substances, notably substance P.

3 Substance P binds with receptors on the walls of arterioles, leading to arteriolar dilatation – the flare response.

4 Substance P also binds with receptors on the surface of mast cells, stimulating them to release *histamine*. The histamine increases capillary permeability and leads to local accumulation of tissue fluid – the wheal response.

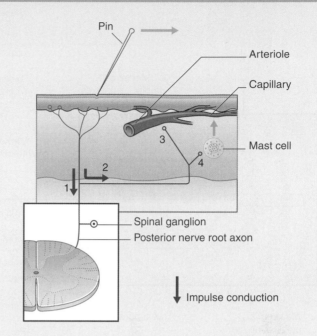

Figure CP 9.1.1 The axon reflex. For the numbers, see text.

Clinical Panel 9.2   Leprosy

The leprosy bacillus enters the skin through minor abrasions. It travels proximally within the perineurium of the cutaneous nerves and kills off the Schwann cells. Loss of myelin segments ('segmental demyelination') blocks impulse conduction in the larger nerve fibers. Later, the inflammatory response to the bacillus compresses all of the axons, leading to Wallerian degeneration of entire nerves and gross thickening of the connective tissue sheaths. Patches of anesthetic skin develop on the fingers, toes, nose, and ears. The protective function of skin sensation is lost and the affected parts suffer injury and loss of tissue. Motor paralyses occur later on, as a consequence of invasion of mixed nerve trunks proximal to the points of origin of their cutaneous branches.

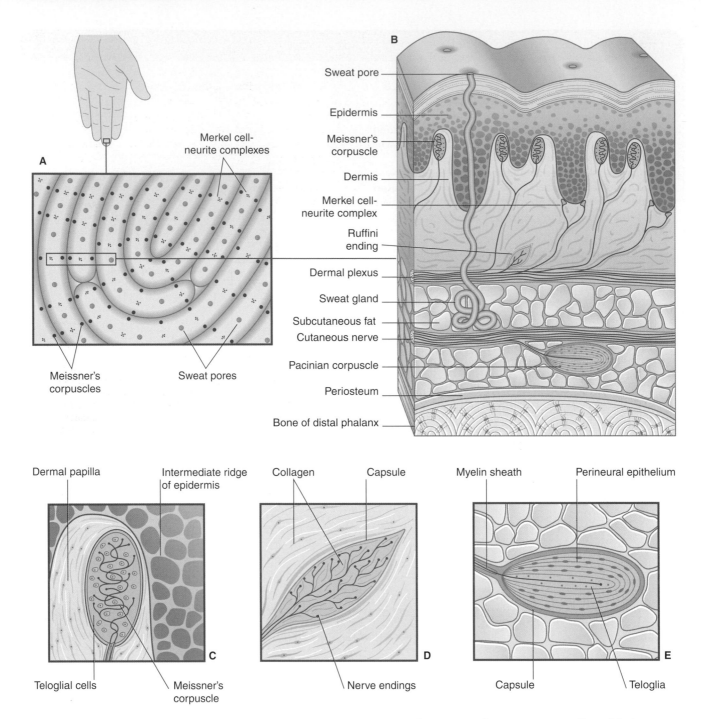

Figure 9.2 Innervation of glabrous skin. **(A)** Finger pad, showing distribution of two types of sensory nerve endings. **(B)** Tissue block from **A** showing positions of four types of sensory nerve endings. **(C)** Meissner's corpuscle. **(D)** Nerve ending of Ruffini. **(E)** Pacinian corpuscle.

Core Information

Cutaneous nerves branch to form a dermal nerve plexus where individual afferent fibers branch and overlap. Each stem fiber and its terminal receptors constitute a sensory unit. The territory of a stem fiber is its receptive field.

Sensory units with free nerve endings include thermoreceptors and both mechanical and thermal nociceptors. Follicular units are rapidly adapting touch receptors, active only when hairs are in motion. Merkel cell–neurite complexes are slowly adapting edge detectors.

The encapsulated endings are mechanoreceptors. Meissner's corpuscles lie beside intermediate ridges in glabrous skin and are rapidly adapting. Ruffini endings lie near hair follicles and fingernails; they are slowly adapting drag receptors. Pacinian corpuscles are subcutaneous, rapidly adapting event detectors and vibration receptors.

Coded information from skin, muscles, and joints is integrated at the level of the posterior parietal lobe of the brain, yielding the faculties of tactile discrimination and stereognosis.

REFERENCES

Cunningham, F.O. and FitzGerald, M.J.T. (1972) Encapsulated nerve endings in hairy skin. *J. Anat.* **112**: 93–97.

Foreman, J.C. (1987) Peptides and neurogenic inflammation. *Br. Med. Bull.* **43**: 386–400.

Iggo, A. (1985) Sensory receptors in the skin of mammals and their sensory functions. *Rev. Neurol.* **141**: 599–615.

James, L.A. (1994) Peripheral mechanisms for touch and proprioception. *Can. J. Physiol. Pharm.* **72**: 484–487.

Johansson, R.S. (1991) How is grasping modified by somatosensory input? In *Motor Control: Concepts and Issues* (Humphrey, D.R. and Freund, H-J., eds), pp. 331–355.

Mitsumoto, H. and Wilburn, A.J. (1994) Causes and diagnosis of sensory neuropathies: a review. *J. Clin. Neurophysiol.* **11**: 553–567.

Stark, B., Carlstedt, T., Hallin, R.G. (1998) Distribution of Pacinian corpuscles in the hand. *J. Hand Surg. (Br)* **23**: 370–372.

Torebjork, A.B., Vallbo, A.B. and Ochoa, J.L. (1987) Intraneural microstimulation in man: its relation to specificity of tactile sensations. *Brain* **110**: 1509–1529.

Autonomic nervous system and visceral afferents

COMPONENTS OF THE AUTONOMIC NERVOUS SYSTEM

The autonomic ('self-regulating') nervous system is distributed to the peripheral tissues and organs by way of outlying autonomic ganglia. Controlling centers in the hypothalamus and brainstem send central autonomic fibers to synapse upon preganglionic neurons located in the gray matter of the brainstem and spinal cord. From these neurons, *preganglionic fibers* (mostly myelinated) project out of the CNS to synapse upon multipolar neurons in the autonomic ganglia. Unmyelinated *postganglionic fibers* emerge and form terminal networks in the target tissues.

Both anatomically and functionally, the autonomic system is composed of sympathetic and parasympathetic divisions.

SYMPATHETIC NERVOUS SYSTEM

The sympathetic system is so called because it acts in sympathy with the emotions. In association with rage or fear, the sympathetic system prepares the body for 'fight or flight': the heart rate is increased, the pupils dilate, and the skin sweats. Blood is diverted from the skin and intestinal tract to the skeletal muscles, and the sphincters of the alimentary and urinary tracts are closed.

The sympathetic outflow from the nervous system is *thoracolumbar*, the preganglionic neurons being located in the lateral gray horn of the spinal cord at thoracic and upper two (or three) lumbar segmental levels. From these neurons, preganglionic fibers emerge in the corresponding anterior nerve roots and enter the paravertebral sympathetic chain. The fibers do one of four things (*Figure 10.1*):

1 Some fibers synapse in the nearest ganglion. Postganglionic fibers enter spinal nerves T1–L2 and supply blood vessels and sweat glands in the territory of these nerves.

2 Some fibers *ascend* the sympathetic chain and synapse in the superior or middle cervical ganglion, or in the stellate ganglion. (The stellate consists of the fused inferior cervical and first thoracic ganglia; it lies in front of the neck of the first rib.) Postganglionic fibers supply the head, neck, and upper limbs; also the heart. Of particular importance is the supply to the dilator muscle of the pupil (*Clinical Panel 10.1*).

3 Some fibers *descend* to synapse in lumbar or sacral ganglia of the sympathetic chain. Postganglionic fibers enter the lumbosacral plexus for distribution to the blood vessels and skin of the lower limbs.

4 Some fibers *traverse* the chain and emerge as the (preganglionic) thoracic and lumbar splanchnic nerves. The thoracic splanchnic nerves (usually called, simply, the splanchnic nerves) pass through the lower eight thoracic ganglia, pierce the diaphragm, and synapse within the abdomen in the celiac and mesenteric prevertebral ganglia, and in renal ganglia. Postganglionic fibers accompany branches of the aorta to reach the gastrointestinal tract, liver, pancreas, and kidneys. Lumbar splanchnic nerves pass through the upper three lumbar ganglia and meet in front of the bifurcation of the abdominal aorta. They enter the pelvis as the hypogastric nerves before ending in pelvic ganglia, from which the genitourinary tract is supplied.

The medulla of the adrenal gland is the homolog of a sympathetic ganglion, being derived from the neural crest. It receives a direct input from fibers of the thoracic splanchnic nerve of its own side (see later).

The sympathetic system exerts tonic (continuous) constrictor activity on blood vessels in the limbs. In order to improve the blood flow to the hands or feet, impulse traffic along the sympathetic system can be interrupted surgically (*Clinical Panel 10.1*).

PARASYMPATHETIC NERVOUS SYSTEM

The parasympathetic system generally has the effect of counterbalancing the sympathetic system. It adapts the eyes for close-up viewing, slows the heart, promotes secretion of salivary and intestinal juices, and accelerates intestinal peristalsis. A notable instance of *concerted* sympathetic and parasympathetic activity occurs during sexual intercourse (*Box 10.4*).

The parasympathetic outflow from the CNS is *craniosacral* (*Figure 10.2*). Preganglionic fibers emerge from the brainstem in four cranial nerves – the oculomotor, facial, glossopharyngeal, and vagus – and from sacral segments of the spinal cord.

Cranial parasympathetic system

Preganglionic parasympathetic fibers emerge in four cranial nerves (*Figure 10.3*):

1 In the oculomotor nerve, to synapse in the **ciliary ganglion**. Postganglionic fibers innervate the sphincter of the pupil and the ciliary muscle. Both muscles act to produce the *accommodation reflex*.

2 In the facial nerve, to synapse in the **pterygopalatine** ganglion, which innervates the lacrimal and nasal

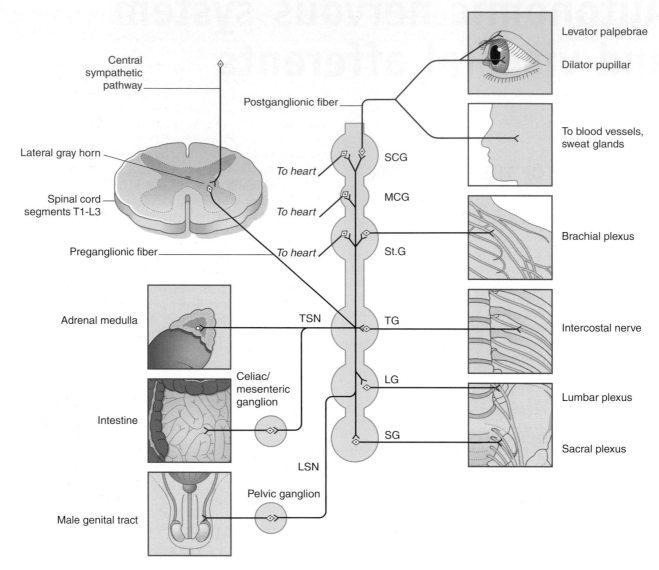

Figure 10.1 General plan of the sympathetic system. Ganglionic neurons and postganglionic fibers are shown in red. LG, lumbar ganglia; LSN, lumbar splanchnic nerve; MCG, middle cervical ganglion; SCG, superior cervical ganglion; SG, sacral ganglia; St.G, stellate ganglion; TG, thoracic ganglia; TSN, thoracic splanchnic nerve.

glands; and in the **submandibular ganglion**, which innervates the submandibular and sublingual glands.

3 In the glossopharyngeal nerve, to synapse in the **otic ganglion**, which innervates the parotid gland.

4 In the vagus nerve, to synapse in **mural** ('on the wall') or **intramural** ('in the wall') ganglia of heart, lungs, lower esophagus, stomach, pancreas, gall bladder, small intestine, and ascending and transverse parts of the colon.

Sacral parasympathetic system

The sacral segments of the spinal cord occupy the conus medullaris (conus terminalis) at the lower extremity of the spinal cord, behind the body of the first lumbar vertebra. From the lateral gray matter of segments S2, S3 and S4, preganglionic fibers descend in the cauda equina within ventral nerve roots. Upon emerging from the pelvic sacral foramina,

the fibers separate out as the pelvic splanchnic nerves. Some fibers of the left and right pelvic splanchnic nerves synapse on ganglion cells in the wall of the distal colon and rectum. The rest synapse in **pelvic ganglia**, close to the pelvic *sympathetic* ganglia already mentioned. Postganglionic parasympathetic fibers supply the detrusor muscle of the bladder; also the tunica media of the internal pudendal artery and of its branches to the cavernous tissue of the penis/clitoris (see later).

NEUROTRANSMISSION IN THE AUTONOMIC SYSTEM

Ganglionic transmission

The preganglionic neurons of the sympathetic and parasympathetic systems are *cholinergic*: the neurons liberate ACh on to the ganglion cells at axodendritic synapses (*Figure 10.4*).

Stellate block

Injection of local anesthetic around the stellate ganglion – *stellate block* – is a procedure used in order to test the effects of sympathetic interruption on blood flow to the hand. Both pre- and postganglionic fibers are inactivated, producing sympathetic paralysis in the head and neck on that side, as well as in the upper limb. A successful stellate block is demonstrated by (a) a warm, dry hand, (b) *Horner's syndrome*, which consists of a constricted pupil owing to unopposed action of the pupillary constrictor, and (c) *ptosis* (drooping) of the upper eyelid owing to paralysis of smooth muscle fibers contained in the levator muscle of the upper eyelid (*Figure CP 10.1.1*).

Dominance of the right stellate ganglion in control of the heart rate is shown by the marked slowing of the pulse following a right, but not a left, stellate block. (*See also Box 10.1.*)

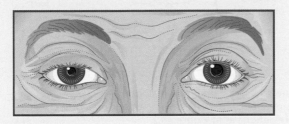

Figure CP 10.1.1 Horner's syndrome, patient's right side. Note the moderate ptosis of the eyelid, and the moderate miosis (pupillary constriction). The affected pupil reacts to light but recovers very slowly.

Functional sympathectomy of the upper limb may be carried out by cutting the sympathetic chain below the stellate ganglion. This is not an anatomical sympathectomy because the ganglionic supply to the limb from the middle cervical and stellate ganglia remains intact. It is a functional one because the ganglionic neurons for the limb are deprived of tonic sympathetic drive. Horner's syndrome is avoided by making the cut at the level of the second rib: the preganglionic fibers for the head and neck enter the stellate direct from the first thoracic spinal nerve.

Two indications for interruption of the sympathetic supply to one or both upper limbs are painful blanching of the fingers in cold weather (*Raynaud phenomenon*), and *hyperhidrosis* (excessive sweating) of the hands – usually an embarrassing affliction of teenage girls.

The sympathetic supply to the eye is considered further in Chapter 18.

Lumbar sympathectomy

In order to improve blood flow in the lower limb, the preganglionic nerve supply may be interrupted by cutting the upper end of the lumbar sympathetic chain. The usual procedure is to remove the second and third lumbar sympathetic ganglia. In males, bilateral lumbar sympathectomy may result in persistent, painful erections (*priapism*) because of interruption of a pathway that maintains the resting, flaccid state of the penis.

The receptors on the ganglion cells are nicotinic, so named because the excitatory effect can be imitated by locally applied nicotine.

Junctional transmission

Postganglionic fibers of the sympathetic and parasympathetic systems form *neuroeffector junctions* with target tissues (*Figure 10.4*). Transmitter substances are liberated from innumerable varicosities strung along the course of the nerve fibers.

The chief transmitter at sympathetic neuroeffector junctions is *norepinephrine* (*noradrenaline*), which is liberated from dense-cored vesicles. The postganglionic sympathetic system in general is described as *adrenergic*. An exception to the adrenergic rule is the *cholinergic* sympathetic supply to the eccrine sweat glands over the body surface.

The chief transmitter at parasympathetic neuroeffector junctions is ACh. The postganglionic parasympathetic system in general is *cholinergic*.

Junctional receptors

The physiological effects of autonomic stimulation depend upon the nature of the *postjunctional receptors* inserted by

target cells into their own plasma membranes. In addition, transmitter release is influenced by *prejunctional receptors* in the axolemmal membrane of the nerve terminals.

Sympathetic junctional receptors (adrenoceptors) (Figure 10.5)

Two kinds of α adrenoceptor and two kinds of β adrenoceptor have been identified for norepinephrine:

1 *Postjunctional α_1 adrenoceptors* initiate contraction of smooth muscle in: peripheral small arteries and large arterioles; the dilator pupillae; the sphincters of the alimentary tract and bladder neck; and the vas deferens.

2 *Prejunctional α_2 adrenoceptors* are present on parasympathetic as well as on sympathetic terminals. They inhibit transmitter release in both cases. On sympathetic terminals, they are called *autoreceptors*.

3 *Postjunctional β_1 adrenoceptors* increase pacemaker activity in the heart and increase the force of ventricular contraction (*Box 10.1*). In response to a severe fall of blood pressure, sympathetic activation of β_1 receptors on the juxtaglomerular cells of the kidney causes secretion

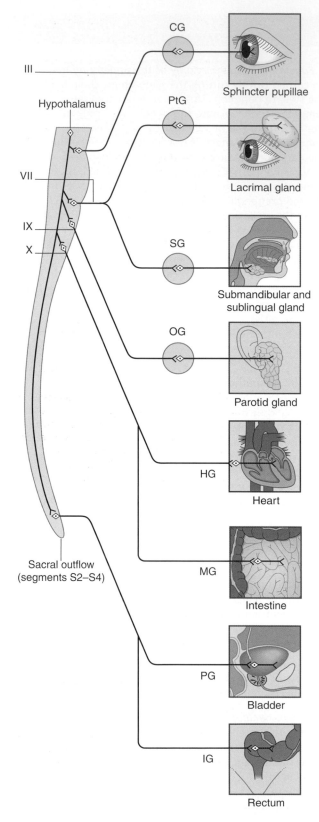

Figure 10.2 General plan of the parasympathetic system. Ganglionic neurons and postganglionic fibers are shown in red. CG, ciliary ganglion; HG, heart ganglia; IG, intramural ganglia; MG, myenteric ganglia; OG, otic ganglion; PtG, pterygopalatine ganglion; SG, submandibular ganglion.

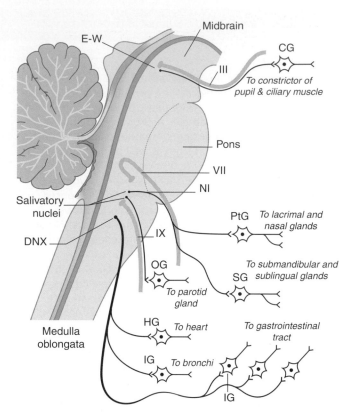

Figure 10.3 Cranial parasympathetic system. E–W, Edinger–Westphal nucleus; DNX, dorsal nucleus of vagus. Other abbreviations as in Figure 10.2.

of renin. Renin initiates production of the powerful vasoconstrictor, angiotensin II.

4 *β₂ receptors* respond to circulating epinephrine (adrenaline) (*Figure 10.6*) in addition to locally released norepinephrine.

Postjunctional β₂ receptors relax smooth muscle, notably in the tracheobronchial tree and in the accommodatory muscles of the eye. Some postjunctional β₂ receptors are on the surface of hepatocytes in the liver, where they initiate glycogen breakdown to provide glucose for immediate energy needs.

Prejunctional β₂ receptors on adrenergic terminals promote release of norepinephrine.

Most of the norepinephrine liberated at sympathetic terminals is retrieved by an *amine uptake pump*. Some is degraded after uptake, by a mitochondrial enzyme, *monoamine oxidase*.

The effects of drugs on the sympathetic system are considered in *Clinical Panel 10.2*.

Parasympathetic junctional receptors

Parasympathetic junctional receptors are called *muscarinic* because they can be mimicked by application of the drug muscarine (*Figure 10.7*). Parasympathetic stimulation produces the following muscarinic effects:

- slowing of the heart in response to vagal stimulation, and diminished force of ventricular contraction (*Box 10.1*)

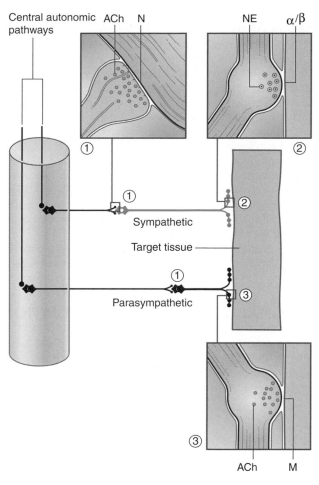

Central autonomic pathways | ACh | N

NE | α/β

① Sympathetic

Target tissue

Parasympathetic

② ③

ACh | M

Figure 10.4 Autonomic transmitters and receptors. Ganglionic neurons and postganglionic fibers are shown in red. ACh, acetylcholine; M, muscarinic receptors; N, nicotinic receptors; NE, norepinephrine.

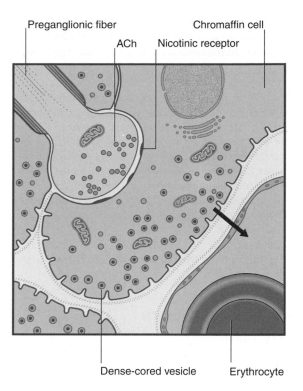

Preganglionic fiber | Chromaffin cell
ACh | Nicotinic receptor

Dense-cored vesicle | Erythrocyte

Figure 10.6 Chromaffin cell of the adrenal medulla receiving a synaptic contact from a preganglionic fiber of the thoracic splanchnic nerve. Acetylcholine (ACh) activates nicotinic receptors. 80% of the cells contain large dense-cored vesicles (represented here) and secrete epinephrine; the arrow indicates release into the capillary bed. 20% contain small dense-cored vesicles and secrete norepinephrine.

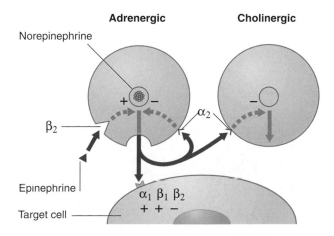

Adrenergic | Cholinergic

Norepinephrine

β_2

α_2

Epinephrine

Target cell

α_1 β_1 β_2
+ + −

Figure 10.5 Adrenergic activity at a neuroeffector junction. Release of norepinephrine is promoted by epinephrine and inhibited by prejunctional α_2 receptors, which also inhibit transmitter release from neighboring parasympathetic varicosities.

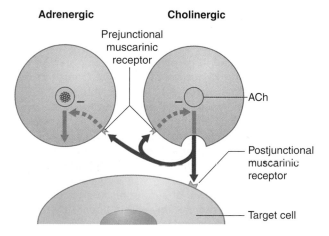

Adrenergic | Cholinergic

Prejunctional muscarinic receptor

ACh

Postjunctional muscarinic receptor

Target cell

Figure 10.7 Cholinergic activity at a neuroeffector junction. Release of excess acetylcholine (ACh) is inhibited by prejunctional muscarinic receptors, which also inhibit transmitter release from neighboring sympathetic varicosities.

- contraction of smooth muscle, with the following effects: intestinal peristalsis (*Box 10.2*), bladder emptying, accommodation of the eye for 'near vision'
- glandular secretion.

In addition to the above postjunctional effects, prejunctional muscarinic receptors located on sympathetic varicosities inhibit release of norepinephrine (*Figure 10.6*).

The effects of *drugs* on the parasympathetic system are considered in *Clinical Panel 10.3*. Drugs having muscarinic effects are described as *cholinergic*. Drugs that prevent access of ACh to junctional receptors are *anticholinergic*.

A major consideration in the use of drugs either to imitate or to suppress sympathetic or parasympathetic activity is the existence of α, β, and muscarinic receptors in the *central* nervous system. In psychiatric practice, in particular, drugs are often chosen for their action at their central rather than peripheral receptors.

Other types of neurons

Non-adrenergic, non-cholinergic (*NANC*) neurons are found in both divisions of the autonomic system. In sympathetic ganglia, small internuncial neurons liberate *dopamine* – a precursor of norepinephrine. Some of the dopamine is secreted into capillaries, the rest binds with dopamine receptors on the main (adrenergic) neurons and exerts a mild inhibitory effect.

NANC neurons are especially numerous among the ganglion cells in the wall of the alimentary tract, and in the pelvic ganglia. More than 50 different *peptide* substances have been identified, either singly or in various combinations, in these neurons. For the most part, they act as *modulators*, acting either pre- or postjunctionally to influence the duration of action of classic transmitters. Some are *cotransmitters*, i.e. released together with ACh.

Vasoactive intestinal polypeptide (VIP) is a cotransmitter in the cholinergic supply to the salivary glands and to sweat glands. VIP is a powerful vasodilator and conveniently opens the local vascular bed (through specific VIP receptors on arterioles) just when the muscarinic ACh receptors are raising glandular metabolism.

Nitric oxide is well established as a transmitter in the parasympathetic system. It is a powerful smooth muscle relaxant.

REGIONAL AUTONOMIC INNERVATION

Box 10.1 describes the autonomic innervation of the heart, *Box 10.2*, the enteric nervous system, *Box 10.3*, lower level bladder controls, and *Box 10.4* and related text, the functional innervation of the genital tract.

Box 10.1 Innervation of the heart

The preganglionic sympathetic supply to the heart arises from the lateral gray horn of cord segments T1–5. The fibers synapse in all three cervical and in the upmost five thoracic ganglia of the sympathetic chain. Postganglionic adrenergic fibers are distributed to the specialized myocardial cells of nodal and conducting tissues, to the general myocardium (of the left ventricle in particular), and to the coronary arteries.

The preganglionic parasympathetic supply arises in the dorsal (motor) nucleus of the vagus (some of these vagal somas may occupy the nucleus ambiguus). The fibers synapse within mural ganglia on the posterior walls of the atria and in the atrioventricular groove (*Figure Box 10.1.1*). Postganglionic cholinergic fibers supply the same tissues as those of the sympathetic although the direct supply to ventricles and coronary arteries is slight.

There is a high level of autonomic interaction where innervation is dense, notably within nodal tissue. Sympathetic nerve endings inhibit parasympathetics in two ways. In the mode depicted in *Figure 10.5*, many also release *neuropeptide Y* which binds to a different specific receptor, with adjuvant inhibitory effect on ACh release.

Many parasympathetic endings, in addition to the effect shown in *Figure 10.6*, co-release VIP which

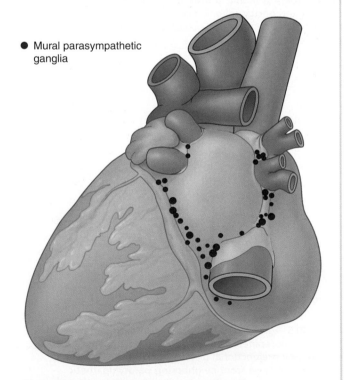

● Mural parasympathetic ganglia

Figure Box 10.1.1 Disposition of mural cardiac parasympathetic ganglia.

Box 10.1 *Continued*

attenuates release of ACh by binding with VIP-specific inhibitory autoreceptors on the endings that release it.

An abundance of NANC neurons modulates the activity of parasympathetic ganglion cells. Also found are scattered adrenergic neurons whose preganglionic supply traverses the sympathetic chain, and bipolar local circuit neurons. Autoregulation of myocardial performance by the intramural ganglionic networks of the normal heart is sufficient to withstand the total extrinsic denervation involved in a cardiac transplant.

A fourth set of neurons is afferent in nature. Unipolar somas in the inferior ganglion of the vagus provide stretch-sensitive nerve endings close to the endocardium – notably in the right atrium where distension produces reflex slowing of the heart rate by way of a central pathway to the dorsal vagal nucleus via the solitary nucleus (Ch. 21). A different set of unipolar somas, in spinal dorsal root ganglia, sends peripheral processes to form chemosensitive nerve endings in the myocardium. Metabolites released by ischemic myocardial cells in response to coronary artery occlusion generate impulse trains which travel along the central processes of these cells to reach the posterior gray horn via *anterior* nerve roots. The central processes synapse upon projection cells of the lateral spinothalamic tract, with consequent perception of referred pain (see main text). A prominent transmitter in the nociceptive neurons is substance P which is released at *both ends simultaneously*: in the gray matter, this peptide is excitatory to spinothalamic projection cells, and in the ischemic tissue it activates specific excitatory receptors on cholinergic endings, thus decelerating the heart.

The cardiac pacemaker (sinuatrial node) is on the right side of the body and mainly innervated by the two right-sided sets of autonomic neurons. The atrioventricular node is on the left side and receives a corresponding preponderance.

The pacemaker tissue of the sinuatrial node is highly responsive to emotional states having their seat of origin in the right, 'emotional' hemisphere (Ch. 29).

The descending pathways concerned are largely ipsilateral and polysynaptic, prior to reaching the lower autonomic nervous system centers of medulla and cord. *Sympathetic* overactivity, in response to 'approach' emotions of sexual or combative nature, may cause the heart to 'miss a beat' (extrasystole) or the 'pulse to race' (tachycardia). *Parasympathetic* overactivity, in response to 'withdraw' (aversive) emotions, usually of olfactory or visual origin, may cause bradycardia – or even cardiac arrest.

The atrioventricular node and Purkinje fibers concordantly increase or reduce the speed of transference of action potentials to the ventricles.

Ventricular contractility, and *synchrony* throughout the ventricular myocardium, are increased by raised sympathetic activity. Both are diminished by the parasympathetic, in this case mainly by autonomic interaction: the scarce cholinergic fibers terminate mainly 'on top' of adrenergic ones without any direct influence on the myocardium.

The coronary arterial tree possesses a considerable degree of autoregulation based on release of myocardial cellular metabolites. However, adrenoceptors are also important. The arterioles ($< 100\mu$ in diameter) are rich in β_2 receptors responsive to neural norepinephrine at the commencement of exercise, and to circulating epinephrine when exercise gets under way. The arteries ($>100\mu$) contain α_1 receptors exerting a restraining effect, directing blood to the *subendocardial* ventricular myocardium, which is vulnerable on two counts: it is the most distal coronary territory; and it is the most compressed myocardial component during systole, receiving blood only during diastole.

Cholinergic coronary nerve endings are scarce, but they have a significant dilator effect on the main arteries – precisely those most at risk of atherosclerosis! It transpires that released ACh acts *indirectly*, by causing release of the potent dilator, nitric oxide, from the vascular endothelium. Progressive devitalization of the endothelium by underlying atherosclerotic plaques leads to more or less complete failure of beneficial nitric oxide production.

Box 10.2 Enteric nervous system

The enteric nervous system (ENS) extends from the midregion of the esophagus all the way to the anal canal. Throughout the length of this tube, it controls peristaltic activity, glandular secretion, and water and ion transfer. In addition, the ENS supplies the pancreas, liver, and gall bladder. The number of intrinsic neurons in the wall of the gastrointestinal tract has been reckoned about the same as in the entire spinal cord. The ENS is sometimes referred to as the 'gut brain' on account of its size and relative functional independence.

The intrinsic neurons of the gut are mainly deployed in two intramural plexuses, namely the **myenteric plexus** (*of Auerbach*) between the longitudinal and circular layers of smooth muscle, and the smaller **submucous plexus** (*of Meissner*). The principal 'drivers' of the muscle and glands belong to the parasympathetic division of the autonomic system. The dorsal (motor) nucleus of the vagus provides the *preganglionic parasympathetic* supply (1) to all parts with the exception of the distal colon and rectum, which receive their preganglionic supply from the *pelvic splanchnic nerves* (having parent neurons in the intermediolateral cell column of cord segments S2–S4). The 'drivers' throughout are *intramural ganglion cells* located in both intramural plexuses. The beaded postganglionic fibers of the myenteric plexus (2) initiate peristaltic waves by simultaneously causing the gut to contract in their own location (3) and to relax distally by activating inhibitory neurons (4). Parasympathetic ganglion cells in the wall of the gall bladder cause expulsion of bile. Those in the submucous plexus (5), and in the pancreas, cause glandular secretion.

Peristaltic activity persists even after total extrinsic denervation because of the intrinsic circuitry and the spontaneous excitability of 'pacemaker' patches of smooth muscle (notably in stomach and duodenum).

The *preganglionic sympathetic* nerve supply originates in lateral horn cells of cord segments T5–T11. The fibers traverse the paravertebral sympathetic chain (6) without synapsing here and terminate in the prevertebral, splanchnic ganglia (7) within the abdomen (celiac, superior and inferior mesenteric). Their beaded postganglionic fibers supply the smooth muscle of the intestine and of blood vessels, which they relax via β_2 receptors.

Visceral afferents reaching the CNS have their unipolar somas in a nodose ganglion of the vagus (8) and in posterior root ganglia at spinal levels T5–T11(9). The spinal afferents reach the posterior gray horn via *anterior* nerve roots. These *ventral root afferents* are of special clinical importance because they include first-order *nociceptive* afferents which synapse centrally upon lateral spinothalamic projection cells providing the principal 'pain pathway' to the brain (*see* Visceral afferents, p. 96).

Intrinsic visceral afferent neurons are in the form of bipolar neurons (10). Some participate in local reflex arcs within the myenteric or submucous plexus. Others (not shown) project as far as the splanchnic ganglia with the potential of exerting more widespread reflex effects.

Transmitters and *modulators* are numerous among the enteric ganglion cells. The principal excitatory transmitter is ACh, with substance P cotransmitted as a modulator. The principal inhibitory transmitters are nitric oxide, GABA γ-aminobutyric acid, and VIP. Large numbers of different peptides have been revealed by means of histochemistry. More often than not, two or more are present within individual cells.

Box 10.2 *Continued*

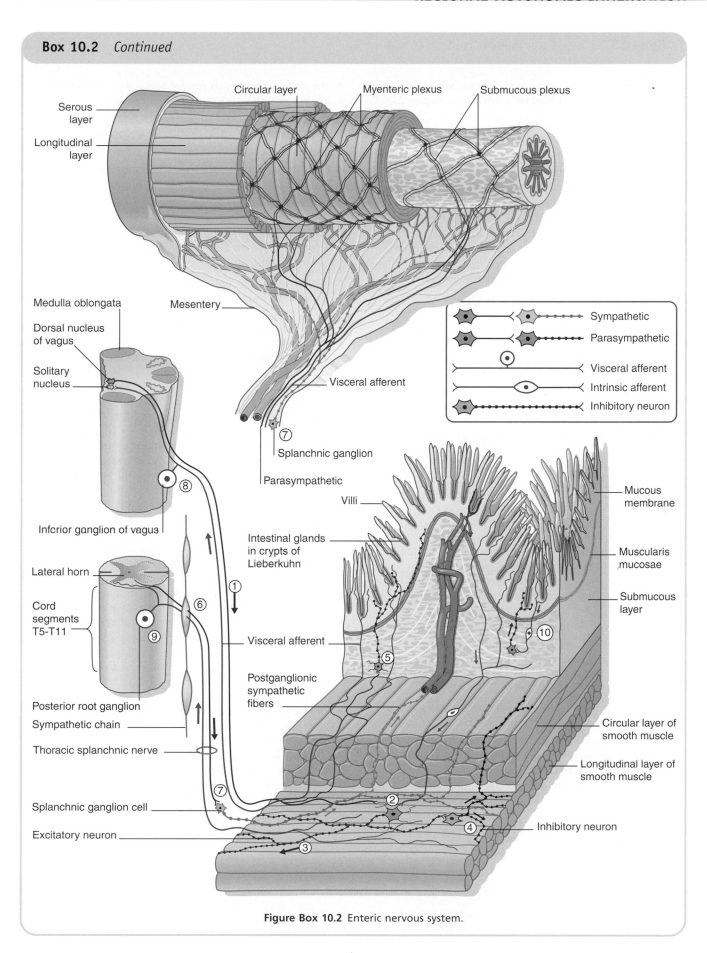

Figure Box 10.2 Enteric nervous system.

Box 10.3 Lower level bladder controls*

The female bladder is selected for this description, and also for higher level bladder controls in Chapter 21.

Relevant anatomical details

- The smooth muscle of the detrusor in the body (corpus) of the bladder is an interwoven meshwork of fasciculi and functions as a unit.

- The bladder neck is surrounded by two layers of longitudinal smooth muscle enclosing a layer of circular muscle, constituting the **internal urethral sphincter**.

- The outer longitudinal fibers descend within the mucous membrane of the urethra. When these fibers contract (along with the rest of the detrusor), they shorten and widen the urethral canal.

- The resting urethral canal is kept closed by a rich encircling web of elastic fibers, a highly vascular mucous membrane, a thin circular layer of smooth muscle, and the striated **external urethral sphincter**.

- The external urethral sphincter is richly endowed with slow-twitch, fatigue-resistant muscle fibers. It comes into play when abdominal pressure is raised either briefly (e.g. during a cough or sneeze) or for longer (e.g. while a heavy load is being carried). The cell group innervating this muscle is the *nucleus of Onuf* in the anterior gray horn at spinal cord levels S2 and S3. Most of the axons travel in the pudendal nerve.

The micturition cycle

1 Immediately prior to the act of micturition, the anterior horn motor neurons to the levator ani and other muscles of the pelvic floor are inhibited by axons descending from the micturition center in the pons (Ch. 21). The neck of the bladder descends passively, and urine trickles into the urethra.

2 Mucosal fibers of the pudendal nerve, sensory to epithelium of trigone and urethra, discharge impulses to the posterior gray horn of cord segments S2–S4.

3 From sacral cord, second-order sensory neurons discharge to the pontine micturition center.

4 Sacral parasympathetic neurons serving the bladder are simultaneously activated by the pontine micturition center and by neurons in the posterior horn at segmental levels S2–S4.

5 The detrusor responds to postganglionic stimulation by contracting uniformly to expel the urine.

6 The external urethral sphincter, slave to Onuf, contracts to expel urine from the urethral canal.

7 Levator ani contracts to resume its supportive role.

8 Bladder filling recommences, whilst the bladder wall is rendered *compliant* by tonic inhibitory β_2 action of the sympathetic system on the detrusor muscle and by α_2 receptors on parasympathetic terminals.

9 When the bladder is half-full, the stretch receptor afferents from the detrusor inform higher level neurons in the brainstem, as described in *Box 21.2*.

Notes on urinary incontinence

Urinary incontinence afflicts about 30% of the female population at one or more periods of their lives. The two chief causes are detrusor instability and stress incontinence.

Detrusor instability ('unstable bladder') is characterized by spontaneous expulsion of urine during the filling phase of the micturition cycle despite conscious attempts to inhibit it. There is as yet no general agreement as to the nature of this problem. Suggestions include: (a) the development of 'pacemaker' patches of detrusor smooth muscle (by analogy with those of the intestine); (b) weakness of the bladder neck allowing urine to escape and excite pudendal nerve endings with a consequent reflex detrusor response; and (c) overreaction of the detrusor to ACh being secreted in small amounts by the pelvic splanchnic nerve. In parous women and elderly nullipara, degeneration of pelvic splanchnic fibers may result in *upregulation* of ACh receptors in the detrusor, whereby the muscle cells have inserted too many additional ACh receptors into their own plasmalemmas.

Parous women are also prone to *stress incontinence*. The underlying problem is *inherent weakness of the pelvic floor*, designed, as it is, to permit passage of the mature fetus. The pelvic floor weakness is often increased during parturition, by injury of the pudendal nerve resulting from its compression against the ischium.

Stress incontinence and urge incontinence also attend advancing age. One or other afflicts about 50% of women in institutional care. The primary problem in the elderly seems to be the progressive loss of striated muscle fibers in the urethral wall and pelvic floor.

In both sexes, disorders of brain function may also be responsible for incontinence (Ch. 29).

---

* For helpful discussions on lower and higher level bladder controls, the authors thank Professor MaryPat FitzGerald, Department of Gynecology, Loyola University School of Medicine, Chicago.

Box 10.3 *Continued*

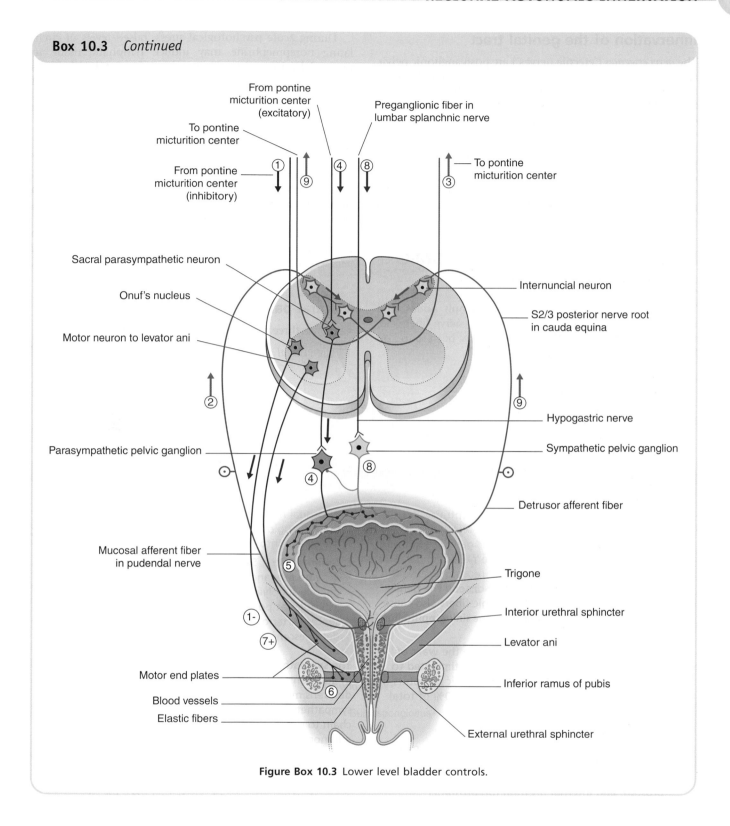

Figure Box 10.3 Lower level bladder controls.

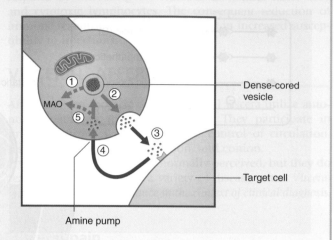
2 *Visceral referred pain*, projected subjectively into the territory of the corresponding somatic nerves

3 *Viscerosomatic pain*, caused by spread of disease to somatic structures.

Pure visceral pain

Pure visceral pain is characteristically vague and deep-seated. It is often accompanied by sweating or nausea. It is experienced as the initial pain in association with inflammation and/or ulceration in the alimentary tract; with obstruction of the intestine, bile duct, or ureter; or when the capsule of a solid organ (liver, kidney, pancreas) is stretched by underlying disease. In marked contrast, the viscera are completely insensitive to cutting or burning.

Visceral referred pain

As its severity increases, visceral pain is 'referred' to somatic structures innervated from the same segmental levels of the spinal cord. For example, the pain of myocardial ischemia is referred to the chest wall ('angina pectoris'), pains of biliary or intestinal origin are referred to the anterior abdominal wall, and labor pains are referred to the sacral area of the back.

According to the generally accepted 'convergence-projection' theory of referred pain, the brain falsely interprets the source of noxious stimulation because visceral and somatic nociceptors have some spinothalamic neurons in common; in previous experience, these neurons habitually signaled somatic pain.

Viscerosomatic pain

The parietal serous membranes (pleura and peritoneum) receive a rich sensory supply from the overlying intercostal nerves, and they are exquisitely sensitive to acute inflammatory exudates. The extension of an inflammatory process to the surface of stomach, intestine, appendix, or gallbladder gives rise to a severe, steady pain in the abdominal wall directly overlying the inflamed organ. With the onset of acute peritonitis, the abdominal wall is 'splinted' by the muscles in a protective reflex.

Tenderness

Tenderness is *pain elicited by palpation*. In the abdomen, it is sought by pressing the hand and fingers against the abdominal wall. The clinician is, in effect, clothing the finger pads with the patient's parietal peritoneum and using this to seek

Clinical Panel 10.3 Drugs and the parasympathetic system

Possible peripheral effects of cholinergic and anticholinergic drugs are listed in *Figure CP 10.3.1*. Some success has been achieved in the search for organ- or tissue-specific drugs. For example, the contribution of the vagus nerve to acid secretion in the stomach involves activation of a muscarinic receptor

(M_1) which is distinct from the receptor type (M_2) found in the heart or on smooth muscle. An M_1 receptor blocker is available for patients suffering from peptic ulcer, for the specific purpose of reducing gastric acidity.

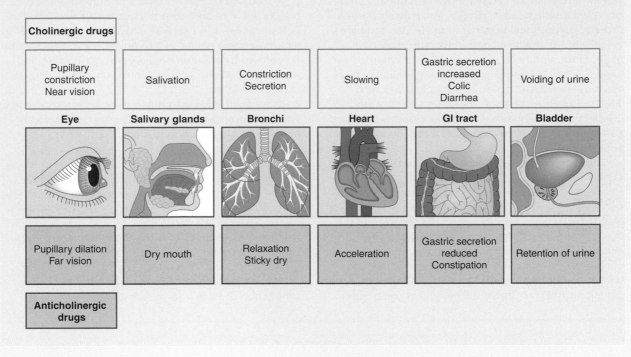

Figure CP 10.3.1 Drugs and the parasympathetic system.

out an inflamed organ. If the organ is mobile, like the appendix, 'shifting tenderness' may be elicited if the patient is willing to roll from one side to the other.

Pain and the mind

Although visceral pain has well-established causative mechanisms (inflammation, spasm of smooth muscle, ischemia, distention), thoracic or abdominal pain may be experienced in the complete absence of visceral disease. Pain that recurs or persists over a long period (months), and is not accounted for by standard investigational procedures, is more likely to have a *psychological* rather than a physical explanation. This is not to deny that the pain is real, but to imply that it originates within the brain itself. An example is the abused child whose abdominal pains represent a cry for help. In adults, recurrent and rather ill-defined pains are a common manifestation of *major depression* (see Ch. 22).

Note on vascular afferents

Two *vascular* sets of unipolar neurons are customarily included in descriptions of the visceral afferent system. One

supplies the carotid sinus and aortic arch with stretch receptors involved in the maintenance of the systemic blood pressure (Ch. 21); the other supplies the carotid body with chemoreceptors and is involved in respiratory control (Ch. 21). There is a progressive tendency to acknowledge *all* vascular afferents as being visceral because those on peripheral blood vessels are morphologically and functionally the same as those serving the heart. They all contain substance P, are 'silent' in health, and subserve pain in the presence of disease or injury – as witness, the 'dragging' leg pains accompanying varicose veins, or the stab of pain when a clumsily inserted antecubital venipuncture needle strikes the brachial artery. The pathway to the posterior nerve roots is still uncertain, but it appears that (to an approximation) perivascular fibers above elbow and knee send impulses by the sympathetic route (but in the reverse direction), and that more peripheral perivascular fibers send messages in company with cutaneous nerves (and in the same direction). The notion of visceral afferents running in cutaneous nerves is reminiscent of their same service with respect to nerve fibers terminating in Golgi tendon organs at wrist and ankle.

Core Information

The autonomic nervous system contains three neuron chains of effector neurons: central neurons project from hypothalamus/brainstem to brainstem/spinal cord preganglionic neurons. These send preganglionic fibers to autonomic ganglion cells which in turn send postganglionic fibers to target tissues.

Sympathetic preganglionic outflow to the sympathetic chain of ganglia is thoracolumbar. Some fibers synapse in nearest ganglia. Some ascend to the superior cervical, middle cervical, or stellate ganglion whence postganglionic fibers innervate head, neck, upper limbs, and heart. Some descend to synapse in lumbar or sacral ganglia whence postganglionic fibers enter the lumbosacral plexus to supply lower limb vessels. Some pass through the chain and synapse instead in central abdominal ganglia (for the supply of gastrointestinal and genitourinary tracts) or in the adrenal medulla.

Parasympathetic preganglionic outflow is craniosacral. Cranial nerve distributions are: oculomotor nerve via ciliary ganglion to sphincter pupillae and ciliaris; facial nerve via pterygopalatine ganglion to lacrimal and nasal glands; facial nerve via submandibular ganglion to submandibular and sublingual glands; glossopharyngeal nerve via otic ganglion to parotid gland; vagus nerve via ganglia on/in walls of heart, bronchi, and alimentary tract to muscle and glands. Sacral nerves 2–4 deliver preganglionic fibers to intramural ganglia of distal colon and rectum, and to pelvic ganglia for supply of bladder and internal pudendal artery.

All preganglionic neurons are cholinergic. They activate nicotinic receptors in the ganglia. All postganglionic fibers end at neuroeffector junctions. In the sympathetic system, these are generally adrenergic, liberating norepinephrine which may activate postjunctional α_1 adrenoceptors on smooth muscle, prejunctional α_2 adrenoceptors on local nerve endings, postjunctional α_1 on cardiac muscle or postjunctional α_2 which are more responsive to epinephrine. Epinephrine is liberated by adrenomedullary chromaffin cells and resultant activation of β_2 receptors on smooth muscle causes relaxation.

Parasympathetic postganglionic fibers are cholinergic. The cholinoceptive receptors on cardiac and smooth muscle and glands are muscarinic.

Visceral afferents

Nociceptive afferents from thoracic and abdominal viscera and from blood vessels use autonomic pathways to reach the CNS. Pure visceral pain is vague and deep-seated. Visceral referred pain is experienced in somatic structures innervated from the same segmental levels. Viscerosomatic pain arises from chemical/thermal irritation of one of the serous membranes: the pain is severe and steady and accompanied by protective contraction of body wall muscles.

REFERENCES

Andersson, K.F. and Wagner, D. (1995) Physiology of penile erection. *Physiol. Rev.* **75**: 191–236.

Ardell, J.L. (1994) Structure and function of mammalian intrinsic cardiac neurons. In *Neurocardiology* (Armour, J.A. and Ardell, J.L., eds), pp. 95–114. New York: Oxford University Press.

Armour, J.A. (1994) Peripheral autonomic neuronal interactions in cardiac regulation. In *Neurocardiology* (Armour, J.A. and Ardell, J.L., eds), pp. 219–244. New York: Oxford University Press.

Armour, J.A., Murphy, D.A., Yuan, B-X., MacDonald, S. and Hopkins, D.A. (1997) Gross and microscopic anatomy of the human intrinsic cardiac nervous system. *Anat. Rec.* **247**: 289–298.

Cardozo, L. (1997) Detrusor instability. In *Gynaecology*, 2nd edn (Shaw, R.W., Soutter, W.P. and Stanton, S.L., eds), pp. 739–752. New York: Churchill Livingstone.

Coupland, R.B. (1989) The natural history of the chromaffin cell. *Arch. Histol. Cytol.* **52**: 331–341.

de Grout, W.C. and Booth, A.M. (1993) Autonomic system to urinary bladder and sexual organs. In *Peripheral Neuropathy*, 3rd edn (Dyck, P.J. and Thomas, P.K., eds), pp. 198–207. Philadelphia: Saunders.

Dixon, J.S., Jen, P.Y.P. and Gosling, J.A. (1998) Structure and autonomic innervation of the human vas deferens: a review. *Micr. Res. Tech.* **42**: 423–432.

Drummond, P.D. (1993) Autonomic innervation of the face. In *Science and Practice of Clinical Neurology* (Gandevia, S.C., Burke, D. and Anthony, M., eds), pp. 223–242. Cambridge: Cambridge University Press.

Feigl, E.O. (1994) Neural control of coronary blood flow. In *Neurocardiology* (Armour, J.A. and Ardell, J.L., eds), pp. 139–164. New York: Oxford University Press.

Gai, W.P. and Blessing, W.W. (1996) Human brainstem preganglionic parasympathetic neurons localized by markers for nitric oxide synthesis. *Brain* **119**: 1145–1152.

Holguin-Acosta, J. (1997) The neurology of dyslexia. *Rev. Neurol.* **141**: 739–743.

Hopkins, D.A., Bieger, D., de Vente, J. and Steinbusch, H.W.M. (1996) Vagal efferent projections: viscerotopy, neurochemistry and effects of vagotomy. In *The Emotional Motor System* (Holstege, G., Bandler, R. and Saper, C.B., eds), pp. 79–96. Amsterdam: Elsevier.

Kinder, M.V., Bastiaanssen, B.H.C., Janknegt, R.A. and Marani, E. (1995) Neuronal circuitry of the lower urinary tract. *Anat. Embryol.* **192**: 195–209.

Leonard, B.E. (1997) *Fundamentals of Psychopharmacology*, 2nd edn. Chichester: Wiley.

Levy, M.N. and Warner, M.R. (1994) Parasympathetic effects on cardiac function. In *Neurocardiology* (Armour, J.A. and Ardell, J.L., eds), pp. 53–76. New York: Oxford University Press.

McLeod, J.G. (1993) Disorders of the autonomic system. In *Science and Practice in Clinical Neurology* (Gandevia, S.C., Burke, D. and Anthony, M., eds) pp. 205–222. Cambridge: Cambridge University Press.

McMahon, S.B., Dmitrieva, N. and Kolzenburg, M. (1995) Visceral pain. *Brit. J. Anaesth.* **75**: 132–144.

Martinotti, E. (1991) Adrenergic subtypes on vascular smooth muscle. *Pharmacol. Res.* **24**: 297–306.

Paintal, A.S. (1986) The visceral sensations – some basic mechanisms. *Prog. Brain Res.* **67**: 3–18.

Panuncio, A.L., De La Pena, S., Gualco, G. and Reisenweber, N. (1999) Adrenergic innervation in reactive human lymph nodes. *J. Anat.* **194**: 143–146.

Perkin, G.D. and Murray-Lyon, I. (1998) Neurology and the gastrointestinal system. *Neurol. Neurosurg. Psychiatry* **65**: 291–300.

Perna, F.M., Schneiderman, N. and LaPierre, A. (1997) Psychological stress, exercise and immunity. *Jnt. J. Sports Med.* **18**(S1): 78–83.

Procacci, P., Zoppi, M. and Maresca, M. (1986) Clinical approach to visceral sensation. *Prog. Brain Res.* **67**: 21–28.

Randall, W.C. (1994) Efferent sympathetic innervation of the heart. In *Neurocardiology* (Armour, J.A. and Ardell, J.L., eds), pp. 77–94. New York: Oxford University Press.

Schott, G.D. (1994) Visceral afferents: their contribution to 'sympathetic-dependent' pain. *Brain* **117**: 397–413.

van Leishout, J.J., Wieling W., Karemaker, J.M. and Eckberg, D.L. (1991) The vasovagal response. *Clin. Sci.* **81**: 575–586.

Wittling, W., Block, A., Genzel, S. and Schweiger, E. (1998) Hemisphere asymmetry in parasympathetic control of the heart. *Neuropsychologia* **36**: 461–468.

Wittling, W., Block, A., Schweiger, E. and Genzel, S. (1998) Hemisphere asymmetry in sympathetic control of the human myocardium. *Brain Cogn.* **38**: 17–35.

Nerve roots

DEVELOPMENT OF THE SPINAL CORD

Cellular differentiation

The neural tube of the embryo consists of a pseudostratified epithelium surrounding the neural canal (*Figure 11.1A*). Dorsal to the sulcus limitans, the epithelium forms the **alar plate**; ventral to the sulcus, it forms the **basal plate**.

The neuroepithelium contains germinal cells which synthesize DNA before retracting to the innermost, **ventricular zone**, where they divide. The daughter nuclei move outward, synthesize fresh DNA, then retreat and divide again. After several such cycles, postmitotic cells round up in the **intermediate zone**. Some of the postmitotic cells are immature neurons; the rest are **glioblasts** which, after further division, become astrocytes or oligodendrocytes. Some of the glioblasts form an ependymal lining for the neural canal.

The microglial cells of the CNS are derived from basophil cells of the blood.

Enlargement of the intermediate zone of the alar plate creates the dorsal horn of gray matter. The dorsal horn receives central processes of dorsal root ganglion cells (*Figure 11.1B*). As explained in Chapter 1, the ganglion cells derive from the neural crest.

Partial occlusion of the neural canal by the developing dorsal gray horn gives rise to the dorsal median septum and to the definitive central canal of the cord (*Figure 11.1C*).

Enlargement of the intermediate zone of the basal plate creates the ventral gray horn and the ventral median fissure (*Figure 11.1C*). Axons emerge from the ventral horn and form the ventral nerve roots.

In the outermost, **marginal zone** of the cord, axons run to and from spinal cord and brain.

Neural cord

The neural tube reaches caudally only to the level of the second lumbar mesodermal somites. Following closure of the posterior neuropore, the ectoderm and mesoderm at the level of the more caudal lumbar and sacral somites blend to form a **neural cord**. This ribbon of cells becomes canalized and links up with the neural tube; it forms the lower end of the spinal cord.

Ascent of the cord   (Figure 11.2)

The spinal cord occupies the full length of the vertebral canal until the end of the 12th postconceptual week. The sixth to eighth are marked by regression of the caudal end of the neural tube, to become a neuroglial thread, the **filum terminale**.

After the 12th week, the vertebral column grows rapidly and drags the cord upward. The tip of the cord is at second or third lumbar level at the time of birth. The adult level (first or second lumbar) is attained 3 weeks later.

In consequence of greater ascent of the lower part of cord compared to the upper part, the spinal nerve roots show an increasing disparity between their segmental levels of attachment to the cord and the corresponding vertebral levels (*Figure 11.3*).

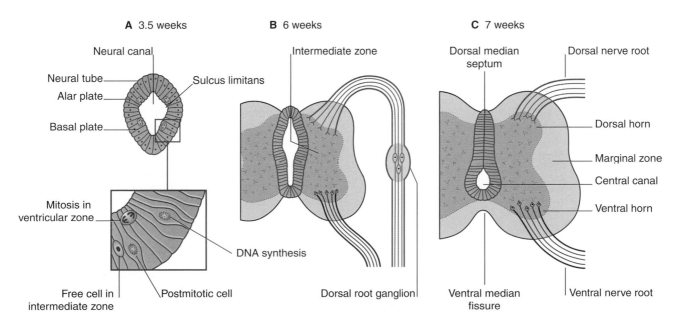

A 3.5 weeks   **B** 6 weeks   **C** 7 weeks

Neural canal · Neural tube · Alar plate · Basal plate · Sulcus limitans · Intermediate zone · Dorsal median septum · Dorsal nerve root · Dorsal horn · Marginal zone · Central canal · Ventral horn · Mitosis in ventricular zone · DNA synthesis · Free cell in intermediate zone · Postmitotic cell · Dorsal root ganglion · Ventral median fissure · Ventral nerve root

Figure 11.1 Cellular differentiation in the embryonic spinal cord.

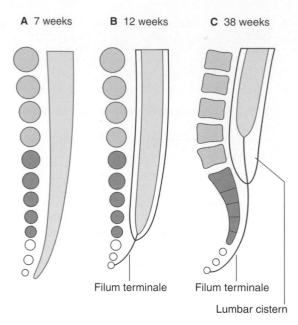

A 7 weeks   **B** 12 weeks   **C** 38 weeks

Filum terminale   Filum terminale

Lumbar cistern

Figure 11.2 (A, B) Regression of coccygeal segments of spinal cord creates the filum terminale. **(C)** Ascent of spinal cord. (*Note:* Recent evidence indicates that (as represented here) the number of embryonic coccygeal vertebrae does not exceed three or four.)

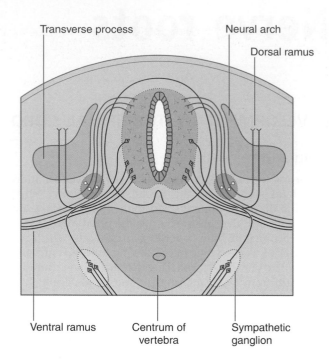

Transverse process   Neural arch

Dorsal ramus

Ventral ramus   Centrum of vertebra   Sympathetic ganglion

Figure 11.4 Normal, bifid stage of neural arch development in an embryo of 8 weeks.

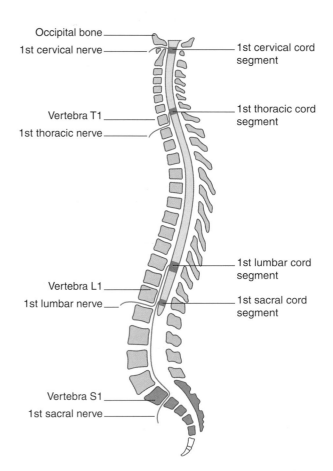

Occipital bone

1st cervical nerve   1st cervical cord segment

Vertebra T1   1st thoracic cord segment

1st thoracic nerve

Vertebra L1   1st lumbar cord segment

1st lumbar nerve   1st sacral cord segment

Vertebra S1

1st sacral nerve

Figure 11.3 Segmental and vertebral levels compared. Spinal nerves 1–7 emerge above the corresponding vertebrae, the remaining spinal nerves emerge below.

Neural arches

During the fifth week, the mesenchymal vertebrae surrounding the notochord give rise to **neural arches** for protection of the spinal cord (*Figure 11.4*). The arches are initially *bifid* (split). Later, they fuse in the midline and form the vertebral spines.

Conditions where the two halves of the neural arches have failed to unite are collectively known as *spina bifida* (*Clinical Panel 11.1*).

ADULT ANATOMY

The spinal cord and nerve roots are sheathed by pia mater and float in cerebrospinal fluid contained in the subarachnoid space. The pial **denticulate ligament** pierces the arachnoid and anchors the cord to the dura mater on each side. Outside the dura is the **extradural (epidural) venous plexus** (*Figure 11.5*) which harvests the vertebral red marrow and empties into the segmental veins (deep cervical, intercostal, lumbar, sacral). These veins are without valves, and reflux of blood from the territory of segmental veins is a *notorious* cause of cancer spread from prostate, lung, breast, and thyroid gland. As example, nerve root compression from collapse of an invaded vertebra may be the presenting sign of cancer in one of these organs.

The respective anterior and posterior nerve roots join at the intervertebral foramina, where the posterior root ganglia are located (*Figure 11.5*). The arachnoid mater blends with the perineurium of the spinal nerve, and the dura mater blends with the epineurium. The nerve roots carry extensions of the subarachnoid space into the intervertebral foramina.

Clinical Panel 11.1 Spina bifida

Among the more common congenital malformations of the CNS are several conditions included under the general heading, spina bifida. The 'bifid' effect is produced by failure of union of the two halves of the neural arches, usually in the lumbosacral region (*Figure CP 11.1.1*)

Spina bifida occulta (**A**) is usually symptom-free, being detected incidentally in lumbosacral radiographs.

In *spina bifida cystica*, a meningeal cyst protrudes through the vertebral defect. In 10% of these cases, the cyst is a *meningocele* containing no nervous elements (**B**). In 90%, unfortunately, the cyst is a *meningomyelocele*, containing either spinal cord or cauda equina (**C**); the lower limbs, bladder and rectum are paralyzed, as in the case illustrated in *Figure CP 11.1.2*, and meningitis is likely to supervene sooner or later. To make matters worse, an *Arnold–Chiari malformation* (Ch. 4) is almost always present as well.

The most severe form of spina bifida is *myelocele* (**D**), where the neural folds have remained open and CSF leaks on to the surrounding skin. The clinical outlook is very poor.

Cauda equina

Cyst

A

B

Cyst

Neural plate

C

D

Figure CP 11.1.1 Varieties of spina bifida. (**A**) Spina bifida occulta. (**B**) Meningocele. (**C**) Meningomyelocele. (**D**) Myelocele.

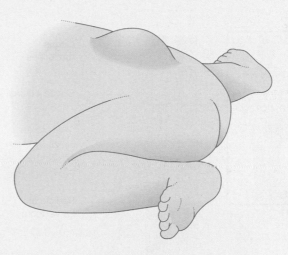

Figure CP 11.1.2 Lumbar meningomyelocele (from a photograph). The 'frog leg' posture is characteristic of combined femoral and sciatic nerve paralysis, with preservation of hip flexion by the iliopsoas.

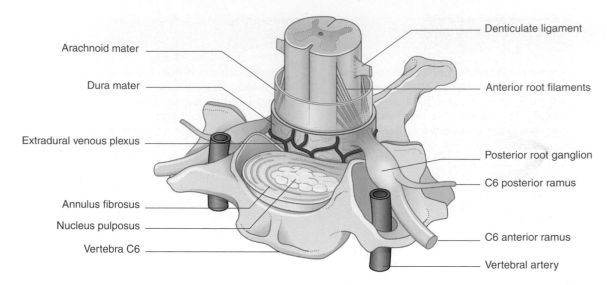

Figure 11.5 Relationships of the sixth cervical spinal nerve.

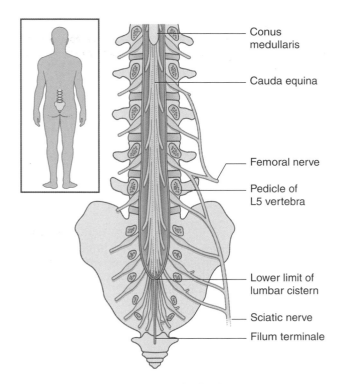

Figure 11.6 The cauda equina in the lumbar cistern. Contributions to the femoral and sciatic nerves are shown on the right side.

Below cord level, nerve roots seeking the lower lumbar and sacral intervertebral foramina constitute the **cauda equina** ('horse's tail'). The cauda equina floats in the lumbar subarachnoid cistern (*Figures 11.6, 11.7*), which reaches to the level of the second sacral vertebra. At its upper end, the

cauda comprises nerve roots L3–S5 of both sides – *a total of 32 roots* (excluding the insignificant coccygeal roots).

In the center of the cauda equina is the unimportant filum terminale, which pierces the meninges to become attached to the coccyx.

DISTRIBUTION OF SPINAL NERVES

Each spinal nerve gives off a *recurrent* branch which provides mechanoreceptors and pain receptors for the dura mater, posterior longitudinal ligament, and intervertebral disc. The synovial *facet* joints between successive articular processes are each supplied by the nearest three spinal nerves. Pain caused by injury or disease of any of the above structures is referred to the cutaneous territory of the corresponding posterior rami (*Figure 11.8*).

Segmental sensory distribution: the dermatomes

A **dermatome** is the strip of skin supplied by an individual spinal nerve. The dermatomes are orderly in the embryo (*Figure 11.9*) but they are distorted by outgrowth of the limbs (*Figure 11.10*). Spinal nerves C5–T1 are drawn into the upper limb, so that C4 dermatome abuts T2 at the level of the sternal angle. Nerves L2–S2 are drawn into the lower limb, so that L2 abuts S3 dermatome over the buttock. Maps like those in *Figure 11.10* fail to portray *overlap* in the cutaneous distribution of successive dorsal nerve roots. On the trunk, e.g., the skin over an intercostal space is supplied by the nerves immediately above and below in addition to the proper nerve.

Segmental motor distribution

In the limbs, the individual muscles are supplied by more than one spinal nerve because of interchange in the

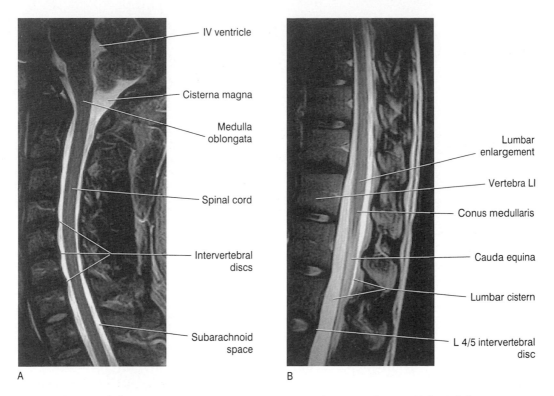

Figure 11.7 Sagittal MRI scans of the vertebral canal, weighted so as to enhance cerebrospinal fluid. **(A)** Brainstem, cerebellum and cervical spinal cord are outlined. **(B)** Lumbosacral spinal cord and cauda are outlined. (From a series kindly provided by Professor J. Paul Finn, Director, MRI Facility, Northwestern University Medical School, Chicago.)

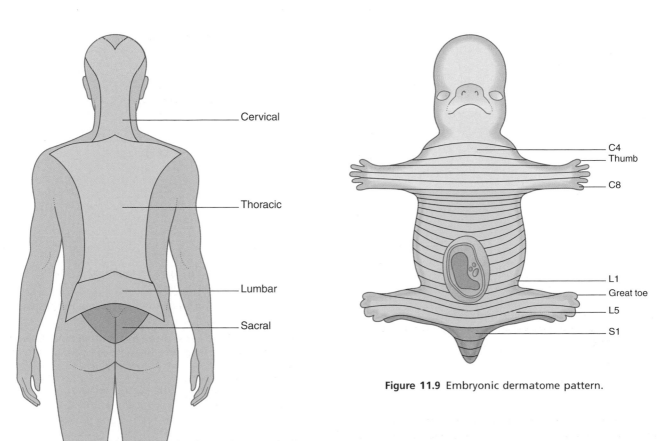

Figure 11.8 Cutaneous distribution of posterior rami of spinal nerves.

Figure 11.9 Embryonic dermatome pattern.

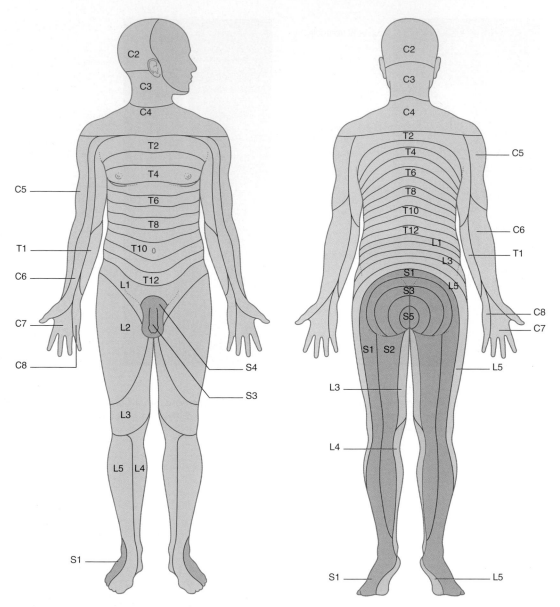

Figure 11.10 Adult dermatome pattern.

brachial and lumbosacral plexuses. The segmental supply of the limbs is expressed in terms of *movements* in *Figure 11.11*.

Segmental sensory inputs and segmental motor outputs are combined during execution of *withdrawal* or *avoidance reflexes* (*Box 11.1*). (The prevalent term, *flexor reflex*, is too limited; e.g. a stimulus applied to the lateral surface of a limb may elicit adduction.)

Nerve root compression syndromes

Nerve root compression within the vertebral canal is most frequent where the spine is most mobile, namely at lower cervical and lower lumbar levels (*Clinical Panel 11.2*). The effects of root compression may be expressed in five different ways:

1 *Pain* perceived in the muscles supplied by the corresponding spinal nerve(s).

2 *Paresthesia* (numbness or tingling) along the respective dermatome(s).

3 *Cutaneous sensory loss* – more likely if two successive dermatomes are involved, because of overlap.

4 *Motor weakness.*

5 *Loss of a tendon reflex* if the segmental level is appropriate (*Table 11.1*).

Lumbar puncture (spinal tap)

The procedure involved in removing a sample of cerebrospinal fluid from the lumbar cistern is described in

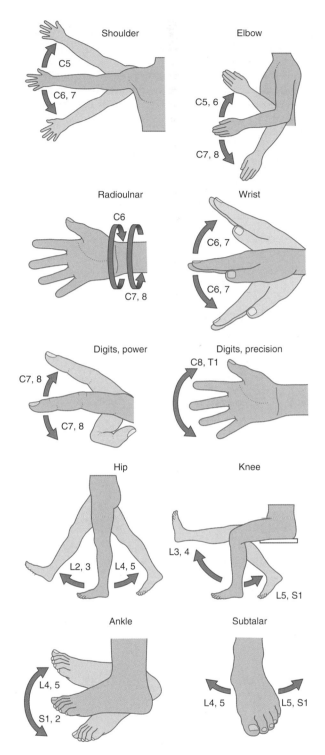

Table 11.1 Segmental levels of tendon reflexes	
Segmental level	**Reflex**
C5,6	Biceps
C5,6	Brachioradialis ('supinator reflex')
C7	Triceps
L3,4	Knee jerk
S1	Ankle jerk

Clinical Panel 11.3. This procedure should not be performed if there is any reason to suspect the presence of raised intracranial pressure. (It *is* performed occasionally when there is some uncertainty, but only under immediate neuro-surgical cover.)

Anesthetic procedures

A so-called *spinal anesthetic* is often given in preference to a general anesthetic, prior to surgical procedures on the prostate in the elderly. A local anesthetic is injected into the lumbar cistern in order to block impulse conduction in the lumbar and sacral nerve roots. Care is taken that the anesthetic does not reach a high level in the subarachnoid space, for fear of paralyzing the intercostal and phrenic nerve root fibers serving respiration.

Anesthesia and childbirth

In skilled hands, pain-free labor can be assured by blocking the lumbar and sacral nerve roots extradurally. For *epidural anesthesia*, local anesthetic is carefully introduced into the extradural space by the lumbar route. For *caudal anesthesia* (rarely performed), the extradural space is approached in an upward direction, through the sacral hiatus. In both proce-dures, the anesthetic diffuses through the dural sheath of the nerve roots where they leave the vertebral canal. Labor may be prolonged because of interruption of excitatory reflex arcs linking perineum to uterus through the lower end of the spinal cord. However, avoidance of general anesthesia is valuable in allowing immediate bonding to take place between mother and child.

Figure 11.11 Segmental control of limb movements. (Adapted from Last, R.J. (1973) *Anatomy: Regional and Applied*, 5th edn. Edinburgh: Churchill Livingstone; and Rosse, C. and Clawson, D.K. (1980) *The Musculoskeletal System in Health and Disease*. Hagerstown: Harper & Row.)

Box 11.1 Lower limb withdrawal reflex

Figure Box 11.1.1 depicts a lower limb *withdrawal reflex* with *crossed extensor thrust*. **(A)** The right foot is about to enter the stance phase of locomotion. **(B)** Contact with a sharp object initiates a withdrawal reflex, together with the crossed extensor response required to support the entire body weight.

Sequence of events

1 Plantar nociceptors send impulse trains along tibial–sciatic afferent fibers (1a) having parent posterior root ganglion somas within the L5–S1 intervertebral foramen. The impulses ascend cauda equina (1b) and enter segment L5 of spinal cord. Some impulses are despatched up and down Lissauer's tract (1c) to activate segments L2–L4 and S1.

2 In all five segments, primary nociceptive afferents excite *flexor reflex internuncials* in the base of the posterior horn (2a). Several internuncials may be interposed, in series, between entering afferents and target motor neurons. Axons of medially placed internuncials cross the midline in the gray commissure, allowing impulse trains to activate contralateral internuncials (2b).

3 On the stimulated side, α and γ motor neurons in cord segments L3–S1 contract iliopsoas (a), hamstrings (b), and ankle dorsiflexors (d). At the same time (not shown here), ipsilateral 1a inhibitory internuncials are recruited to silence the antigravity motor neurons.

4 On the contralateral side, α and γ motor neurons in cord segments L2–L5 contract gluteus maximus (not visible here) and quadriceps femoris (c).

Note: Not shown in the figure are *lateral spinothalamic tract* relay neurons (see Ch. 12). These neurons receive inputs from nociceptive afferent fibers in Lissauer's tract and they relay impulses to brain sites able to decode the location and nature of the initial stimulus.

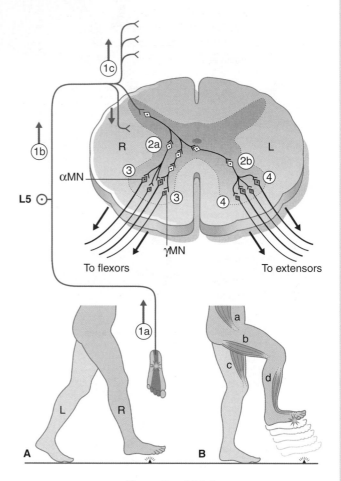

Figure Box 11.1.1

Clinical Panel 11.2   Nerve root compression

Cervical roots

The intervertebral discs and synovial joints of the neck are subject to degenerative disease (*cervical spondylosis*) in 50% of 50-year-olds and in 70% of 70-year-olds. Although any or all of the joints may deteriorate, problems are most frequent in relation to vertebra C6, which provides the fulcrum for flexion/extension movements of the neck. Spinal nerve C6 (above) or C7 (below) may be pinched by extruded disc material or by bony outgrowths (*osteophytes*) beside the synovial joints (*Figure CP 11.2.1*). Sensory, motor, and reflex disturbances may result in accordance with the data in *Figures 11.9* and *11.10* and *Table 11.1*.

Lumbosacral roots

One important cause of low-back pain is a *prolapsed intervertebral disc* (*herniated nucleus pulposus*). Fully 95% of all disc prolapses occur immediately above or below the last lumbar vertebra. The typical herniation is *posterolateral*, with compression of the nerve roots passing to the *next* intervertebral foramen (*Figure CP 11.2.2*).

Symptoms include backache caused by rupture of the annulus fibrosus, and pain in the buttock/thigh/leg caused by pressure on posterior root fibers contributing to the sciatic nerve. The pain is increased by stretching the affected root, e.g. by having the straightened leg raised by the examiner.

An L4–L5 disc prolapse produces pain/paresthesia over the L5 dermatome. Motor weakness may be detected during dorsiflexion of the great toe (later, of all toes and of the ankle), and during eversion of the foot. Abduction of the hip may also be weak; this movement is tested with the patient lying on one side.

With an L5–S1 prolapse (the commonest of all), symptoms are felt in the back of the leg/sole of foot (S1 dermatome). Plantar flexion may be weak and the ankle jerk reduced or absent.

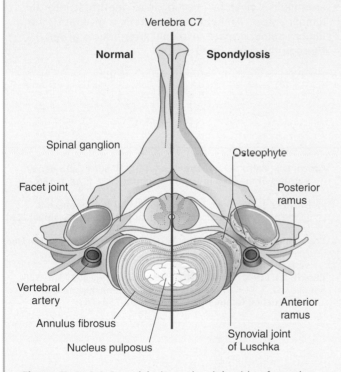

Figure CP 11.2.1 Spondylosis on the right side of vertebra C7. Osteophytes are pinching C7 spinal nerve trunk.

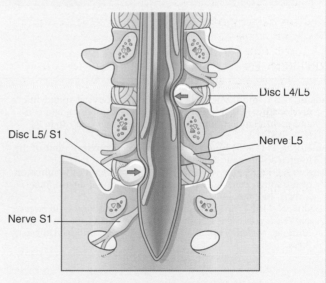

Figure CP 11.2.2 Nerves compressed (arrows) by posterolateral prolapse of the two lowest intervertebral discs.

Core Information

The neuroepithelium of the embryonic cord undergoes mitotic activity in the inner, ventricular zone. Daughter cells move into the intermediate zone and become either neuroblasts or glioblasts. The developing dorsal horn receives central processes of neural crest-derived spinal ganglion cells. The ventral horn issues axons that form ventral nerve roots. The outer, marginal zone contains the axons of developing nerve pathways. The caudal end of the cord develops separately, from the neural cord, which links up with the neural tube. After the 12th week, rapid growth of the vertebral column drags the cord up the vertebral canal; the lower tip of the cord is at L2–L3 level at birth and at L1–L2 level 3 weeks later. The result is a progressive disparity between segmental levels of nerve root attachment to the cord and intervertebral levels of exit of spinal nerves. The neural arches are dorsal projections of vertebral mesenchyme; the initial bifid arrangement is normally lost by fusion of the projections to form spines.

The mature cord and nerve roots are sheathed by pia mater and float in the subarachnoid space, anchored to dura by the denticulate ligament. The extradural space contains valveless veins which drain vertebral bone marrow into segmental veins and provide potential avenues for spread of cancer cells. Below the level of the cord, the cauda equina comprises paired nerve roots L3–S5 of both sides. As it emerges from the intervertebral foramen (occupied by the posterior root ganglion), each spinal nerve gives a recurrent branch supplying ligaments and dura mater.

Segmental sensory distribution is shown by the regular dermatomal pattern of skin innervation by the posterior roots (via the mixed peripheral nerves). Segmental motor supply is expressed in the form of movements performed by specific muscle groups. Nerve root compression, e.g. by a prolapsed disk, may be expressed segmentally by muscle pain, dermatomal paresthesia, cutaneous sensory loss, motor weakness, or loss of a tendon reflex.

Lumbar puncture (spinal tap) is performed by passing a careful needle between spines at L3–L4 or L4–5 – but not if raised intracranial pressure is suspected. A spinal anesthetic is given by injecting local anesthetic into the lumbar cistern. An epidural anesthetic is given into the lumbar epidural space. A caudal anesthetic is given through the sacral hiatus.

REFERENCES

Adams, C.B.T. and Logue, V. (1971) Studies in cervical spondylitic myelopathy. 1. Movement of the cervical roots, dura, and cord, and their relation to the course of extrathecal roots. *Brain* **94**: 557–568.

Auteroche, P. (1983) Innervation of the zygapophyseal joints of the lumbar spine. *Anat. Clin.* **5**: 17–28.

Barson, A.J. and Logue, V. (1970) The vertebral level of termination of the spinal cord during normal and abnormal development. *J. Anat.* **106**: 489–497.

Bogduk, N. (1993) Spinal pain: backache and neck pain. In *Science and Practice in Clinical Neurology* (Gandevia, S.C., Burke, D. and Anthony, M., eds), pp. 39–60. Cambridge: Cambridge University Press.

Groen, D.J., Baljet, R. and Drukker, J. (1990) Nerves and nerve plexuses of the human vertebral column. *Am. J. Anat.* **188**: 282–296.

Holsheimer, J., den Boer, J.A., Strujik, J.J. and Rozeboom, A.R. (1994) MR assessment of the normal position of the spinal cord in the spinal canal. *Am. J. Neuroradiol.* **15**: 951–959.

Postacchini, F. and Rauschning, W. (1999) Anatomy. In *Lumbar Disc Herniation* (Postacchini, F., ed.) pp. 17–58. Berlin: Springer-Verlag.

Russell, E.J. (1990) Cervical disc disease. *Radiology* **177**: 313–325.

Sunderland, S. (1974) Meningeal–dural relationships in the intervertebral foramen. *J. Neurosurg.* **40**: 756–763.

Spinal cord: ascending pathways

GENERAL FEATURES

The arrangement of gray and white matter at different levels of the spinal cord is shown in *Figure 12.1*. The cervical and lumbosacral enlargements are produced by expansions of the gray matter required to service innervation of the limbs. White matter is most abundant in the upper reaches of the cord, which contain the sensory and motor pathways serving all four limbs. In the posterior funiculus, e.g., the gracile fasciculus carries information from the lower limb and is present at cervical as well as lumbosacral segmental levels, whereas the cuneate fasciculus carries information from the upper limb and is not seen at lumbar level.

Although it is convenient to refer to different levels of the spinal cord in terms of numbered segments, corresponding to the sites of attachment of the paired nerve roots, the cord shows no evidence of segmentation internally. The nuclear groups seen in transverse sections are in reality cell columns, most of them spanning several segments (*Figure 12.2*).

Types of spinal neurons

The smallest neurons (soma diameters 5–20 μm) are *propriospinal*, being entirely contained within the cord. Some are confined within a single segment; others span two or more segments by way of the neighboring **propriospinal tract**. Many of the smallest neurons participate in spinal reflexes. Others are intermediate cell stations interposed between fiber tracts descending from the brain and motor neurons projecting to the locomotor apparatus. Others again are so placed as to influence sensory transmission from lower to higher levels of the CNS.

Medium-sized neurons (soma diameters 20–50 μm) are found in all parts of the gray matter except the substantia gelatinosa. Most are *relay (projection) cells* receiving inputs from posterior root afferents and projecting their axons to the brain. The projections are in the form of *tracts*, a tract being defined as a functionally homogeneous group of fibers. As will be seen, the term 'tract' is often used loosely because many projections originally thought to be 'pure' contain more than one functional class of fiber.

The largest neurons of all are the **alpha motor neurons** (soma 50–100 μm) for the supply of skeletal muscles. Scattered among them are small, **gamma motor neurons** supplying muscle spindles. In the medial part of the anterior horn are **Renshaw cells**, which exert tonic inhibition upon alpha motor neurons.

Spinal reflex arcs originating in muscle spindles and tendon organs have been described in Chapter 8, and the withdrawal reflex in Chapter 9.

In thick sections of the spinal cord, the nerve cells exhibit a laminar (layered) arrangement. True lamination is confined to the posterior horn (*Figure 12.3*), but 10 laminae of Rexed have been defined in the gray matter as a whole in order to correlate findings from animal research in different laboratories.

Spinal ganglia

The spinal or posterior root ganglia are located in the intervertebral foramina, where the anterior and posterior roots come together to form the spinal nerves. Thoracic ganglia contain about 50 000 unipolar neurons, and those serving the limbs contain about 100 000. The individual ganglion cells are invested with modified Schwann cells called **satellite cells** (*Figure 12.4*). The common stem axon of each cell bifurcates, sending a centrifugal process into one or other ramus of the spinal nerve (or into the recurrent branch) and a centripetal ('center-seeking') process into the spinal cord. Following stimulation of the peripheral sensory receptors, trains of nerve impulses traverse the point of bifurcation without interruption, although the cell body is also depolarized. The initial segment of the stem axon does not normally generate impulses but it may do so if the adjacent part of the posterior root is compressed, e.g. by a prolapsed intervertebral disc.

Traditionally, the centripetal axons of all spinal ganglion cells have been thought to enter posterior nerve roots. It is now known that many visceral afferents (in particular) enter the cord by way of ventral roots and work their way to the posterior gray horn (Ch. 10). This feature accounts for the frequent failure of *posterior rhizotomy* (surgical section of posterior roots) to relieve pain originating from intra-abdominal cancer.

Central terminations of posterior root afferents
(Figure 12.5)

In the *dorsal root entry zone* close to the surface of the cord, the afferent fibers become segregated into medial and lateral streams. The medial stream comprises medium and large fibers which divide within the posterior funiculus into ascending and descending branches. The branches swing into the posterior gray horn and synapse in laminae II, III and IV. The largest ascending fibers run all the way to the posterior column nuclei (gracilis/cuneatus) in the medulla oblongata. These long fibers form the bulk of the gracile and cuneate fasciculi.

The lateral stream comprises small (Aδ and C) fibers which, upon entry, divide into short ascending and descending branches within the **posterolateral tract** *of Lissauer*. They synapse upon neurons in the marginal zone (lamina I) and in the substantia gelatinosa (lamina II); some fibers synapse upon dendrites of cells belonging to laminae III–V.

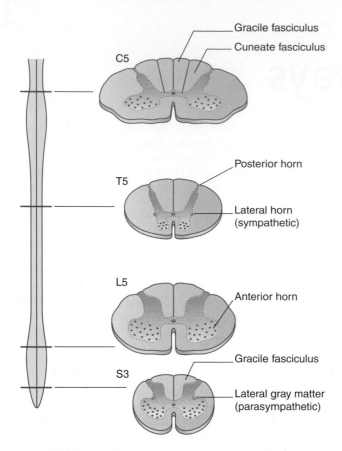

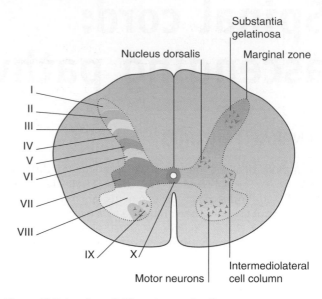

Figure 12.1 Representative transverse sections of the spinal cord.

Figure 12.3 Laminae (I–X) and named cell groups at mid-thoracic level.

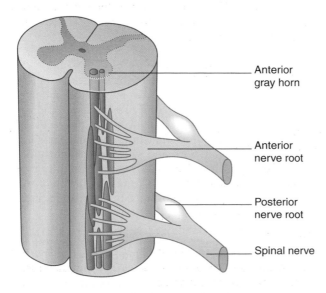

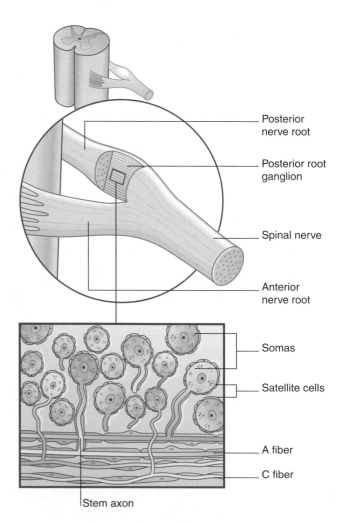

Figure 12.2 Two segments of the spinal cord, showing cell columns in the anterior gray horn.

Figure 12.4 Posterior root ganglion. In bottom figure, note T-shaped bifurcation of stem fibers.

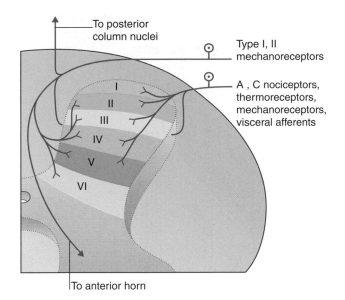

Figure 12.5 Targets of primary afferent neurons in the posterior gray horn.

ASCENDING SENSORY PATHWAYS

Categories of sensation

In accordance with the flowchart in *Table 12.1*, neurologists speak of two kinds of sensation, conscious and nonconscious (unconscious). Conscious sensations are perceived at the level of the cerebral cortex. Nonconscious sensations are not perceived; they have reference to the cerebellum (see later).

Conscious sensations

There are two kinds of conscious sensation: *exteroceptive* and *proprioceptive*. Exteroceptive sensations come from the external world; they impinge either on somatic receptors on the body surface or on telereceptors serving vision and hearing. Somatic sensations include touch, pressure, heat, cold, and pain.

Conscious proprioceptive sensations arise within the body. The receptors concerned are those of the locomotor system (muscles, joints, bones) and of the vestibular labyrinth. The pathways to the cerebral cortex form the substrate for position sense when the body is stationary, and for *kinesthetic sense* during movement.

Nonconscious sensations

These also are of two kinds. *Nonconscious proprioception* is the term used to describe afferent information reaching the cerebellum through the spinocerebellar pathways. This information is essential for smooth motor co-ordination. Second, *enteroception* (*Gr.* enteron, gut) is a little-used term referring to unconscious afferent signals involved in visceral reflexes.

Sensory testing

Routine assessment of *somatic exteroceptive sensation* includes tests for:

- touch, by grazing the skin with the finger tip or a cotton swab

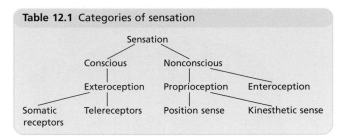

Table 12.1 Categories of sensation

	Sensation		
	Conscious	Nonconscious	
	Exteroception	Proprioception	Enteroception
Somatic receptors	Telereceptors	Position sense	Kinesthetic sense

- pain, by applying the point of a pin
- thermal sense, by applying warm or cold test-tubes to the skin.

In alert and co-operative patients, active and passive tests of conscious proprioception can be performed. Active tests examine the patient's ability to execute set-piece activities with the eyes closed:

- in the erect position, stand still, and 'toe the line' without swaying
- in the seated position, bring the index finger to the nose from the extended position of the arm (finger-to-nose test)
- in the recumbent position, place the heel of the foot on the opposite knee (heel-to-knee test).

Passive tests of conscious proprioception include:

- *Joint sense.* The clinician grasps the thumb or great toe by the sides and moves it while asking the patient to name the direction of movement ('up' or 'down'). Joint sense is mediated in part by articular receptors but mainly by passive stretching of neuromuscular spindles. (If the nerves supplying a joint are anesthetized, or if the joint is completely replaced by a prosthesis, joint sense is only slightly impaired. Alternatively, activation of spindles by means of a vibrator creates the illusion of movement when the relevant joint is stationary.)
- *Vibration sense.* The clinician assesses the patient's ability to detect the vibrations of a tuning fork applied to the radial styloid process or to the shin.

SOMATIC SENSORY PATHWAYS

Two major pathways are involved in somatic sensory perception. They are the *posterior column–medial lemniscal pathway* and the *spinothalamic pathway*. They have the following features in common (*Figure 12.6*):

- Both comprise first-order, second-order, and third-order sets of sensory neurons.
- The somas of the first-order neurons, or *primary afferents*, occupy posterior root ganglia.
- The somas of the second-order neurons occupy CNS gray matter on the same side as the first-order neurons.
- The second-order axons *cross the midline* and then ascend to terminate in the thalamus.
- The third-order neurons project from the thalamus to the somatic sensory cortex.

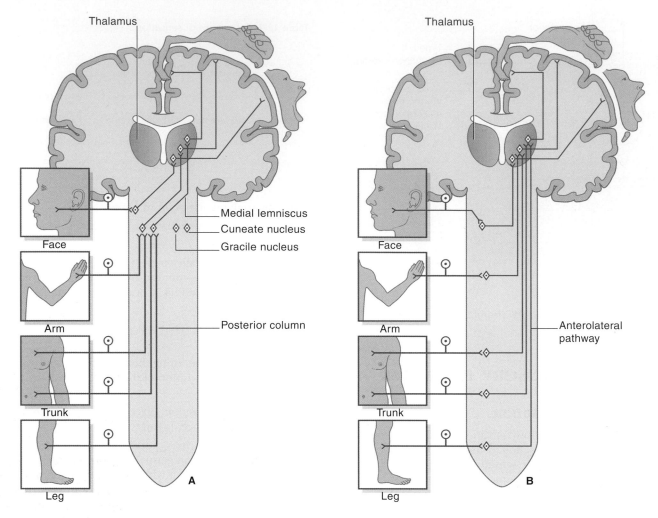

Figure 12.6 Basic plans of **(A)** posterior column–medial lemniscal pathway; **(B)** spinothalamic pathway.

- Both pathways are *somatotopic:* an orderly map of body parts can be identified experimentally in the gray matter at each of the three loci of fiber termination.

- Synaptic transmission from primary to secondary neurons, and from secondary to tertiary, can be modulated (inhibited or enhanced) by other neurons.

Posterior column–medial lemniscal pathway

The first-order afferents include the largest somas in the posterior root ganglia. Their peripheral processes receive information from the largest sensory receptors: Meissner's and Pacinian corpuscles, Ruffini endings and Merkel cell–neurite complexes, neuromuscular spindles, and Golgi tendon organs. The centripetal processes from cells supplying the lower limb and lower trunk give branches to the gray matter before ascending as the **gracile fasciculus (fasciculus gracilis)** to reach the gracile nucleus in the medulla oblongata (*Figure 12.7*). The corresponding collaterals from the upper limb and upper trunk run in the **cuneate fasciculus (fasciculus cuneatus)** to reach the cuneate nucleus.

The second-order afferents commence in the posterior column nuclei, namely the **nucleus gracilis** and **nucleus cuneatus**. They pass ventrally in the tegmentum of the medulla oblongata before intersecting their opposite

numbers in the great **sensory decussation**. Having crossed the midline, the fibers turn rostrally in the **medial lemniscus**.

The medial lemniscus diverges from the midline as it ascends through the tegmentum of the pons and midbrain. It terminates in the lateral part of the ventral posterior nucleus of the thalamus (**ventral posterolateral nucleus**).

Terminating in the medial part of the same nucleus (**ventral posteromedial nucleus**) is the *trigeminal lemniscus*, which serves the head region.

The third-order afferents project from the thalamus to the somatic sensory cortex (see Ch. 24 for details).

Functions

The chief functions of the posterior column–medial lemniscal pathway are those of *conscious proprioception* and *discriminative touch*. Together, these attributes provide the parietal lobe with an instantaneous body image so that we are constantly aware of the position of body parts both at rest and during movement. Without this informational background, the execution of movements is severely impaired.

In humans, disturbance of posterior column function is most often observed in association with demyelinating diseases such as multiple sclerosis. The classic symptom is known as *sensory ataxia*. This term signifies a movement dis-

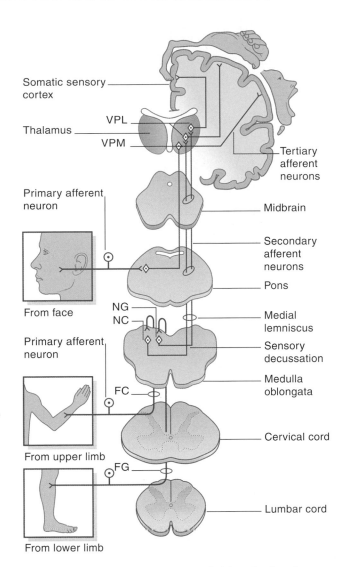

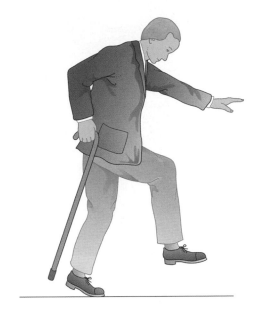

Figure 12.8 The 'stamp and stick' gait of sensory ataxia.

Figure 12.7 The posterior column–medial lemniscal pathway. FC, fasciculus cuneatus; FG, fasciculus gracilis; NC, nucleus cuneatus; NG, nucleus gracilis. VPL, VPM, ventral posterior lateral, ventral posterior medial nuclei of thalamus.

order resulting from sensory impairment, in contrast to *cerebellar ataxia*, in which a movement disorder results from a lesion within the motor system. The patient with a severe sensory ataxia can stand unsupported only with the feet well apart and with the gaze directed downward to include the feet. The gait is broad-based, with a stamping action that maximizes any conscious proprioceptive function that remains (*Figure 12.8*).

Sensory testing in posterior column disease reveals severe swaying when the patient stands with the feet together and the eyes closed. This is *Romberg's sign*. (Inability to 'toe the line' with the eyes closed is tandem Romberg's sign.) The finger-to-nose and/or heel-to-knee tests may reveal loss of kinesthetic sense. Joint sense and vibration sense may also be impaired. (*Note:* Romberg's sign may also be elicited in patients suffering from vestibular disorders (Ch. 16); in cerebellar disorders, there may be instability of station whether the eyes are open or closed (Ch. 22).)

Tactile, painful and thermal sensations are preserved, but

there is impairment of tactile discrimination. The patient has difficulty in discriminating between single and paired stimuli applied to the skin ('two-point discrimination test'); in identifying numbers traced on to the skin by the examiner's finger; and in distinguishing between objects of similar shape but of different textures.

A difficulty in assigning specific functional deficits to posterior column disease is the rarity of pathology affecting the posterior funiculi *alone*. In particular, the posterior part of the lateral funiculus is likely to be involved as well. Postmortem findings from patients having different degrees of pathology in the posterior and lateral funiculi suggest that kinesthetic sense from the lower limb may be mediated in part by fibers that leave the gracile fasciculus at thoracic level and relay rostrally in the posterior part of the lateral funiculus.

Spinothalamic pathway

The spinothalamic pathway consists of second-order sensory neurons projecting from laminae I, III, IV, and V of the posterior gray horn to the contralateral thalamus (*Figure 12.9*). The cells of origin receive excitatory and inhibitory synapses from neurons of the substantia gelatinosa; these have important 'gating' (modulatory) effects on sensory transmission, as explained in Chapter 21.

The axons of the spinothalamic pathway cross the midline in the anterior commissure at all segmental levels. Having crossed, they run upward in the anterolateral part of the cord. This *anterolateral pathway* (as it is usually called) is divisible into an **anterior spinothalamic tract** located in the anterior funiculus and a **lateral spinothalamic tract** located in the lateral funiculus. The two tracts merge in the brainstem as the **spinal lemniscus**. The spinal lemniscus is joined by trigeminal afferents from the head region, and it accompanies the medial lemniscus to the ventral posterior nucleus of the thalamus, terminating immediately behind the medial lemniscus. Third-order sensory neurons

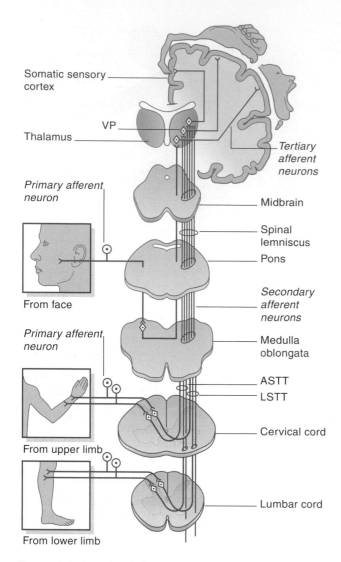

Figure 12.9 The spinothalamic pathway. ASTT, anterior spinothalamic tract; LSTT, lateral spinothalamic tract. VP, ventral posterior nucleus of thalamus.

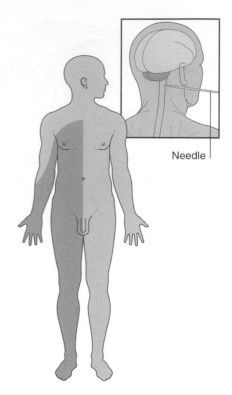

Figure 12.10 Usual extent of analgesia (shaded) following cordotomy at C1–C2 segmental level.

project from the thalamus to the somatic sensory cortex (Ch. 24).

Functions

The functions of the spinothalamic pathway have been elucidated by the procedure known as *cordotomy*, whereby the spinothalamic pathway is interrupted on one or both sides for the relief of intractable pain. For a *percutaneous cordotomy*, the patient is sedated and a needle is passed between the atlas and the axis, into the subarachnoid space. Under radiological guidance, the needle tip is advanced into the anterolateral region of the cord.

A stimulating electrode is passed through the needle. If the placement is correct, a mild current will elicit paresthesia (tingling) on the opposite side of the body. The anterolateral pathway is then destroyed electrolytically. Afterwards, the patient is insensitive to *pinprick, heat,* or *cold* applied to the opposite side (*Figure 12.10*). Sensitivity to *touch* is reduced. The effect commences several segments below the level of the procedure because of the oblique passage of spinothalamic fibers across the white commissure.

Cordotomy is sometimes performed for patients terminally ill with cancer. It is not used for benign conditions because the analgesic (pain-relieving) effect wears off after about a year. This functional recovery may be due to nociceptive transmission either in uncrossed fibers of the spinoreticular system (see later) or in C-fiber collaterals sent to the posterior column nuclei by some axons of the lateral root entry stream.

The internal anatomy of the human spinothalamic pathway has been worked out from postoperative sensory testing and is shown in *Figure 12.11*. The picture is one of *modality segregation*. The lateral spinothalamic tract mediates noxious and thermal sensations separately, and the anterior spinothalamic tract mediates touch. The lateral tract is somatotopically arranged, the neck being represented at the front and the leg at the back. The anterior tract is likely (though not proven) to be somatotopic also.

A rare but classical condition illustrating dissociated sensory loss is illustrated in *Clinical Panel 12.1*.

Spinoreticular tracts

The spinoreticular tracts are the phylogenetically oldest somatosensory pathways. The reticular formation of the brainstem has scant regard for the midline, being often bilaterally distributed in terms of its ascending and descending connections. Spinoreticular fibers originate in laminae V–VII and accompany the spinothalamic pathway as far as the brainstem (*Figure 12.12*). Postmortem studies of

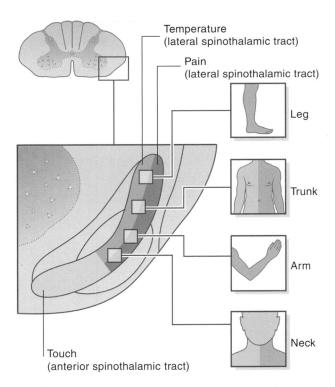

Figure 12.11 Sensory modalities in spinothalamic pathway at upper cervical level.

Temperature
(lateral spinothalamic tract)

Pain
(lateral spinothalamic tract)

Leg

Trunk

Arm

Neck

Touch
(anterior spinothalamic tract)

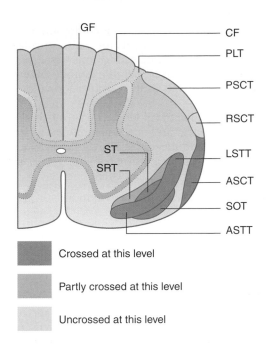

Crossed at this level

Partly crossed at this level

Uncrossed at this level

Figure 12.12 Ascending pathways at upper cervical level. ASCT, anterior spinocerebellar tract; ASTT, anterior spinothalamic tract; CF, cuneate fasciculus; GF, gracile fasciculus; LSTT, lateral spinothalamic tract; PLT, posterolateral tract; PSCT, posterior spinocerebellar tract; RSCT, rostral spinocerebellar tract; SOT, spino-olivary tract; SRT, spinoreticular tract; ST, spinotectal tract.

Clinical Panel 12.1 Syringomyelia

Syringomyelia is a disorder of uncertain etiology, characterized by development of a *syrinx* (fusiform cyst) in or beside the central canal, usually in the cervical region (*Figure CP 12.1.1*). Initial symptoms arise from obliteration of spinothalamic fibers decussating in the white commissure.

The early clinical picture is one of *dissociated sensory loss*: sensitivity is lost to painful and thermal stimuli whereas sensitivity to touch is retained because the posterior column–medial lemniscal pathway is preserved. Typically, the patient develops ulcers on the fingers arising from painless cuts and burns. The joints of the elbow, wrist, and hand may become disorganized over time, or even dislocated, owing to loss of warning sensation from stretched joint capsules.

Progressive expansion of the syrinx may compromise conduction in the long ascending and descending pathways.

Syrinx

Figure CP 12.1.1 Syringomyelia. Shading shows distribution of analgesia.

nerve fiber degeneration following cordotomy procedures indicate that at least half of the spinoreticular fibers may be uncrossed. Accurate estimations based on axonal degeneration are difficult because some spinothalamic fibers give off collaterals to the reticular formation as they pass by.

The spinoreticular tracts terminate at all levels of the brainstem and they are not somatotopically arranged. Impulse traffic is continued rostrally to the thalamus in the *ascending reticular activating system* (Ch. 21). Briefly, the spinoreticular system has two interrelated functions:

1 to arouse the cerebral cortex, i.e. to induce or maintain the waking state

2 to report to the limbic cortex of the anterior cingulate gyrus about the nature of the stimulus. The emotional response may be pleasurable (e.g. to stroking) or aversive (e.g. to pinprick).

In summary, the phylogenetically old, 'paleospinothalamic' pathways through the reticular formation are concerned with the arousal and affective (emotional) aspects of somatic sensory stimuli. In contrast, the direct, 'neospinothalamic' pathway is analytical, encoding information about modality, intensity, and location.

Spinocerebellar pathways

Four fiber tracts run from the spinal cord to the cerebellum. They are:

- posterior spinocerebellar
- cuneocerebellar
- anterior spinocerebellar
- rostral spinocerebellar.

The first two are principally concerned with nonconscious proprioception. The second two report continuously about the state of play among the internuncial neurons of the spinal cord.

Nonconscious proprioception

Nonconscious proprioception is served by the posterior spinocerebellar tract for the lower limb and lower trunk, and by the cuneocerebellar tract for the upper limb and upper trunk. Both are uncrossed, in keeping with the known control by each cerebellar hemisphere of its own side of the body.

The posterior spinocerebellar tract originates in the **posterior thoracic nucleus** (formerly, *dorsal nucleus, Clarke's column*) in lamina VII at the base of the posterior gray horn (*Figure 12.3*). The nucleus extends from T1 through L1 segmental levels and the primary afferents from the lower limb enter the gracile fasciculus to reach it (*Figure 12.13*). It receives primary afferents of all kinds from the muscles and joints, including an intense input from muscle spindle primaries. It also receives collaterals from cutaneous sensory neurons. The fibers of the posterior spinocerebellar tract are the largest in the entire CNS, measuring 20 μm in external diameter. Very fast conduction is required to keep the cerebellum informed about ongoing movements. The tract ascends close to the surface of the

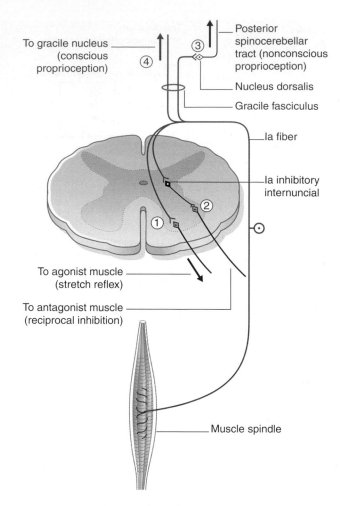

Figure 12.13 Functional anatomy of a spindle primary afferent from the lower limb. **(1)** Stretch reflex; **(2)** Ia internuncial serving reciprocal inhibition; **(3)** nonconscious proprioception; **(4)** kinesthesia.

cord (*Figure 12.13*) and enters the inferior cerebellar peduncle.

The **cuneocerebellar tract** comes from the **accessory cuneate nucleus**, which lies above and outside the cuneate nucleus. The primary afferent inputs are of the same nature as those for the posterior thoracic nucleus; they reach it through the cuneate fasciculus. The cuneocerebellar tract enters the inferior cerebellar peduncle.

Information from reflex arcs

Two tracts originate in the intermediate gray matter of the cord. Although they receive some primary afferents of a similar nature to those already mentioned, their main function is to monitor the state of activity of spinal reflex arcs.

From the lower half of the cord, the pathway is the **anterior spinocerebellar tract** (*Figure 12.13*). The component fibers cross initially and run close to the surface as far as the midbrain. They then turn into the *superior* cerebellar peduncle and re-cross within the cerebellar white matter.

From the upper half of the cord, the **rostral spinocerebellar tract** ascends without crossing and enters (mainly) the inferior cerebellar peduncle.

Core Information

The unipolar neurons of the spinal ganglia are first-order (primary) sensory neurons. They send a centrifugal process to peripheral tissues and a centripetal process into the cord. They serve all categories of somatic and visceral sensation, conscious and nonconscious.

Conscious proprioception and discriminative touch are served by large centripetal processes that ascend to the posterior column nuclei in the medulla where second-order neurons project via the sensory decussation to the contralateral thalamus; third-order neurons project to the somatic sensory cortex.

Painful, thermal, and more crude tactile sensations are served by fine processes that enter Lissauer's tract and end in the posterior gray horn; second-order neurons project across the midline at all segmental levels, coalescing as the spinothalamic tract (anterior and lateral) which is similarly relayed by the thalamus.

The spinoreticular tract projects to the brainstem reticular formation of both sides; it has an arousal function and is concerned with qualitative aspects of stimuli.

First-order neurons serving unconscious proprioception from the lower body end in the posterior thoracic nucleus, for relay to the ipsilateral cerebellum by the posterior spinocerebellar tract; from the upper body, they run via cuneate fasciculus to accessory cuneate nucleus for relay by the cuneocerebellar tract.

Information about activity in spinal reflex arcs is relayed (partly crossed) by the anterior and rostral spinocerebellar tracts.

The spinotectal tract (tactile function, crossed) runs to the superior colliculus for integration with visual data. The spino-olivary tract runs to the inferior olivary nucleus.

OTHER ASCENDING PATHWAYS

The **spinotectal tract** runs alongside the spinothalamic pathway (*Figure 12.13*), which it resembles in its origin and functional composition. It ends in the superior colliculus, where it joins crossed visual inputs involved in turning the eyes/head/trunk toward sources of sensory stimulation (**spinovisual reflex**).

The **spino-olivary tract** sends tactile information to the **inferior olivary nucleus** in the medulla oblongata. The inferior olivary nucleus has an important function in *motor learning* through its action on the contralateral cerebellar cortex (Ch. 22). The spino-olivary tract may have a role in modifying olivary discharge when a moving part encounters an obstacle (e.g. if the toe is stubbed while climbing a stairway).

A *spinocervical tract* is well developed in the cat, where the spinothalamic pathways are small. It seems to be vestigial or absent in humans.

REFERENCES

Cervero, F. (1986) Dorsal horn neurons and their sensory inputs. In *Spinal Afferent Processing* (Yaksh, T.L., ed.), pp. 197–216. New York: Plenum Press.

Coggeshall, R.E. (1990) Unmyelinated primary afferent fibers in the dorsal column, a possible alternate ascending pathway for noxious information. In *Recent Achievements in Restorative Neurology 3: Altered Sensation and Pain* (Dimitrijivic, S. et al., eds), pp. 128–131. Basel: Karger.

Dykes, R.W. (1983) Parallel processing of somatosensory information: a theory. *Brain Res. Rev.* **6**: 47–115.

Nathan, P.W., Smith, M.C. and Cook, A.W. (1986) Sensory effects in man of lesions of the posterior columns and of some other afferent pathways. *Brain* **109**: 1003–1041.

Smith, M.C. and Deacon, P. (1984) Topographical anatomy of the posterior columns of the spinal cord in man. *Brain* **107**: 671–698.

Willis, W.D. (1985) Ascending somatosensory systems. In *Spinal Afferent Processing* (Yaksh, T.L., ed.), pp. 243–274. New York: Plenum Press.

Spinal cord: descending pathways

ANATOMY OF THE ANTERIOR GRAY HORN

Cell columns

Each of the columns of motor neurons in the anterior gray horn supplies a group of muscles having similar functions. The individual muscles are supplied from cell groups (nuclei) within the columns. Axial (trunk) muscles are supplied from medially placed columns, proximal limb segment muscles from the midregion, and distal limb segment musculature from lateral columns (*Figure 13.1*). Columns supplying extensor muscles lie anterior to columns supplying flexors; hence the presence of ventromedial and dorsomedial columns for the trunk, and ventrolateral and dorsolateral columns for the limbs. A retrodorsolateral nucleus is devoted to the intrinsic muscles of the hand and foot. An isolated, central nucleus supplies the diaphragm.

The segmental levels of the six somatomotor cell columns are listed in *Table 13.1*. The autonomic nervous system is represented by the intermediolateral cell column.

Cell types

Large, **α (alpha) motor neurons** supply the extrafusal fibers of the skeletal muscles. Interspersed among them are small, **γ (gamma) motor neurons** supplying the intrafusal fibers of neuromuscular spindles.

Tonic and phasic motor neurons

The α motor neurons have large dendritic trees receiving some 10 000 excitatory boutons from propriospinal neurons and from supraspinal pathways descending from the cerebral cortex and brainstem. (The term 'supraspinal' refers to any pathway descending to the cord from a higher level.) The somas of α motor neurons receive some 5000 inhibitory boutons, mostly from propriospinal sources.

Two principal types of α motor neurons are recognized, tonic and phasic. Tonic α motor neurons innervate slow, oxidative–glycolytic (SOG) muscle fibers; they are readily depolarized and have relatively slowly conducting axons with small spike amplitudes. Phasic α motor neurons innervate squads of fast, oxidative (FO) and fast, oxidative–glycolytic (FOG) muscle fibers. The phasic neurons are larger, have higher thresholds, and have rapidly conducting axons with large spike amplitudes.

Tonic neurons are usually the first recruits when voluntary movements are initiated, even if the movement is to be fast.

Renshaw cells

The axons of the α motor neurons give off recurrent branches which form excitatory, cholinergic synapses upon inhibitory internuncial neurons called *Renshaw cells* in the medial part of the anterior horn. The Renshaw cells form inhibitory, glycinergic synapses upon the α motor neurons. This is a classic example of *negative feedback*, or *recurrent inhibition*, through which the discharges of α motor neurons are self-limiting (see *Clinical Panel 13.1*).

Segmental-level inputs to α motor neurons

At each segmental level, α motor neurons receive powerful excitatory and inhibitory inputs. Note that any inhibitory effect produced by activity in dorsal nerve root fibers requires interpolation of inhibitory internuncials, since all primary afferent neurons are excitatory in nature.

Segmental-level inputs to a flexor α motor neuron include the following:

- Type Ia and Type II afferents from spindles in the flexor muscles provide the afferent limb of the monosynaptic stretch reflex (e.g. the biceps reflex).
- Type Ia afferents from spindles in extensor muscles exert reciprocal inhibition upon the flexor motor neurons via Ia inhibitory internuncials.
- Type Ib afferent from Golgi tendon organs in the flexor muscles exert autogenetic inhibition upon the flexor motor neurons.
- Type Ib afferents from Golgi tendon organs in extensor muscles exert reciprocal excitation of flexors via excitatory internuncials.
- Afferents from the flexor aspect of relevant synovial joints are stimulated when the capsule becomes taut in extension. They initiate an articular protective reflex, as described in Chapter 9.
- In execution of the *withdrawal reflex* described in Chapter 11, large numbers of excitatory, 'flexor reflex' internuncials are activated over several spinal segments on the same side as the stimulus, as well as inhibitory internuncials supplying motor neurons to antagonist muscles.
- Renshaw cells.

A reciprocal list can be drawn up for extensor motor neurons, with substitution of extensor thrust inputs for flexor reflex internuncials.

DESCENDING MOTOR PATHWAYS

Important pathways descending to the spinal cord are the following:

- corticospinal (pyramidal)
- reticulospinal (extrapyramidal)
- vestibulospinal

Clinical Panel 13.1 Strychnine poisoning

Strychnine is a glycine receptor blocker. The victim of strychnine poisoning suffers agonizing convulsions because of liberation of α motor neurons from the tonic inhibitory control of Renshaw cells. The convulsions resemble those induced by the tetanus toxin, described in Chapter 6. This is no surprise because tetanus toxin prevents the release of glycine from Renshaw cells. Postmortem studies of normal human brain, using radiolabeled strychnine, have shown glycine receptors to be especially abundant on internuncial neurons in the nucleus of the trigeminal nerve supplying the jaw muscles, and in the nucleus of the facial nerve supplying the muscles of facial expression. These two muscle groups are especially affected in both types of convulsive attack.

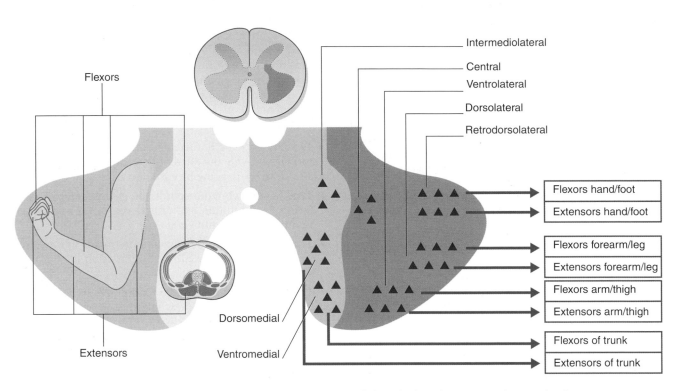

Figure 13.1 Cell columns in the anterior gray horn of the spinal cord: somatotopic organization.

Table 13.1 The somatomotor cell columns

Cell column	Muscles
Ventromedial (all segments)	Erector spinae
Dorsomedial (T1–L2)	Intercostals, abdominals
Ventrolateral (C5–C8, L2–S2)	Arm/thigh
Dorsolateral (C6–C8, L3–S3)	Forearm/leg
Retrodorsolateral (C8, T1, S1–S2)	Hand/foot
Central (C3–C5)	Diaphragm

- raphespinal
- aminergic
- autonomic.

Corticospinal tract

The corticospinal tract is the great voluntary motor pathway. Some 60–80% of its fibers take their origin from the primary motor cortex in the precentral gyrus. Other sources include the supplementary motor area on the medial side of the hemisphere, the premotor cortex on the lateral side, the somatic sensory cortex, and the superior parietal lobule (*Figure 13.2*). The contributions from the two sensory areas mentioned terminate in sensory nuclei of the brainstem and spinal cord, where they modulate sensory transmission.

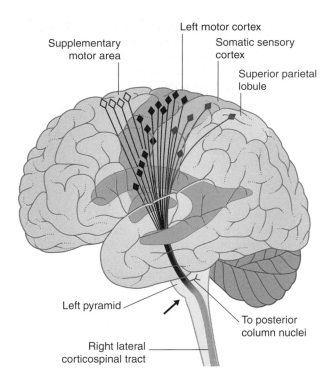

Figure 13.2 Pyramidal tract visualized from the left side. The supplementary motor area is on the medial surface of the hemisphere. Arrow indicates level of pyramidal decussation. Non-motor neurons are shown in blue.

The corticospinal tract descends through the corona radiata and internal capsule to reach the brainstem. It continues through the crus of the midbrain and the basilar pons to reach the medulla oblongata. Here it forms the **pyramid** (hence the synonym, pyramidal tract).

During its descent through the brainstem, the corticospinal tract gives off fibers which activate motor cranial nerve nuclei, notably those serving the muscles of the face, jaw, and tongue. These fibers are called *corticonuclear* (*Figure 13.3*). (The term *'corticobulbar'* is sometimes used, but 'bulb' is open to different interpretations.)

Just above the spinomedullary junction (*Figure 13.4*):

- About 80% of the pyramidal fibers cross the midline in the **pyramidal decussation**.
- These fibers descend on the contralateral side of the spinal cord as the **lateral corticospinal tract** (crossed corticospinal tract, LCST).
- About 10% enter the **anterior corticospinal tract**, which occupies the anterior funiculus at cervical and upper thoracic levels. These fibers cross in the white commissure and supply motor neurons serving deep muscles in the neck.
- About 10% of the pyramidal fibers enter the lateral corticospinal tract on the same side.

The corticospinal tract contains about one million nerve fibers. The average conduction velocity is 60 m/s, indicating an average fiber diameter of 10 µm ('rule of six' in Ch. 6). About 3% of the fibers are extra large (up to 20 µm); they arise from **giant neurons (cells of Betz)**, located mainly in

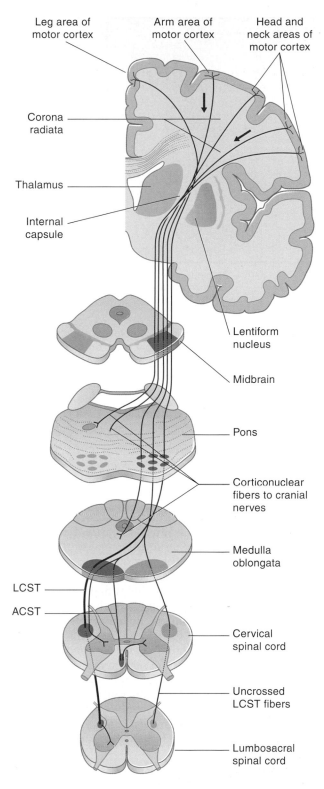

Figure 13.3 The pyramidal tract. ACST, anterior corticospinal tract; LCST, lateral corticospinal tract. *Note*: Only the motor components are shown; the parietal lobe components are omitted.

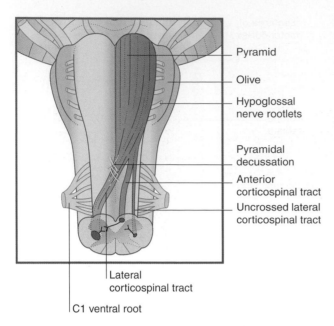

Pyramid

Olive

Hypoglossal
nerve rootlets

Pyramidal
decussation

Anterior
corticospinal tract

Uncrossed lateral
corticospinal tract

Lateral
corticospinal tract

C1 ventral root

Figure 13.4 Ventral view of medulla oblongata and upper spinal cord, showing the three spinal projections of the left pyramid.

the leg area of the motor cortex (Ch. 26). All corticospinal fibers are excitatory and appear to use glutamate as their transmitter substance.

Targets of the lateral corticospinal tract

Distal limb motor neurons

In the anterior gray horn, LCST axons synapse upon the dendrites of α and γ motor neurons supplying limb muscles, notably in the upper limb. A unique property of these *corticomotoneuronal fibers* of LCST is that of *fractionation*, whereby small groups of neurons can be selectively activated. This is most obvious in the case of the index finger, which can be flexed or extended quite independently, although three of its long tendons arise from muscle bellies devoted to all four fingers. Fractionation is essential for the execution of skilled movements such as buttoning a coat or tying shoe laces. Skilled movements are lost, and seldom recover completely, following damage to the corticomotoneuronal system anywhere from the motor cortex to the spinal cord.

Although fractionation is a manifestly important function, even simple voluntary movements, such as flexion of the elbow or abduction of the shoulder, are initiated by corticomotoneuronal fibers.

As mentioned already in Chapter 8, the α and γ motor neurons are coactivated by the LCST during a given movement, so that spindles in the prime movers are signaling active stretch while those in the antagonists are signaling passive stretch.

Renshaw cells

The number of possible functions served by LCST synapses on Renshaw cells is large because some of the cells synapse mainly upon Ia inhibitory internuncials, and others upon other Renshaw cells. Probably the most important function

is to permit *co-contraction* of prime movers and their antagonists, in order to fix one or more joints, e.g. when a chopping or shoveling action is required of the hand. Co-contraction is achieved by inactivation of Ia inhibitory internuncials by Renshaw cells.

Excitatory internuncials

In the intermediate gray matter and the base of the anterior horn, motor neurons supplying axial (vertebral) and proximal limb muscles are recruited mainly indirectly by the LCST, by way of excitatory internuncials.

Ia inhibitory internuncials

Also located in the intermediate gray matter are the Ia inhibitory internuncials, and these are the *first* neurons to be activated by the LCST during voluntary movements. Activity of the Ia internuncials causes the antagonist muscles to relax before the prime movers (agonists) contract. In addition, it renders the antagonists' motor neurons refractory to stimulation by spindle afferents passively stretched by the movement. The sequence of events is shown in *Figure 13.5* and its caption for voluntary flexion of the knee.

(*Note on terminologies*: During quiet standing, the knees are 'locked' in slight hyperextension and the quadriceps is inactive, as indicated by the patellae being 'loose'. Any tendency of one or both knees to go into flexion is counteracted by a twitch of quadriceps in response to passive stretching of dozens of muscle spindles there. Because the flexion movement is resisted in this way, the reflex concerned is called a *resistance reflex*. During voluntary flexion of the knee, on the other hand, the movement is helped along in the manner described in the caption to *Figure 13.5*, through an *assistance reflex*. The *change of sign* (from negative to positive) is called *reflex reversal*.)

Presynaptic inhibitory neurons serving the stretch reflex

Consider a sprinter. At each stride, gravity pulls the body out of the air onto a knee extended by the quadriceps muscle. At the moment of impact, all of the muscle spindles in the contracted quadriceps are thrown into active stretch. The obvious danger is that the quadriceps may rupture. Golgi tendon endings (Ch. 8) offer some protection through autogenetic inhibition, but the main protection seems to be through presynaptic inhibition by the LCST of spindle afferents close to their contact points with motor neurons. At the same time, preservation of the ankle jerk is advantageous in this situation, giving immediate recruitment of calf motor neurons for the next take-off. The extent of suppression of the stretch reflex by the LCST in fact appears to depend upon the particular motor program being executed.

Presynaptic inhibition of first-second-order afferents

In the posterior gray horn, there is some suppression of sensory transmission into the spinothalamic pathway during voluntary movement. This is brought about by activation of inhibitory internuncials synapsing upon primary afferent nerve terminals.

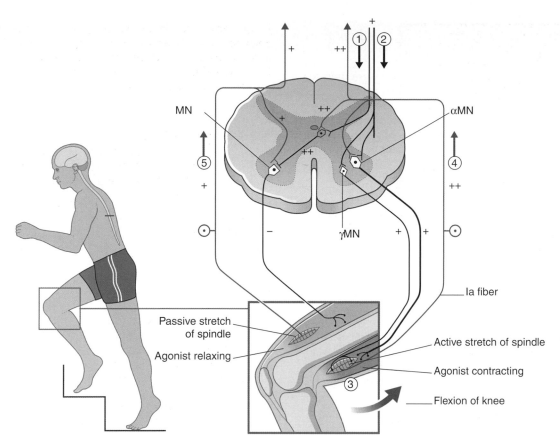

Figure 13.5 Sequence of events in a voluntary movement (flexion of the knee). **(1)** Activation of Ia internuncials to inhibit antagonist α motor neurons (αMN); **(2)** activation of agonist α and γ motor neurons; **(3)** activation of extrafusal and intrafusal muscle fibers; **(4)** feedback from actively stretched spindles increases excitation of agonist α motor neurons and inhibition of antagonist α motor neuron; **(5)** Ia fibers from passively stretched antagonist spindles find the respective α motor neurons refractory. *Note*: The sequence, γ motor neuron–Ia fiber–α motor neuron, is known as the *gamma loop*.

Modulation is more subtle at the level of the gracile and cuneate nuclei, where pyramidal tract fibers (after crossing) are capable of either enhancing sensory transmission during slow, exploratory movements, or reducing it during rapid movements.

Upper and lower motor neurons

In the context of disease, clinicians refer to the corticospinal (and corticonuclear) neurons as upper motor neurons (*Clinical Panel 13.2*), and those of the brain stem and spinal cord as lower motor neurons (*Clinical Panel 13.3*).

Reticulospinal tracts

The reticulospinal tracts originate in the reticular formation of the pons and medulla oblongata. They are partially crossed.

The **pontine reticulospinal tract** descends ipsilaterally in the anterior funiculus, and the **medullary reticulospinal tract** descends, partly crossed, in the lateral funiculus (*Figure 13.6*). Both tracts act, via internuncials shared with the corticospinal tract, upon motor neurons supplying axial (trunk) and proximal limb muscles. Information from animal experiments indicates that the pontine reticulospinal tract acts

upon extensor motor neurons and the medullary reticulospinal tract upon flexor motor neurons. Both pathways exert reciprocal inhibition.

The reticulospinal system is involved in two different kinds of motor behavior: *locomotion* and *postural control*.

Locomotion

Walking and running are rhythmical events involving all four limbs. Movements of the two sides are reciprocal with respect to flexor and extensor contractions and relaxations. In lower animals, locomotion is regulated by a hierarchical system in which the lowest members are internuncial neurons on both sides at cervical and lumbosacral levels, activating the flexors and extensors of the individual limbs. They are called *pattern generators*. Co-ordinating the pattern generators for the individual limbs is a further generator situated in the intermediate gray matter at the upper end of the spinal cord; it is capable of initiating rhythmical movements after section of the neuraxis at the spinomedullary junction. Locomotion is initiated from a *locomotor center* stretched across the upper part of the pons. In anesthetized animals, electrical stimulation of the locomotor center with pulses of increasing frequency

Clinical Panel 13.2   Upper motor neuron disease

Upper motor neuron disease is a clinical term used to denote interruption of the corticospinal tract somewhere along its course. If the lesion occurs above the level of the pyramidal decussation, the signs will be detected on the opposite side of the body; if it occurs below the decussation, the signs will be detected on the same side.

Sudden interruption of the corticospinal tract is characterized by the following features:

1 The affected limb(s) show an initial flaccid (floppy) paralysis with loss of tendon reflexes. Normal muscle tone – defined as the resistance to passive movement (e.g. flexion/extension of the knee by the examiner) – is lost.

2 After several days or weeks, some return of voluntary motor function can be expected. At the same time, muscle tone increases progressively. The typical long-term effect on muscle tone is one of *spasticity*, with abnormally brisk reflexes (*hyperreflexia*). Classically, spasticity in the leg is 'claspknife' in character: after initial strong resistance to passive flexion of the knee, the joint gives way.

3 *Clonus* can often be elicited at the ankle/wrist. It consists of rhythmic contraction of the flexor muscles 5–10 times per second in response to sudden passive dorsiflexion.

4 *Babinski sign* (*extensor plantar response*) consists of dorsiflexion of the great toe and fanning of the other toes in response to a scraping stimulus applied to the sole of the foot. The normal response is flexion of the toes (*Figure CP 13.2.1*).

5 *The abdominal reflexes* are absent on the affected side. A normal abdominal reflex consists of brief contraction of the abdominal muscles when the overlying skin is scraped.

The above features are most commonly observed after a vascular *stroke* interrupting the corticospinal tract on one side of the cerebrum or brainstem. The usual picture here is one of initial flaccid *hemiplegia* ('half-paralysis'), followed by a permanent spastic *hemiparesis* ('half-weakness'). As illustrated in Chapter 30, *Clinical Panel 30.2*, the spasticity following a stroke characteristically affects the antigravity muscles. In the lower limb, these are the extensors of the knee and the plantar flexors of the foot; in the upper limb, they are the flexors of the elbow and of the wrist and fingers. Following complete transection of the spinal cord, on the other hand, there may be a *paraplegia in flexion* of the lower limbs, owing to concurrent interruption of the vestibulospinal tract (*Clinical Panel 13.4*).

The 'positive' signs listed under **2**, **3**, and **4** cannot be explained on the basis of interruption of the corticospinal tract alone. In the rare cases in which the human pyramid has been transected surgically,

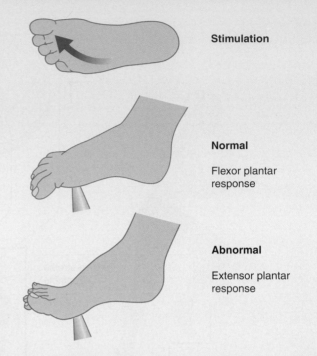

Stimulation

Normal

Flexor plantar response

Abnormal

Extensor plantar response

Figure CP 13.2.1 The plantar reflex.

spasticity and hyperreflexia have not been prominent later on, although a Babinski sign has been present.

Spasticity and hyperreflexia are largely explained by the fact that stretch reflexes in spastic muscle groups are hyperactive. Electromyograph (EMG) records of spastic muscles show enhanced motor unit activity in response to relatively slow rates of stretch, e.g. slow passive elbow extension. However, this is not the sole basis of explanation. In patients with spastic hemiparesis, the ankle flexors show increased tone (resistance to passive dorsiflexion) even with very slow rates of stretch – too slow to elicit any EMG response. The resistance takes several weeks to become pronounced. It is called 'passive stiffness' and may be caused by progressive accumulation of collagen within the muscles affected. In addition, biochemical changes within paretic muscle leads to increasing change of fast-twitch to slow-twitch fibers, accounting for progressively greater difficulty in execution of rapid movements.

Why are motor neurons hyperexcitable?
In paraplegic patients, spasticity and hyperreflexia are often accompanied by increased cutaneomuscular reflex excitability, through polysynaptic propriospinal pathways. Pulling on a pair of trousers may be enough to produce spasms of the hip and knee flexors, sometimes accompanied by autonomic effects (sweating, hypertension, emptying of the bladder). Where the requisite technical facilities exist, the

situation can be dramatically improved by perfusion of the lumbar CSF cistern with minute amounts of *baclofen*, a GABA-mimetic (imitative) drug. The first inference is that the drug diffuses through the pia-glial membrane of the spinal cord, activates GABA receptors located on the surface of primary afferent nerve terminals, and dampens impulse traffic by means of presynaptic inhibition. The second inference is that the resident population of GABA neurons in the substantia gelatinosa has fallen silent in these cases through loss of tonic supraspinal 'drive'. The normal source of supraspinal drive seems to derive in part from the corticospinal tract, and in part from corticoreticulospinal fibers that reach the spinal cord via the tegmentum of the brainstem rather than via the pyramids.

Figure CP 13.2.2 shows the distribution of inhibitory nerve endings derived from Renshaw cells. Not alone do they normally have a tonic breaking action on α and γ motor neurons at their own segmental level: they also tonically inhibit heteronymous motor neurons (i.e. those serving other muscle groups). For example, they act simultaneously upon motor neurons controlling knee and ankle movements, as part of the executive arm of central motor programs regulating successive muscle engagements and disengagements during locomotion. Locomotion is controlled by reticulospinal rather than corticospinal neurons, and any reduction in reticulospinal drive will render motor neurons hyperexcitable, and accounts for the frequent occurrence of ill-timed contractions produced by heteronymous motor neurons.

How do voluntary movements recover?

The simplest explanation for the return of voluntary movement on the affected side would be a progressive increase in influence of the *ipsilateral* (unaffected) motor cortex on the 10% of *uncrossed* fibers in the pyramidal tract. Radiological studies of cortical metabolic activity (Ch. 24) indicate that ipsilateral motor areas do in fact become more active. It is of

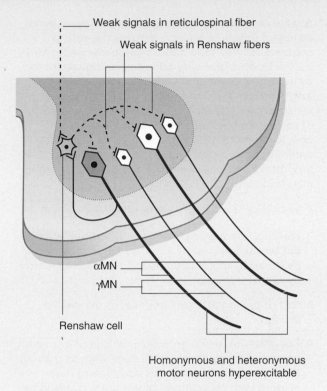

Figure CP 13.2.2 Impaired Renshaw cell activity in spasticity. MN, motor neurons.

interest in this context that in right-handed individuals, i.e. where the left hemisphere is dominant (a) right hemiplegias are usually more disabling than left hemiplegias; and (b) patients with right hemiplegia more often report some clumsiness of skilled movement on the *left* side. The inference seems to be that in right-handers the left cortical motor areas normally make a significant contribution to motor function on the ipsilateral side.

(For recovery of *automatic* locomotion, see Ch. 26.)

Clinical Panel 13.3 Lower motor neuron disease

Disease of lower motor neurons may be caused by a variety of infectious agents – notably the virus of poliomyelitis. The term *motor neuron disease*, or MND, is used to describe a symptom complex characterized by degeneration of upper and lower motor neurons in late middle age. The etiology is unknown; the variable manifestations of the disease are suggestive of more than one cause. During the first year or two, lower motor neurons alone may be involved, especially in the upper limbs. This phase is called *progressive muscular atrophy* and it has the following manifestations:

1 *Weakness* of the muscles affected, together with

2 *Wasting*. The wasting is not merely a disuse atrophy but results from loss of a trophic (nourishing) factor produced by motor neurons and conveyed to muscle by axonal transport.

3 *Loss of tendon reflexes* (areflexia) in the wasted muscles.

4 *Fasciculations*, which are visible twitchings of small groups of muscle fibers in the early stage of wasting. They arise from spontaneous discharge of motor neurons with activation of motor units. It should be stressed that fasciculations are sometimes observed in healthy muscle, especially after exercise.

5 *Fibrillations*, which are minute contractions detectable only by needle electromyography (a recording electrode in the form of a needle is inserted into the muscle). Fibrillations are the result of denervation supersensitivity: following denervation, additional ACh receptors develop along the surface of muscle fibers, to the extent that the fibers respond to minute amounts of free ACh in the circulating blood.

6 Sooner or later, signs of upper motor neuron disease appear. The lower limbs become weak, with increased muscle tone and brisk reflexes. This condition is called *amyotrophic lateral sclerosis*. Motor cranial nerve nuclei in the pons and medulla oblongata may be involved from the start (*progressive bulbar palsy*, Ch. 15) or only terminally. Death, from respiratory complications, usually occurs within 5 years of onset.

The search for etiological clues is intense. Damage to motor neurons by free radicals has long been suspected, and it is of interest that mutation of a free-radical scavenging enzyme has been detected in some of the 10% of patients who inherit MND in an autosomal dominant mode. Other research targets concern the numbers and nature of neurofilaments, the question of autoimmune disorder, and possible benefits of administering neurotrophic (nerve growth) factors.

---

produces walking movements, then trotting, and finally, galloping.

Although the basic locomotor patterns are inbuilt, they are modulated by sensory feedback from the terrain. Overall control of the motor output resides in the premotor cortex, which has direct projections to the pontine and medullary neurons that give rise to the reticulospinal tracts. The tracts are used to steer the animal as it walks or runs and to override the spinal generators, e.g. in scaling a wall.

Human locomotion is less 'spinal' than that of quadrupeds. However, the general neuroanatomical framework has been conserved during higher evolution, and the basic physiology seems to be in place as well. In particular, a bilaterally organized motor system controlling proximal and axial muscles *must* exist to account for the return of near-perfect locomotor function following removal of an entire cerebral hemisphere during childhood or adolescence. Such people never recover manual skill on the contralateral side, and this reinforces the belief among physical therapists that two distinct pathways are involved in motor control: *pyramidal* and '*extrapyramidal*'. The latter term denotes the reticulospinal pathway and its controls upstream in the cerebral cortex and basal ganglia.

Higher-level locomotor controls are described in Chapter 21.

Posture

Definitions of posture vary with the context in which the term is used. In the general context of standing, sitting, and recumbency, posture may be defined as the position held between movements. In the local context of a single hand or foot, the term denotes *postural fixation* – the immobilization of proximal limb joints by co-contraction of the surrounding muscles, leaving the distal limb parts free to do voluntary business. As will be noted in Chapter 26, there is reason to believe that the human premotor cortex is programmed to select appropriate proximal muscle groups by way of the reticulospinal tracts, to set the stage for any particular movement of the hand or foot.

The interpolation of internuncial neurons between the two main motor pathways acting upon motor neurons serving axial and proximal limb muscles means that either pathway may be in command for a particular movement sequence – the extrapyramidal (reticulospinal) pathway for routine tasks such as walking along a clear path, the pyramidal pathway for tasks requiring close attention, e.g. picking one's way along a path strewn with rubble.

Tectospinal tract

The tectospinal tract is a crossed pathway descending from the tectum of the midbrain to the medial part of

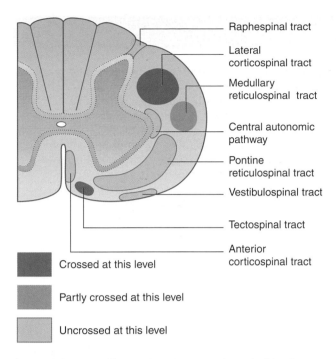

Raphespinal tract

Lateral corticospinal tract

Medullary reticulospinal tract

Central autonomic pathway

Pontine reticulospinal tract

Vestibulospinal tract

Tectospinal tract

Anterior corticospinal tract

Crossed at this level

Partly crossed at this level

Uncrossed at this level

Figure 13.6 Descending pathways at upper cervical level. *Notes*: The anterior corticospinal tract crosses completely at cervical and upper thoracic levels to engage anterior horn cells. Some 10% of lateral corticospinal tract fibers descend ipsilaterally.

the anterior gray horn at cervical and upper thoracic levels. It is strategically placed for access to axial motor neurons (*Figure 13.6*).

The tectospinal tract is an important motor pathway in the reptilian brain, being responsible for orienting the head/trunk toward sources of visual stimulation (superior colliculus) or auditory stimulation (inferior colliculus). It is likely to have similar automatic functions in humans.

Vestibulospinal tract

The vestibulospinal tract is an important uncrossed pathway whereby the tone of appropriate antigravity muscles is automatically increased when the head is tilted to one side. It descends in the anterior funiculus (*Figure 13.6*) and its function is to keep the center of gravity between the feet. It originates in the vestibular nucleus in the medulla oblongata. (*Note*: As explained in Chapter 16, there are in fact two vestibulospinal tracts on each side. The unqualified term refers to the lateral vestibulospinal tract.)

Raphespinal tract

The raphespinal tract originates in and beside the raphe nucleus situated in the midline in the medulla oblongata. It descends on both sides within the posterolateral tract of Lissauer. Its function is to modulate sensory transmission between first- and second-order neurons in the posterior gray horn – particularly with respect to pain (see Ch. 21).

Aminergic pathways

Aminergic pathways descend from specialized cell groups in the pons and medulla oblongata (Ch. 19). The principal neurotransmitters involved are *norepinephrine* and *serotonin*, both of which are classed as *biogenic amines*. The aminergic pathways descend in the outer parts of the anterior and lateral funiculi, and are distributed widely in the spinal gray matter. In general terms, they have inhibitory effects on sensory neurons and facilitatory effects on motor neurons.

Central autonomic pathways

Central sympathetic and parasympathetic fibers descend beside the intermediate gray matter (*Figure 13.6*). They originate in part from autonomic control centers in the hypothalamus and in part from several nuclear groups in the brainstem. They terminate in the intermediolateral cell columns that give rise to the preganglionic sympathetic and parasympathetic fibers of the peripheral autonomic system.

The central sympathetic pathway is required for normal *baroreceptor reflex* activity. If the spinal cord is crushed in a neck injury, the patient loses consciousness if raised from the recumbent position within the first week or so because a fall of blood pressure in the carotid sinus on sitting up normally causes a compensatory increase in sympathetic activity in order to maintain blood flow to the brain.

The central parasympathetic pathway is required for normal bladder (and rectal) function. The fibers concerned originate in the reticular formation, mainly at the level of the pons (Ch. 21). The pontine micturition center has a tonic inhibitory action on the sacral parasympathetic system. Severe injury to the spinal cord or cauda equina results in reflex voiding when the bladder is only half full (*Clinical Panel 13.4*).

Note on the rubrospinal tract
The rubrospinal tract is an important motor pathway in cats and dogs, where it arises in the contralateral red nucleus and descends in front of the corticospinal tract. In monkeys this tract is small and in humans it is quite negligible.

BLOOD SUPPLY OF THE SPINAL CORD

Arteries

Close to the foramen magnum, the two vertebral arteries give off **anterior** and **posterior spinal** branches. The anterior branches fuse to form a single **anterior spinal artery** in front of the anterior median fissure (*Figure 13.7*). Branches are given alternately to the left and right sides of the spinal cord. The posterior spinal arteries descend along the line of attachment of the dorsal nerve roots on each side.

The three spinal arteries are boosted by several **radiculospinal branches** from the vertebral arteries and from intercostal arteries. They are distinguishable from the small **radicular arteries** which enter every intervertebral foramen to nourish the nerve roots. The largest radiculospinal

Clinical Panel 13.4   Spinal cord injury

In the industrialized world, automobile accidents are the commonest cause of spinal cord injury. More than half of the victims are between 15 and 30 years old, and the cervical cord is most commonly affected.

Injury at thoracic or lumbar segmental level results in *paraplegia* (paralysis of lower limbs). Injury at cervical level causes *tetraplegia* (*quadriplegia*), in which the extent of upper limb paralysis depends on the number or level of cervical segments involved.

Spinal shock

The following features are found below the segmental level of the injury in the first few days following a complete cord transection:

- Paralysis of movement. The limbs are flaccid and tendon reflexes are absent.
- Anesthesia (loss of all forms of sensation).
- Paralysis of the bladder and rectum.

Spinal shock is currently attributed to a generalized hyperpolarization of spinal neurons below the level of the lesion, perhaps because of large-scale release of the inhibitory transmitter, glycine. In addition, the patient develops *postural hypotension* when raised from the recumbent position, owing to interruption of the baroreceptor reflex. Wearing an abdominal binder may be sufficient to compensate for the lost reflex.

Return of spinal function

Several days or weeks later, reflex functions of the cord become progressively restored, and 'upper motor neuron signs' appear. Muscle tone becomes excessive (spastic). Tendon reflexes become abnormally brisk. A Babinski sign can be elicited on both sides. Ankle clonus is commonly seen when a patient's leg is lifted into contact with the footplate of a wheelchair.

If extensor spasticity in the lower limbs is dominant, the patient develops *paraplegia in extension*; if flexor spasticity is dominant, *paraplegia in flexion*. An extended posture may permit *spinal standing*; it is promoted by appropriate passive placement of the limbs, and it is the rule following cord injury which is either incomplete or low. A flexed posture is promoted by repetitive mass flexor reflexes involving the ankles, knees, and hips; mass reflexes can follow any cutaneous stimulation of the legs if the flexor reflex internuncial neurons of the cord are already sensitized by afferent discharges from a pressure sore or from an infected bladder.

The condition of the bladder is of great importance because of the twin dangers of infection and formation of bladder stones. For the initial, *atonic* bladder, a sterile catheter is inserted in order to ensure unobstructed drainage. Later, the bladder becomes *automatic*, emptying itself every 4–6 hours through a reflex arc involving the sacral autonomic center in the conus medullaris.

In animals, much of the damage done to the cord by injury has been shown to be secondary to local shifts in electrolyte concentrations, and to vascular changes including arterial spasm and venous thrombosis. Modest success is being achieved in counteracting these effects. Another line of experimental research is to implant *embryonic* spinal gray matter at the site of injury. These grafts often survive and establish local synaptic connections, but the goal of functional recovery has not been attained.

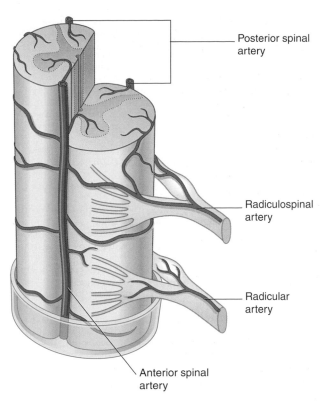

Figure 13.7 Arteries of spinal cord and spinal nerve roots.

Posterior spinal artery

Radiculospinal artery

Radicular artery

Anterior spinal artery

artery is the **artery of Adamkiewicz**, which arises from a lower intercostal artery or upper lumbar artery on the left side and supplies the lumbar enlargement and conus medullaris.

Vascular disorders of the spinal cord are quite rare. As part of a generalized atherosclerosis, a branch of the anterior spinal artery may become occluded, causing necrosis of the anterior half of the cord on one side. The clinical picture has some resemblance to a one-sided amyotrophic lateral sclerosis owing to destruction of anterior horn motor neurons and diminished function in the lateral corticospinal tract on the same side. However, arterial disease should be suspected here because of the relatively abrupt onset of symptoms and because concurrent damage to the spinothalamic pathway produces loss of pain and of thermal sense on the opposite side, below the level of the lesion.

The artery of Adamkiewicz has to be borne in mind by the vascular surgeon attempting to deal with an abdominal aortic aneurysm. If a clamp is placed across the aorta and the artery happens to arise below that level, the patient is at risk of postoperative paraplegia with incontinence!

Veins

The venous drainage of the cord is by means of anterior and posterior spinal veins, which drain outward along the nerve roots. Any obstruction to the venous outflow is liable to produce edema of the cord, with progressive loss of function.

Core Information

Fibers of the corticospinal tract (CST) governing voluntary movement originate in motor, premotor, and supplementary motor areas of the cerebral cortex; fibers governing sensory transmission during movement originate in the parietal lobe. The CST includes corticonuclear fibers innervating motor cranial nerve nuclei. The lateral CST innervates anterior horn cells supplying trunk and limb muscles; 90% of these fibers cross in the pyramidal decussation, 10% are entirely ipsilateral. Lateral CST targets include alpha and gamma motor neurons, Ia inhibitory internuncials, and Renshaw cells.

Clinically, the CST is the upper motor neuron. Damage (e.g. in hemiplegia from stroke) is characterized by initial flaccid paralysis, later by spasticity, brisk reflexes, clonus, and Babinski sign. Lower motor neuron (anterior horn cell) disease is characterized by muscle weakness, wasting, fasciculation, and loss of related segmental reflexes. Spinal cord transection is characterized by initial flaccid paraplegia/tetraplegia with areflexia, atonic bladder, and (permanent) anesthesia below the segmental level involved; later, by spasticity, hyperreflexia, clonus,

Babinski sign, and automatic bladder.

Reticulospinal tracts are activated by the premotor cortex. For locomotion, they originate in a pontine locomotor center and travel to pattern generators in the cord. For postural fixation, they originate in pons and medulla and supply motor neurons via internuncials.

The tectospinal tract descends (crossed) from colliculi to anterior horn; it operates to direct the gaze toward visual/auditory/tactile stimuli. The (lateral) vestibulospinal tract (uncrossed) increases antigravity tone on the side to which the head is tilted. The raphespinal tract descends from the medullary raphe nucleus to the posterior horn via Lissauer's tract; it modulates sensory transmission, especially for pain.

A central sympathetic pathway from hypothalamus/brain stem to the lateral horn includes the efferent limb of the baroreflex. A central parasympathetic pathway activates the bladder and rectum.

The cord receives spinal branches from the vertebral arteries, boosted by radiculospinal arteries at segmental levels. Venous drainage is into segmental veins.

REFERENCES

Burne, A. and Lippold, O.C.J. (1996) Reflex inhibition following electrical stimulation over muscle tendons in man. *Brain* **119**: 1107–1114.

Busches, A. and El Manira, A. (1998) Sensory pathways and their modulation in the control of locomotion. *Current Opin. Neurobiol.* **8**: 733–739.

Crone, C. and Nielson, J. (1994) Central control of disynaptic inhibition in humans. *Acta Physiol. Scand.* **152**: 351–363.

Davidoff, R.A. (1990) The pyramidal tract. *Neurology* **40**: 332–339.

Dietz, V. (1996) Spastic gait disorder. In *Clinical Disorders of Balance Posture and Gait* (Bronstein, A.M., Brandt, T. and Woollacott, M., eds), pp. 1–16. London: Arnold.

Jeanmonod, D. (1991) Neuroanatomical bases of spasticity. In *Neurosurgery for Spasticity* (Sindou, M., Abbott, R., and Keravel, Y., eds), pp. 3–14. New York: Springer-Verlag.

Katz, R. and Pierrot-Deseilligny, E. (1998) Recurrent inhibition in man. *Prog. Neurobiol.* **57**: 325–355.

Levin, M.L. and Feldman, A.G. (1994) The role of stretch reflex threshold regulation in normal and impaired motor control. *Brain Res.* **657**: 23–30.

Martaens de Nordhout, A., Rapisarda, G., Bogacz, D., Gerard, P., De Pasqua, V., Pennisi, G. and Delwaide, P.J. (1999) Corticomotoneural synaptic connections in man. *Brain* **122**: 1327–1340.

Mazzocchio, R. and Rossi, A. (1997) Involvement of spinal recurrent inhibition in spasticity. *Brain* **120**: 991–1003.

Meinck, H.M., Benecke, R., Kuster, S. and Konrad, B. (1983) Cutaneomuscular (flexor) reflex organization in normal man and in patients with motor disorders. In *Motor Control Systems in Health and Disease* (Desmedt, J.E., ed.), pp. 787–796. New York: Raven Press.

Mitz, A.R. and Winstein, C. (1993) The motor system. 1, lower centers. In *Neuroscience for Rehabilitation* (Cohen, M., ed.), pp. 141–175. Philadelphia: Lippincott.

Nacimiento, W. and Noth, J. (1999) What, if anything, is spinal shock? *Arch. Neurol.* **53**: 1033–1035.

Nathan, P.W. and Smith, M.C. (1982) The rubrospinal and central tegmental tracts in man. *Brain* **105**: 223–269.

Nathan, P.W., Smith, M. and Deacon, P. (1996) Vestibulospinal, reticulospinal and descending propriospinal nerve fibers in man. *Brain* **119**: 1809–1833.

Schoenen, J. and Faull, R.L.M. (1990) Spinal cord: cytoarchitectural, dendroarchitectural, and myeloarchitectural organization. In *The Human Nervous System* (Paxinos, G., ed.), pp. 19–54. San Diego: Academic Press.

Ugawa, Y., Uesaka, Y., Terao, Y., Hanajima, R. and Kanazawa, I. (1994) Magnetic stimulation of corticospinal pathways at the foramen magnum level in humans. *Ann. Neurol.* **36**: 618–624.

Brainstem

GENERAL ARRANGEMENT OF CRANIAL NERVE NUCLEI

In the thoracic region of the developing spinal cord, four distinct cell columns can be identified in the gray matter on each side (*Figure 14.1A,B*). In the basal plate, the *general somatic efferent column* supplies the striated muscles of the trunk and limbs. The *general visceral efferent column* contains preganglionic neurons of the autonomic system. In the alar plate, the *general visceral afferent column* receives afferents from thoracic and abdominal organs. A *general somatic afferent* column receives afferents from the body wall.

In the brainstem, these four cell columns can be identified, but they are fragmented, and not all contribute to each cranial nerve. Their connections are as follows:

- *General somatic efferent column:* supplies the striated musculature of the orbit (via the oculomotor, trochlear, and abducens nerves) and tongue (via the hypoglossal nerve).
- *General visceral efferent column:* gives rise to the cranial parasympathetic system introduced in Chapter 10. The target ganglia are the ciliary, pterygopalatine, otic, and submandibular ganglia in the head, and the vagal ganglia in the thorax and abdomen.
- *General visceral afferent column:* receives from the visceral territory of the glossopharyngeal and vagus nerves.
- *General somatic afferent column:* receives from skin and mucous membranes, mainly in trigeminal nerve territory whose most important components are the skin and mucous membranes of the oro-naso-facial region, and the dura mater.

Three additional cell columns (*Figure 14.1C,D*) serve branchial arch tissues and the inner ear, as follows:

- *Special visceral (branchial) efferent column:* to branchial arch musculature of face, jaws, palate, larynx, and pharynx (via facial, trigeminal, glossopharyngeal, and vagus nerves). These striated muscles have visceral functions in relation to food and air intake (hence, *visceral*).
- *Special visceral afferent column:* receives from taste buds located in the endoderm lining the branchial arches.
- *Special sense afferent column:* receives vestibular (balance) and cochlear (hearing) from the inner ear.

Figure 14.2 shows the position of the various nuclei in a dorsal view of the brainstem.

In this chapter, details of the internal anatomy of the brainstem accompany nine representative transverse sections and their captions. Connections (direct or indirect) with the *right* cerebral hemisphere have been highlighted in accordance with information to be provided.

BACKGROUND INFORMATION

As stated earlier, exteroceptive and conscious proprioceptive information are transferred (by spinothalamic and dorsal column–medial lemniscal pathways, respectively) from left trunk and limbs to right cerebral hemisphere. It was also explained that corticospinal fibers of the pyramidal tract arising from motor areas of the cerebral cortex supply contralateral anterior horn cells and give a small ipsilateral supply of similar nature; and that those arising from the parietal lobe project to the contralateral posterior gray horn.

The same arrangement holds good for the brainstem. The pyramidal tract fibers terminating in the brainstem are *corticonuclear*. As shown in *Figure 14.3*, their distribution is predominantly contralateral to somatic and branchial motor nuclei, and entirely contralateral to the somatic sensory nuclei. The only motor exception is the lower part of the facial nucleus (serving the lower part of the face), where the corticonuclear supply is *entirely contralateral.*

Absent from this figure are the three pairs of motor ocular nuclei. Why? Because these do not receive a direct corticonuclear supply. Instead, their predominantly contralateral supply synapses upon adjacent cell groups known as *gaze centers* having the function of synchronizing conjugate (conjoint parallel) movements of the eyes.

For a basic understanding of neural relationships in the brainstem, it is also essential to appreciate hemisphere linkages to the inferior olivary nucleus and to the cerebellum (*Figure 14.4*).

The general layout of the **reticular formation** (*Figure 14.5*) is taken from a figure in Chapter 21 which is devoted to this topic. It may be consulted when reading under this heading in successive descriptions.

Figure 14.6 depicts the main components of the **medial longitudinal fasciculus** (MLF). This fiber bundle extends the entire length of the brainstem, changing its fiber composition at different levels. This figure, too, may be consulted during study of the brainstem sections to be described, following inspection of C1 segment of the spinal cord.

Study guide

The presentation departs from the traditional method, which is to describe photographs or diagrams at successive levels in ascending order without highlights. In the present approach:

1 The various nuclei and pathways are highlighted and labeled on the side having primary affiliation with one cerebral hemisphere. The right hemisphere has been chosen.

2 The nuclei and pathways are color-coded by systems, e.g. red for motor, blue for sensory, green for connections of cerebellum and reticular formation.

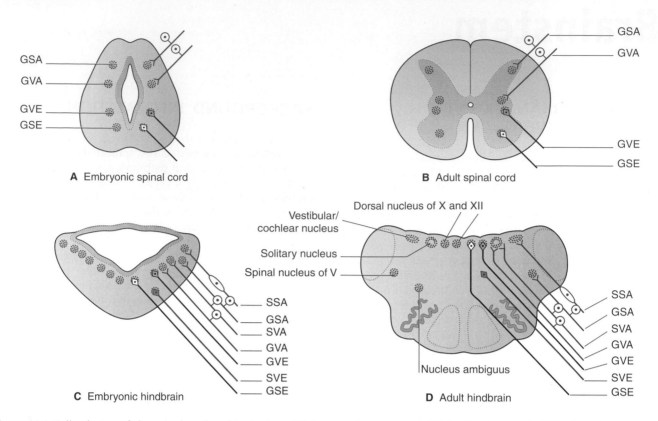

Figure 14.1 Cell columns of the spinal cord and brainstem. **(A)** Embryonic spinal cord. **(B)** Adult spinal cord. **(C)** Embryonic hindbrain. **(D)** Adult hindbrain. *Afferent cell columns*: GSA, general somatic afferent; GVA, general visceral afferent; SSA, special somatic afferent; SVA, special visceral afferent. *Efferent cell columns*: GSE, general somatic efferent; GVE, general visceral efferent; SVE, special visceral efferent.

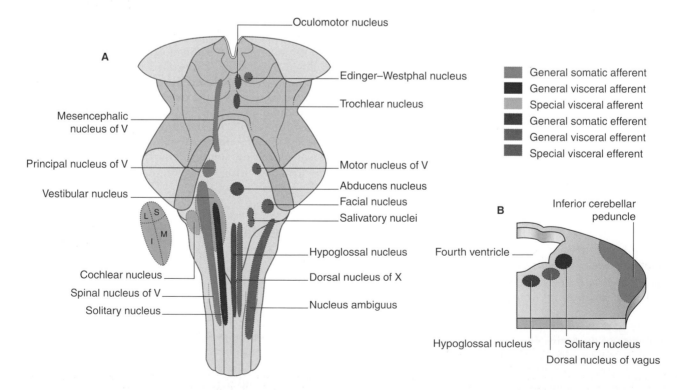

Figure 14.2 Posterior view of adult brainstem showing position of cranial nerve cell columns. L, S, I, M, lateral, superior, inferior, medial vestibular nuclei.

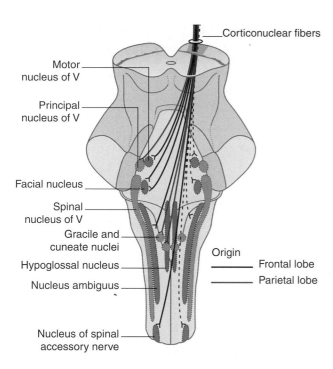

Figure 14.3 Posterior view of brainstem showing distribution of corticonuclear fibers from the right cerebral cortex.

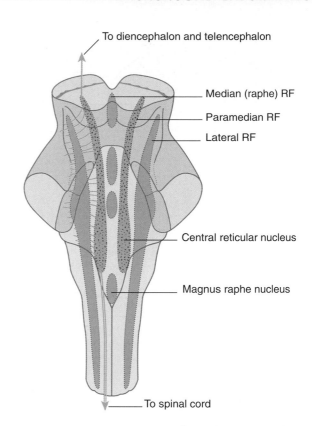

Figure 14.5 Layout of the reticular formation (RF).

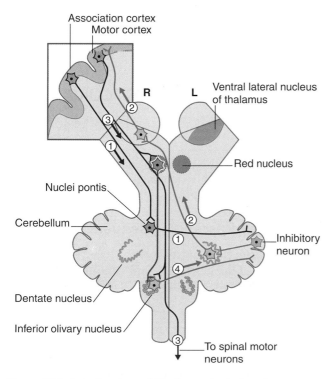

Figure 14.4 Anterior view of the four principal motor decussations of the brainstem. Pathways are numbered in accordance with their sequence of activation in voluntary movements. **(1)** Corticopontocerebellar; **(2)** Dentatothalamocortical; **(3)** Corticospinal; **(4)** Olivocerebellar. Also shown is the rubro-olivary connection.

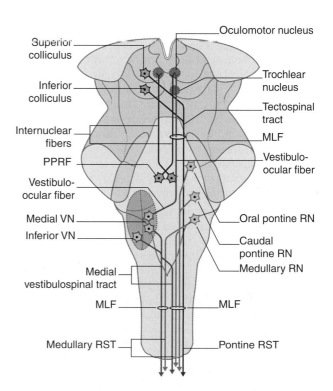

Figure 14.6 Main fiber composition of the medial longitudinal fasciculus (MLF). PPRF, paramedian pontine reticular formation; RN, reticular nucleus; RST, reticulospinal tract; VN, vestibular nucleus.

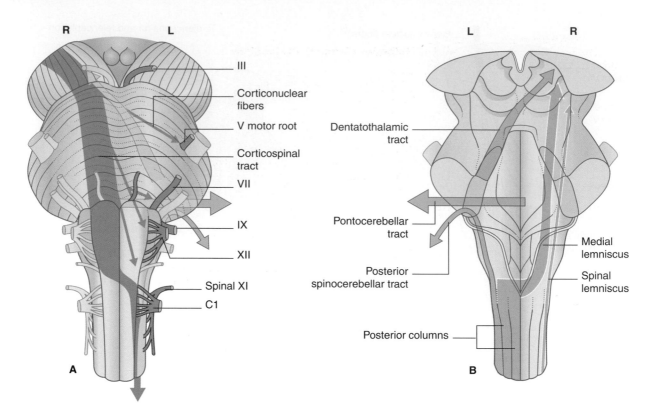

Figure 14.7 (A) Anterior and **(B)** posterior view of brainstem showing disposition of some major pathways.

3 Highlighting together with color-coding makes it possible to study individual systems in vertical, 'multiple window' mode. The descriptive text related to the brainstem sections enables a logical sequence of study whereby afferent pathways can be followed from below upward to thalamic level (commencing with Figure 14.10) and efferent pathways can be followed from above downward (commencing with Figure 14.19). This accounts for the 'First figure' and 'Last figure' headings in relation to level C1. It must be emphasized that, following study in the vertical mode, a horizontal approach must be undertaken, of the various systems to be studied together at each level. This is because occlusion of a small artery of supply to the brainstem may affect function in a patch which may include several distinct nuclei/pathways.

At each level, miniature replicas of the diagrams in *Figure 14.7* are inserted to assist left–right orientation.

Special note: Readers unfamiliar with the internal anatomy of the brainstem may be disconcerted by the amount of new information contained in the series of sections to be described. It may be reassuring to know that *all* of the information will come up again in later chapters. Therefore a sensible approach could be to undertake an initial browse through the sections and to recheck the location of individual items during later reading.

Overview of three pathways in the brainstem

Figure 14.8 shows the *posterior column–medial lemniscal* and *anterolateral pathways* already described in Chapter 12. Recall that the latter comprises the lateral spinothalamic tract

serving pain and temperature, and the anterior spinothalamic tract serving touch. Within the brainstem the two are combined as the **spinal lemniscus**.

The corticospinal tract, treated in Chapter 13, is shown in *Figure 14.9*. Also included are corticonuclear projections to the facial and hypoglossal nuclei.

C1 SEGMENT OF SPINAL CORD

(Figure 14.10)

Landmarks

Immediately below the pyramidal decussation, the lateral corticospinal tract (6) is crossing to occupy the lateral funiculus of the spinal cord.

First figure of ascending sequence

Afferent nuclei and pathways

The positions of the **gracile** (1) and **cuneate** (2) **fasciculi**, and of the **anterolateral pathway** (15) are unchanged from lower levels (Ch. 12).

The inner three laminae of the posterior gray horn are compressed. The outer three laminae constitute the **spinal nucleus of the trigeminal nerve** (3). The **spinal tract of the trigeminal nerve** (4) is at this level conveying posterior root axons from nerves C2 and C3 to the spinal nucleus. (C1 usually lacks a posterior root.)

Cerebellar connections (ascending)

Of the four spinocerebellar pathways (posterior, anterior and rostral spinocerebellar, and cuneocerebellar), only the pos-

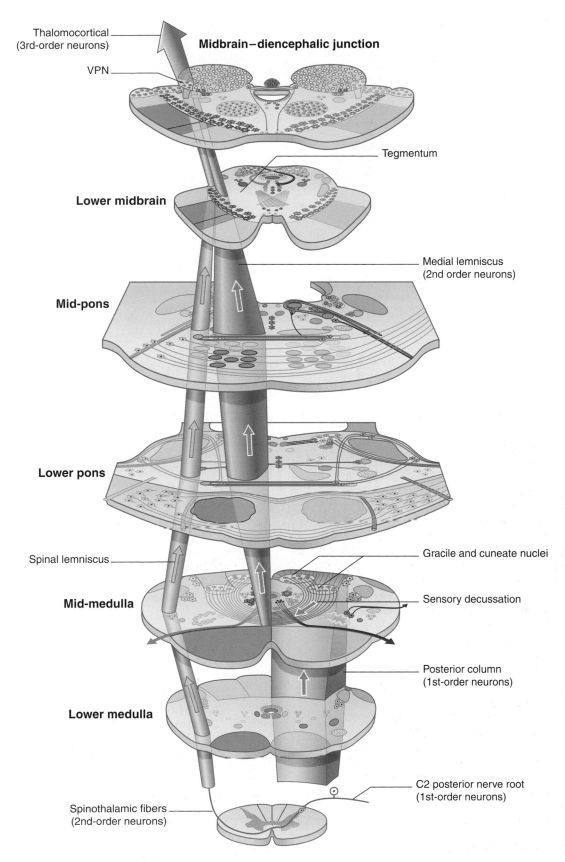

Thalomocortical
(3rd-order neurons)

VPN

Midbrain–diencephalic junction

Tegmentum

Lower midbrain

Medial lemniscus
(2nd order neurons)

Mid-pons

Lower pons

Spinal lemniscus

Gracile and cuneate nuclei

Mid-medulla

Sensory decussation

Posterior column
(1st-order neurons)

Lower medulla

C2 posterior nerve root
(1st-order neurons)

Spinothalamic fibers
(2nd-order neurons)

Figure 14.8 Posterior column–medial lemniscal and anterolateral pathways. VPN, ventral posterior nucleus of thalamus.

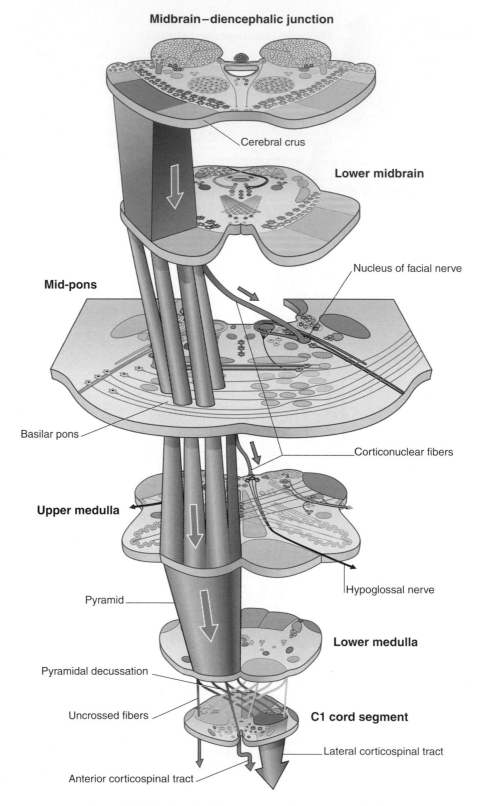

Midbrain–diencephalic junction

Cerebral crus

Lower midbrain

Nucleus of facial nerve

Mid-pons

Basilar pons

Corticonuclear fibers

Upper medulla

Hypoglossal nerve

Pyramid

Lower medulla

Pyramidal decussation

Uncrossed fibers

C1 cord segment

Lateral corticospinal tract

Anterior corticospinal tract

Figure 14.9 Corticospinal tract; two corticonuclear projections.

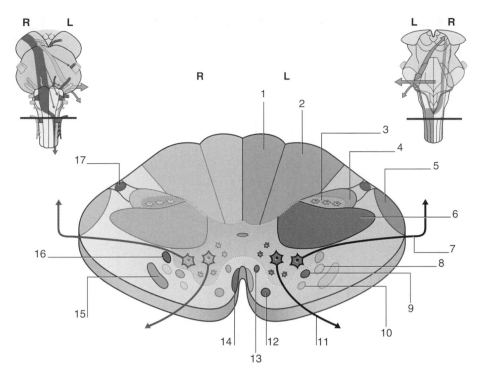

Figure 14.10 C1 segment of spinal cord. (Modified from Noback et al. (1996) *The Human Nervous System: Structure and Function*. Baltimore: Williams & Wilkins.)

terior spinocerebellar tract (5) is shown in this series. Its position is unchanged from lower levels (Ch. 12).

Final figure of descending sequence

Efferent nuclei and pathways
The medial part of the anterior horn of gray matter gives rise to the anterior root of nerve C1 (11). The lateral part gives rise to the uppermost root (7) of the spinal accessory nerve.

The highlighted lateral corticospinal tract (6) has not quite completed its journey from the right pyramid of the medulla to the left lateral funiculus of the spinal cord. Fibers of the anterior corticospinal tract (14) will cross in the anterior commissure to supply deep muscles in the left side of the neck. The highlighted tectospinal tract (12) arose in the right midbrain tectum (*Figure 14.20*). Both medial vestibulospinal tracts (13) are highlighted because each medial vestibular nucleus sends axons into both tracts.

Reticular formation
The pontine reticulospinal tract (10) is descending ipsilaterally to supply motor neurons innervating antigravity muscles. The medullary reticulospinal tract (8), partly crossed, will supply flexor motor neurons.

The raphespinal tract (16) arises in the midline of the upper medulla oblongata, descends bilaterally within the posterolateral tract of Lissauer, and terminates in the posterior gray horn at all segmental levels.

Autonomic system
The central autonomic pathway (16) conveys sympathetic and parasympathetic fibers from the ipsilateral hypothalamus to the lateral gray horn of the cord at appropriate levels (Ch. 10).

SPINOMEDULLARY JUNCTION
(Figure 14.11)

Landmarks
The central canal and central gray matter (1) occupy the midregion. The remainder of the spinal gray matter is broken into discrete cranial nerve nuclei, as will be seen at all higher levels. Ventral to (1) is (19), the **medial longitudinal fasciculus**, whose contents at this level are shown in *Figure 14.6*.

Afferent nuclei and pathways
Dorsally, the left **gracile fasciculus** (2) and **cuneate fasciculus** (4) are highlighted. They subserve conscious proprioception and discriminative touch for the left limbs and trunk.

The right spinal lemniscus (16) is highlighted. This is the brainstem continuum of the anterolateral pathway (anterior and lateral spinothalamic tracts, Ch. 12). Included within the spinal lemniscus is the small, crossed, spinotectal tract which accompanies it all the way to the tectal plate of the midbrain.

The spinal tract and nucleus (5) of the trigeminal nerve are seen again.

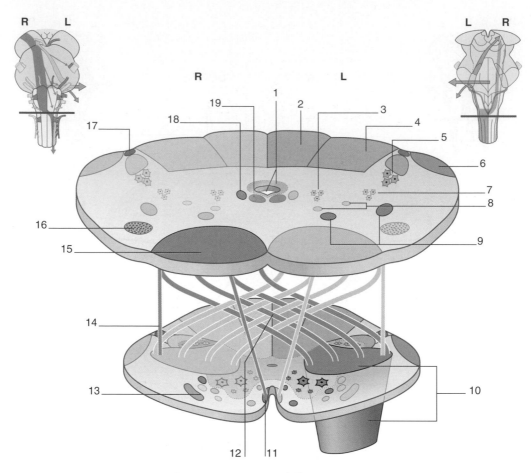

Figure 14.11 Spinomedullary junction.

Cerebellar connections (ascending)
The position of the posterior spinocerebellar tract (6) is unchanged.

Efferent nuclei and pathways
In the ventral region, fibers of the right pyramidal tract (15) are passing through the **pyramidal decussation** (12). Some have emerged from the decussation and are proceeding to the lateral funiculus of the spinal cord as the **lateral (crossed) corticospinal tract** (10). Also seen are fibers entering the ipsilateral **anterior corticospinal tract** (11) to cross lower down, and a bundle (14) representing the 10% of fibers that remain uncrossed.

Dorsal to the pyramids are the lateral and medial vestibulospinal tracts (8 and 9).

Reticular formation
Somas of the paramedian (3) and lateral (7) columns of the reticular formation are seen; also the pontine and medullary reticulospinal tracts (8) and the raphespinal tracts (19).

Autonomic system
Central autonomic fibers (18) are descending from the hypothalamus to autonomic cell stations in the spinal cord.

MIDDLE OF MEDULLA OBLONGATA
(Figure 14.12)

Landmarks
The central canal and central gray matter (1) are beginning to move dorsally.

Afferent nuclei and pathways
A striking feature at this level is the great **sensory decussation** (17). The fibers concerned arise in the **gracile nucleus** (4) and **cuneate nucleus** (10), having received their inputs from the respective fasciculi (3, 6). Dorsal to these nuclei are some fascicular fibers passing ventrally to enter them. The sensory decussation is formed by the decussation of **internal arcuate fibers** (16) emerging from the nuclei and sweeping around the central gray matter. The highlighted left set, having crossed the midline, turn upward immediately, as the right **medial lemniscus** (19). Each lemniscus belongs to the second-order pathway from the periphery to the contralateral thalamus. (The third-order pathway extends from thalamus to somatic sensory cortex.)

Another second-order somatic sensory pathway here is the spinal lemniscus (22) already encountered. The spinal tract and nucleus of the trigeminal nerve (9) are also seen again.

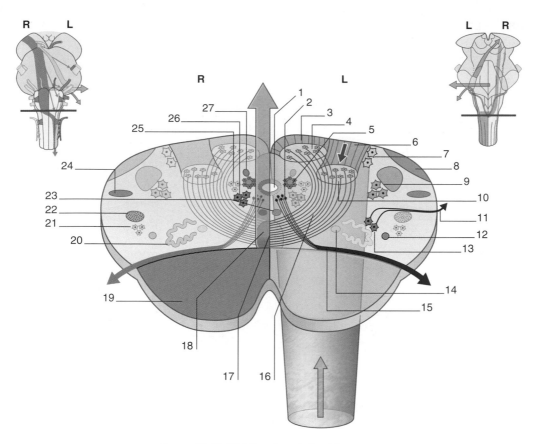

Figure 14.12 Middle of medulla oblongata.

The solitary tract and nucleus (5) will be considered with the next section.

Cerebellar connections (ascending)

The posterior spinocerebellar tract is unchanged. Fibers (not shown) separate from the cuneate fasciculus and synapse in the **accessory cuneate nucleus** (7) which projects cuneocerebellar fibers into the inferior cerebellar peduncle just above this level. This pathway was seen in Chapter 12 to be the upper limb counterpart of the posterior spinocerebellar tract.

The inferior olivary nucleus (20) will be considered with the next section.

Efferent nuclei and pathways

Two pairs of nuclei are associated with cranial nerves. The *somatic efferent* **hypoglossal nucleus** (2) sends the **hypoglossal nerve** (15) to the muscles on its own side of the tongue. The *branchial efferent* nucleus ambiguus (13) sends the **cranial accessory nerve** (11) for distribution (via the vagus nerve) to muscles of the palate, larynx, and pharynx. Lateral to the nucleus ambiguus is the lateral vestibulospinal tract (12).

Reticular formation

Close to the arch of internal arcuate fibers is the paramedian reticular formation (25). The somas seen send the medullary reticulospinal tract the full length of the spinal cord (partly crossed) to participate in withdrawal reflexes (Ch. 13).

Embedded in the lateral reticular formation (21) are cells important for control of the sympathetic nervous system. Variously designated as the *superficial ventrolateral area, vasomotor center,* and *vasopressor center,* it contains numerous noradrenergic and adrenalinergic neurons involved in the control of arterial blood pressure (Ch. 21).

The pontine reticulospinal tract (14) is lateral to the hypoglossal nerve.

The raphespinal tract (24) is moving toward the surface.

Autonomic system

The dorsal nucleus of vagus (26) will be considered with the next section. Dorsal to the sensory decussation is the MLF (23). Autonomic fibers (27) continue their descent from the hypothalamus in the dorsal longitudinal fasciculus (DLF).

UPPER PART OF MEDULLA OBLONGATA (Figure 14.13)

Landmarks

The central canal has opened into the fourth ventricle (1). The central gray matter in the floor of the ventricle contains cranial nerve nuclei.

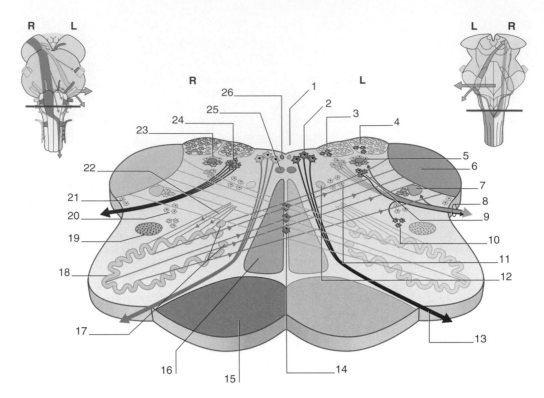

Figure 14.13 Upper medulla oblongata.

Afferent nuclei and pathways

The **medial** (3) and **inferior** (4) **vestibular nuclei** are prominent. These are two of four nuclei in receipt of incoming terminals from the vestibular division of the eighth cranial nerve.

Afferents in the **glossopharyngeal nerve** (8) include general visceral afferent fibers from the oropharynx, terminating in the **solitary nucleus** (5). Some of these fibers provide the afferent limb of the swallowing reflex. Others provide the afferent limb of the baroreceptor reflex arc (Ch. 21). Also seen are glossopharyngeal fibers entering the spinal tract and nucleus of the trigeminal nerve (7); these are activated by inflammation of the oropharynx.

On the right side of the medulla are the medial lemniscus (16) and spinal lemniscus (19).

Cerebellar connections (ascending)

A striking feature at this level is the wrinkled **inferior olivary nucleus** (18). The principal cells of the inferior olivary nucleus, and of the small **accessory olivary nuclei** (17), give rise to the **olivocerebellar tract** (marked by eight arrows), which intersects with its opposite number before entering the opposite **inferior cerebellar peduncle** (6). The right nuclei and tract are highlighted because the main input to their nucleus is from the ipsilateral red nucleus (*Figure 14.4*). Here the rubro-olivary fibers (22) are fanning prior to termination.

Efferent nuclei and pathways

Motor neurons highlighted in the medial and inferior vestibular nuclei give rise to the **medial vestibulospinal**

tract which enters the MLF (25) for ultimate distribution to anterior horn cells in the cervical spinal cord (see head-righting reflexes in Ch. 16). The medial vestibular nucleus also sends fibers to the contralateral motor ocular nuclei (*Figure 14.6*) to participate in the vestibulo-ocular reflex described in Chapter 16.

In the ventral tegmentum, the nucleus ambiguus (10) sends branchial efferent fibers into the glossopharyngeal nerve to innervate the stylopharyngeus. Fibers from the hypoglossal nucleus (2) are emerging in a rootlet of the hypoglossal nerve (13).

Reticular formation

In the midline is the **magnus raphe nucleus** (14) which sends a fountain of serotoninergic fibers into both raphespinal tracts. They seek the posterolateral tract of Lissauer, extend the full length of the cord, and are significant in relation to 'gate control' of pain (Ch. 21).

Cells of the paramedian reticular formation at this level (11) give rise to the (partly crossed) medullary reticulospinal tract seen at lower levels.

The pontine reticulospinal tract (12) will be considered with the pontomedullary junction.

The **retroambiguus nucleus** (20) is the *expiratory center*. The *inspiratory center* is a group of reticular neurons in the solitary nucleus (23).

The *chemoreceptive area* (21) contains neurons sensitive to the carbonic acid levels in the overlying cerebrospinal fluid.

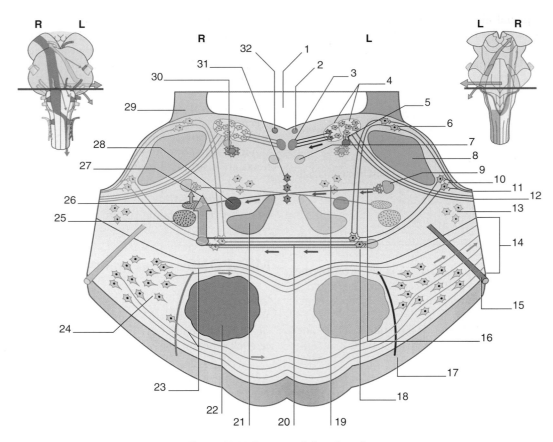

Figure 14.14 Pontomedullary junction.

Autonomic system

Ventral to the medial vestibular nucleus is the **dorsal (motor) nucleus of the vagus** (24, sometimes referred to as the *DMX*). This is the *general visceral efferent* motor nucleus supplying preganglionic fibers to autonomic ganglia in the walls of the thoracic and abdominal viscera (Ch. 10). (Information from animal experiments suggests that some vagal neurons, serving the heart, are lodged in the nucleus ambiguus.)

The small, *general visceral efferent* **inferior salivatory nucleus** (9) provides the preganglionic parasympathetic secretomotor supply for the parotid gland (Ch. 19).

The slender **dorsal longitudinal fasciculus** (26) is at its level of termination. DLF fibers travel from the limbic lobe and hypothalamus to central autonomic nuclei in the medulla and spinal cord.

PONTOMEDULLARY JUNCTION

(Figure 14.14)

Landmarks

The tegmentum of the pons extends from the floor of the fourth ventricle to the posterior set of transverse fibers (23). The transverse fibers and pyramidal tract (22) occupy the basilar pons.

Afferent nuclei and pathways

The **cochlear** and **vestibular** divisions of the eighth cranial nerve are present. Both comprise *bipolar* neurons whose somas are housed in sensory ganglia within the temporal bone (Ch. 16). The cochlear nerve (11) terminates by synapsing upon the *special sense afferent* **dorsal** (6) and **ventral** (10) **cochlear nuclei**, respectively located on the dorsal and lateral aspects of the inferior cerebellar peduncle (8). Many second-order afferents follow the general plan of sensory pathways and project across the midline – in this instance within the **trapezoid body** (20) – and run upward in the **lateral lemniscus** (27). Others synapse in the ipsilateral **superior olivary nucleus** (18) to be relayed either to the opposite lateral lemniscus or into the *ipsilateral* one. The presence of ipsilateral fibers in these ensures bilateral representation of hearing at higher levels (Ch. 17).

The bipolar neurons of the vestibular nerve (12) synapse in the special sense afferent **lateral** and **superior vestibular nuclei** (4) as well as upon those of the medial and inferior vestibular nuclei previously identified.

The **medial lemniscus** (21) is taking up a more lateral position. Lateral to the lateral lemniscus is the **trigeminothalamic tract** (26). This tract comprises axons that originate in the spinal nucleus of the trigeminal nerve and cross (16) to accompany the spinal lemniscus. It is the homologue, for the head and upper neck regions, of the lateral spinothalamic tract, signaling painful and/or thermal stimulation of peripheral nerve endings. The spinal nucleus sends fibers across to the tract at all brainstem levels of that nucleus.

Also seen are the spinal lemniscus (25) and the solitary tract and nucleus (30).

Cerebellar connections (ascending)

The inferior cerebellar peduncle (8) contains the olivocerebellar tract seen in the previous section; also the posterior spinocerebellar tract.

The **superior cerebellar peduncle** (29) will be seen again at higher levels.

Efferent nuclei and pathways

The pyramidal tract (22) occupies the midregion of the basilar pons on each side.

The **lateral vestibulospinal tract** (5) is given off by the lateral vestibular nucleus and descends in the anterior funiculus of the cord to motor neurons supplying antigravity muscles.

The emergent fibers of the **facial nerve** (15) and **abducens nerve** (17) are seen in the basilar pons.

Cerebellar connections (descending)

The nature of the nuclei pontis (24) and transverse fibers (23) is the same as in *Figure 14.15*.

Reticular formation

The **caudal pontine reticular nucleus** (19), together with the oral pontine nucleus at a higher level, gives rise to the pontine reticulospinal tract which will be seen in the next section. Somas of the lateral reticular nucleus (13) are also seen.

The **central tegmental tract** (28), containing rubro-olivary fibers, continues its descent from the ipsilateral red nucleus to the inferior olivary nucleus.

From the pontine raphe nucleus (31), serotoninergic fibers are distributed to pons and cerebellum.

Autonomic system

Fibers of hypothalamic origin (32) are descending in the DLF (2).

MID-PONS (Figure 14.15)

Landmarks

The facial colliculus (3) is in the floor of the fourth ventricle (1). The ventricle is bounded laterally by the superior cerebellar peduncles (6).

Afferent nuclei and pathways

Previously seen are the spinal tract and nucleus of the trigeminal nerve (10), now at their highest level, the medial

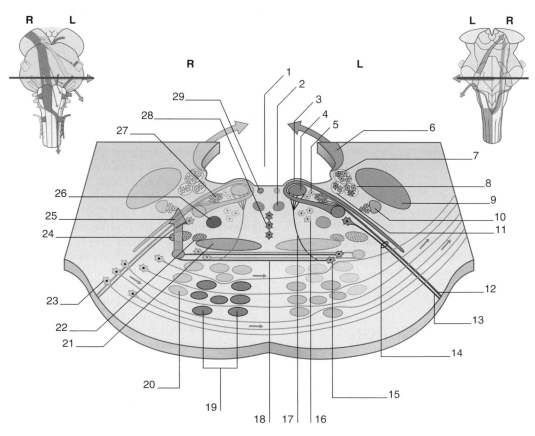

Figure 14.15 Mid-pons.

(21) and spinal (24) lemnisci and the trigeminothalamic tract (22). The superior olivary nucleus (15) continues to send fibers through the trapezoid body (18) into the contralateral lateral lemniscus (25).

Gustatory (taste) fibers (12) leave the nervus intermedius to enter the uppermost part of the solitary tract and nucleus.

Cerebellar connections (ascending)
The inferior cerebellar peduncle (9) is embedded in cerebellar white matter. The superior cerebellar peduncles (6) are converging (arrows).

Efferent nuclei and pathways
The facial colliculus is created by the *somatic efferent* **abducens nucleus** (4) from which the **abducens nerve** (17) passes through the tegmentum. From the *branchial efferent* **facial nucleus**, the **facial nerve** (3) loops mediolaterally around the abducens nucleus before traveling forward through the tegmentum.

The pyramidal tract (19) is parceled into fascicles by transverse fibers.

Cerebellar connections (descending)
Corticopontine fibers (20) continue to synapse upon pontine nuclei (23) which send pontocerebellar tract fibers through the contralateral middle cerebellar peduncle.

Reticular formation
Close to the abducens nucleus is the **paramedian pontine reticular formation** (PPRF, 5) or *pontine gaze center*

(Ch. 20), which enables *saccades* (glances) toward the same side.

In the medial tegmentum are cells of the paramedian reticular formation (16).

In the midline, the pontine raphe nucleus (28) is sending serotoninergic fibers to supply the pons and cerebellum.

Autonomic system
The **superior salivatory nucleus** is sending secretomotor fibers (13) alongside the gustatory fibers identified earlier. Together, the two sets constitute the **nervus intermedius** (14), which will accompany the facial nerve into the internal acoustic meatus.

The DLF (29) contains autonomic fibers descending from the hypothalamus.

UPPER PONS (Figure 14.16)

Landmarks
The fourth ventricle (1) is being narrowed by convergence of the superior cerebellar peduncles (5). The DLF (2) lies in its floor.

Afferent nuclei and pathways
Previously encountered are the medial (16), spinal (18), and lateral (19) lemnisci; also the trigeminothalamic tract (20).

The **sensory root** (10) of the trigeminal nerve (11) terminates in the **principal** (*pontine*) **nucleus** (8) which serves a tactile function for the face, mouth, and other areas supplied by the sensory root. The nucleus projects second-order

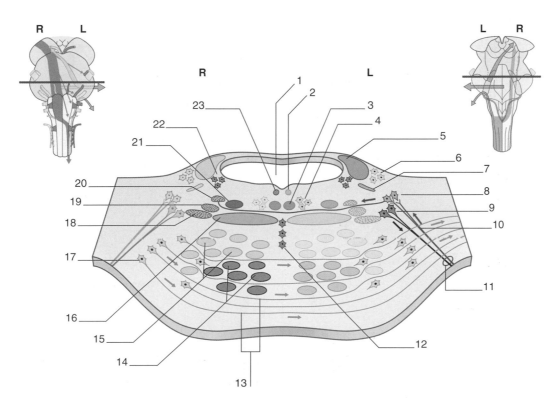

Figure 14.16 Upper pons.

fibers across the midline to join those of the trigeminothalamic tract. Above this level, the crossed pair are called the **trigeminal lemniscus**.

Dorsal to the principal sensory nucleus lies the **mesencephalic tract** (7) of the trigeminal nerve. The parent nucleus is in the midbrain.

Cerebellar connections (ascending)

The superior cerebellar peduncles (5) again form the side walls of the fourth ventricle. They are composed mainly of a projection from the dentate nucleus of cerebellum to the thalamus contralateral.

Efferent nuclei and pathways

The *branchial efferent* **motor nucleus** of the **trigeminal nerve** (9) sends the **motor root** through tegmentum and basilar pons to its point of emergence from the brainstem. Its main targets are the muscles of mastication (chewing).

The trigeminal nerve is used to indicate the demarcation line between pons proper and middle cerebellar peduncle.

The tectospinal tract has been incorporated into the MLF (3).

The pyramidal tract (14) has been parceled into fascicles by transverse fibers (13).

Cerebellar connections (descending)

The corticopontine fibers descended from the crus cerebri synapse upon millions of somas which make up the **nuclei pontis** (17). The nuclei send their axons to the contralateral cerebellar cortex via **transverse fibers** (13) which enter the cerebellum through the middle cerebellar peduncle.

Reticular formation

In the upper, lateral part of the fourth ventricle on each side is the **cerulean nucleus** (22). It contains the largest group of noradrenergic neurons in the brain. It distributes long, fine, beaded axons to all parts of the cerebellar and cerebral cortex (*see* Ch. 21).

The DLF contains autonomic fibers (23) descending from the ipsilateral hypothalamus.

LOWER MIDBRAIN (Figure 14.17)

Landmarks

The central canal (2) is the **cerebral aqueduct** (*aqueduct of Sylvius*), which in life contains cerebrospinal fluid pouring down from the third ventricle to the fourth. In the lateral part of the **periaqueductal gray matter** (PAG) are *enkephalinergic* neurons (3) projecting to the magnus raphe nucleus

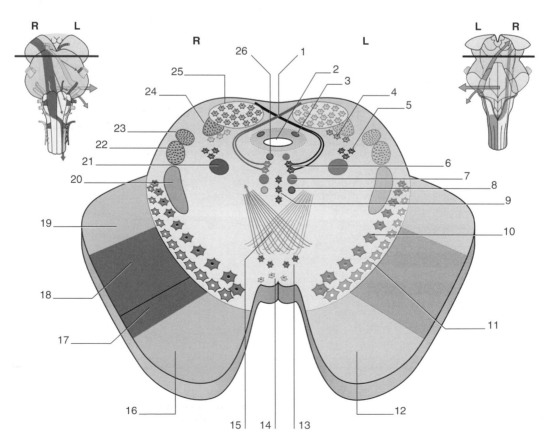

Figure 14.17 Lower midbrain.

of the medulla with a significant role in the suppression of pain sensation (*see* Ch. 21).

Afferent nuclei/pathways

In the most ventral tegmentum are the **compact** (10) and **reticular** (11) parts of the **substantia nigra**. The compact part, comprising pigmented *dopaminergic neurons*, is the source of the *nigrostriatal pathway* to the corpus striatum. The nigrostriatal pathway loses both pigment and cells progressively, in those unfortunates bound for *Parkinson's disease* (Ch. 28). The reticular part comprises GABAergic neurons.

The **ventral tegmental nuclei** (13) contain *mesocortical* dopaminergic neurons projecting to the frontal cortex, and *mesolimbic* dopaminergic neurons projecting to the nucleus accumbens (a ventral part of the corpus striatum). Both elements are clinically significant (Ch. 29).

In the lateral tegmentum are the medial (20), spinal (22), and trigeminal (23) lemnisci. The lateral lemniscus (24) is terminating in the **inferior colliculus** (25), the subcortical center for hearing.

The **mesencephalic nucleus** of the trigeminal nerve (4) is anatomically unique in the central nervous system: it is entirely composed of *unipolar neurons* that remained within the pons and midbrain at the time (third week of embryonic life) when homologous precursors elsewhere moved outside, within the neural crest (Ch. 1), to form posterior root ganglion cells. The nucleus and tract serve proprioception in the trigeminal territory.

Cerebellar connections (ascending)

The most prominent feature at this level is the **decussation of the superior cerebellar peduncles** (15). The highlighted fibers originated mainly in the dentate nucleus of the left cerebellar hemisphere (*Figure 14.4*).

Efferent nuclei and pathways

From the *somatic efferent* **trochlear nucleus** (6), the **trochlear nerve** skirts PAG and decussates (1) prior to emergence on the dorsum of the brainstem.

The corticonuclear (17) and corticospinal (18) fibers are unchanged.

Cerebellar connections (descending)

The two sets of corticopontine fibers (16, 19) are unchanged. The red nucleus is giving rise to rubro-olivary fibers which descend within the central tegmental tract (21) to synapse in the ipsilateral inferior olivary nucleus.

Reticular formation

The interpeduncular nucleus (14) occupies the most ventral tegmentum.

Autonomic system

The DLF (26) contains ipsilateral descending autonomic fibers.

UPPER MIDBRAIN   (Figure 14.18)

Landmarks

The cerebral aqueduct and PAG (1) are unchanged, as are the compact and reticular parts of the substantia nigra (8,9).

Afferent nuclei and pathways

The medial (21), trigeminal (22), and spinal (23) lemnisci continue to move dorsally as they near the thalamus. Fibers leaving the spinal lemniscus are fellow travelers that have reached their station. They have emerged as the small **spinotectal tract** (24) to enter the **superior colliculus** (25).

Cerebellar connections (ascending)

Dentatothalamic fibers (20) of the crossed superior cerebellar peduncle have bypassed the red nucleus. Some dentate fibers (not shown here) enter the red nucleus; their significance is discussed in Chapter 22. *Rubrothalamic* fibers (19) ascend in the central tegmental tract.

Efferent nuclei and pathways

Close to the midline is the *somatic efferent* **oculomotor nucleus** (2). Vestibulo-ocular and internuclear fibers leave the MLF (5) and enter the nucleus.

The **oculomotor nerves** traverse the red nuclei prior to emergence in the interpeduncular fossa (11).

The **tectospinal tract** crosses the midline before descending (7). This tract belongs to the efferent limb of the *spino-visual reflex*, which turns the head toward something glimpsed. Behaviors such as these are better called *responses* because reaction is optional.

Unchanged from *Figure 14.19* are corticopontine (15, 18), corticonuclear (16), and corticospinal (17) fibers.

Reticular formation

The interpeduncular nucleus (13) is unchanged. The **midbrain raphe nucleus** (14) sends an enormous *serotoninergic* projection to both cerebral hemispheres via the medial forebrain bundle (Ch. 21).

The **cuneiform nucleus** (3) projects upward within the central tegmental tract (4) to participate in *arousal* mechanisms at thalamic level (Ch. 21).

Autonomic system

Lateral to the oculomotor nucleus is the tiny general visceral efferent **anteromedial** (*Edinger–Westphal*) **nucleus** (26) which contributes parasympathetic fibers to the oculomotor nerve. The DLF (27) contains autonomic fibers descending to lower levels.

MIDBRAIN–THALAMIC JUNCTION

(Figure 14.19)

Landmarks

The bulky **thalamus** (3) lies above the upper extremity of the midbrain tegmentum. In the midline is the overhanging **pineal gland** (1). The central canal is opening into the **third ventricle** (2).

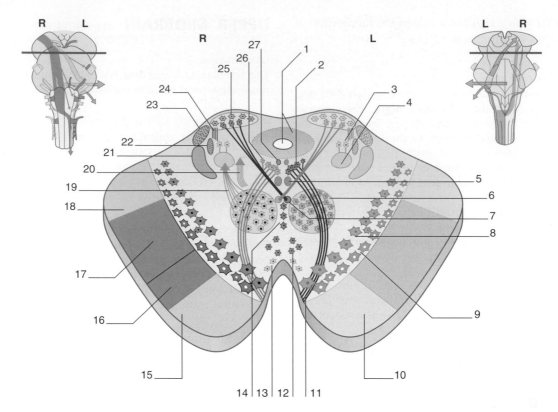

Figure 14.18 Upper midbrain.

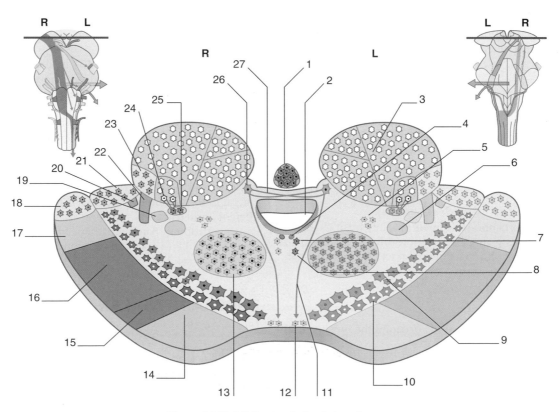

Figure 14.19 Midbrain–thalamic junction.

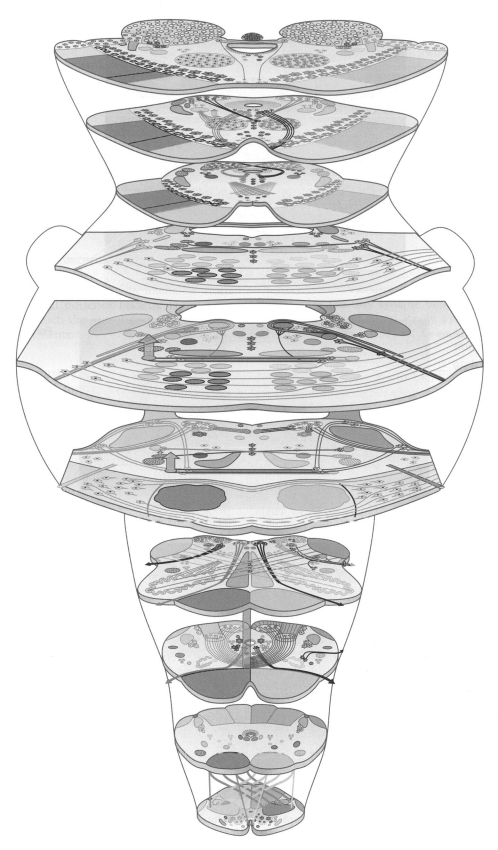

Figure 14.20 Brainstem review.

Core Information

Cell columns

Cranial nerve cell columns and their representations are as follows:

- *General somatic efferent*, represented in the medulla by the hypoglossal nucleus, in the pons by the abducens nucleus, and in the midbrain by the oculomotor and trochlear nuclei;
- *Special visceral efferent*, supplying muscles of branchial arch origin, represented in the medulla by the nucleus ambiguus and in the pons by trigeminal and facial motor nuclei;
- *General visceral efferent*, represented in the medulla by dorsal nucleus of the vagus and in the medulla and in the pons by the salivatory nucleus;
- *General visceral afferent*, represented in the medulla by the inferior solitary nucleus;
- *Special visceral afferent*, represented in the pons by the superior solitary nucleus;
- *General somatic afferent*, represented by trigeminal sensory nuclei: spinal in the medulla, principal sensory in the pons, and mesencephalic in the midbrain;
- *Special sense afferent*, represented at the pontomedullary junction by the cochlear and vestibular nuclei.

Ascending pathways

The gracile and cuneate nuclei send internal arcuate fibers across the midline to form the medial lemniscus, which goes through pons and midbrain to reach the thalamus. The spinal trigeminal nucleus sends fibers across the midline to form the trigeminothalamic tract. The posterior spinocerebellar and cuneocerebellar tracts send their fibers into the ipsilateral inferior cerebellar peduncle, where they mingle with olivocerebellar fibers crossing from the inferior and accessory olivary nuclei. The (crossed) anterior spinocerebellar tract enters the superior cerebellar peduncle; its fibers cross a second time within the cerebellar white matter.

The spinal lemniscus is formed of the anterior and lateral spinothalamic tracts. It is accompanied first by trigeminothalamic fibers, later by the lateral lemniscus and by fibers crossing from the principal trigeminal nucleus completing the trigeminal lemniscus.

The cochlear nuclei project fibers across the trapezoid body to form the lateral lemniscus which ascends to the inferior colliculus. Some fibers synapse instead in a superior olivary nuclear relay to the ipsilateral inferior colliculus. Third-order neurons of the inferior colliculus project via inferior brachium to the medial geniculate body. The medial and superior vestibular nuclei send fibers to the oculomotor nucleus to execute the vestibulo-ocular reflex.

The upper part of the central tegmental tract contains fibers of the ascending reticular activating system.

In the ventral tegmentum of the midbrain are the pigmented (compact) substantia nigra giving rise to the nigrostriatal pathway, and the ventral tegmental nucleus giving rise to the mesocortical and mesolimbic pathways. The nonpigmented (reticular) nigral neurons are inhibitory.

Descending pathways other than reticulospinal

Corticonuclear fibers from motor areas of the cerebral cortex are distributed preferentially to contralateral motor cranial nerve nuclei excepting the ocular motor slaves of gaze centers. Corticonuclear fibers from sensory areas synapse in contralateral trigeminal and posterior column nuclei and posterior gray horn of spinal cord.

Prior to the initiation of a voluntary movement on the left side of the body, the left cerebellar hemisphere is notified by discharges from association areas of the right cerebral cortex, along the corticopontocerebellar pathway. The left cerebellum responds via the dentatothalamocortical pathway, to the right primary motor cortex. Then the right pyramidal tract discharges and on its way down notifies the cerebellum a second time by activating the right red nucleus which in turn activates the right olivocerebellar tract.

Corticospinal fibers pass through the middle three-fifths of the cerebral crus and through the basilar pons (where they are segregated into bundles by transverse fibers), finally creating the pyramid of the medulla before four-fifths enter the pyramidal decussation.

The lateral vestibular nucleus gives rise to the lateral vestibulospinal tract having an antigravity function. The medial and inferior vestibular nuclei give rise to the medial vestibulospinal tract involved in head-righting reflexes. The tectospinal tract belongs to the spinovisual reflex arc. The dorsal longitudinal fasciculus contains ipsilateral central autonomic fibers.

A sleep-related pathway from the septal area reaches the interpeduncular nucleus by way of the habenular nucleus and fasciculus retroflexus.

Reticular formation

In the uppermost midbrain are the upward and downward gaze centers. (The lateral gaze centers adjoin the abducens nucleus in the pons.) The midbrain also contains an upgoing, 'arousal' projection from the cuneiform nucleus, a downgoing, pain-suppressant projection from the peri-aqueductal gray matter, and a locomotor generator, the pedunculopontine nucleus.

The pons contains the noradrenergic, cerulean nucleus; also the oral and caudal pontine reticular nuclei which send ipsilateral pontine reticulospinal tracts to extensor motor neurons. The medullary reticulospinal tract is partly crossed and supplies flexor motor neurons. Three respiratory reticular nuclei also occupy the medulla.

The lowest four cranial nerves

HYPOGLOSSAL NERVE

The hypoglossal nerve (cranial nerve XII) contains somatic efferent fibers for the supply of the extrinsic and intrinsic muscles of the tongue. Its nucleus lies close to the midline in the floor of the fourth ventricle and extends almost the full length of the medulla (*Figure 15.1*). The nerve emerges as a series of rootlets in the interval between the pyramid and the olive. It crosses the subarachnoid space and leaves the skull through the hypoglossal canal. Just below the skull, it lies close to the vagus and spinal accessory nerves (*Figure 15.2*). It descends on the carotid sheath to the level of the angle of the mandible, then passes forward on the surface of the hyoglossus muscle where it gives off its terminal branches.

In the neck, proprioceptive fibers enter the nerve from the cervical plexus, to accept afferents from about 100 muscle spindles in the same half of the tongue.

Phylogenetic note

In reptiles, the lingual muscles, the geniohyoid muscle, and the infrahyoid muscles develop together from the uppermost mesodermal somites. The somatic efferent neurons supplying this *hypobranchial muscle sheet* form a continuous ribbon of cells extending from lower medulla to the third cervical spinal segment. In mammals, the hypoglossal nucleus is located more rostrally and its rootlets emerge separately from the cervical rootlets. However, the caudal limit of the hypoglossal nucleus remains linked to the cervical motor cell column by the *supraspinal nucleus*, from which the thyrohyoid muscle is supplied via the first cervical ventral root. In rodents, some of the intrinsic muscle fibers of the tongue receive their motor supply indirectly, from axons which leave the most caudal cells of the hypoglossal nucleus and emerge in the first cervical nerve to join the hypoglossal nerve trunk in the neck. Whether this arrangement holds for primates is not yet known.

Supranuclear supply to the hypoglossal nucleus

The hypoglossal nucleus receives inputs from the reticular formation, whereby it is recruited for stereotyped motor routines in eating and swallowing. For delicate functions including articulation, most of the fibers from the motor cortex cross over in the upper part of the pyramidal decussation; some remain uncrossed and supply the ipsilateral hypoglossal nucleus.

Supranuclear, nuclear, and infranuclear lesions of the hypoglossal nerve are described together with lesions of the accessory nerve (see *Clinical Panels 15.1–15.3*).

SPINAL ACCESSORY NERVE

The spinal accessory nerve (cranial nerve XI) is a purely motor nerve attached to the uppermost five segments of the spinal cord. The nucleus of origin is a column of α and γ motorneurons in the basolateral anterior gray horn.

The nerve runs upward in the subarachnoid space, behind the denticulate ligament. It enters the cranial cavity through the foramen magnum and leaves it again through the jugular foramen. While in the jugular foramen, it shares a dural sheath with the cranial accessory nerve, but there is no exchange of fibers (*Figure 15.3*). Upon leaving the cranium, it crosses the transverse process of the atlas and enters the sternomastoid muscle, in company with twigs from roots C2 and C3 of the cervical plexus. It emerges from the posterior border of the sternomastoid and crosses the posterior triangle of the neck to reach the trapezius. It pierces the trapezius in company with twigs from roots C3 and C4 of the cervical plexus. In the posterior triangle, the nerve is vulnerable, being embedded in prevertebral fascia and covered only by investing cervical fascia and skin.

The spinal accessory nerve provides the extrafusal and intrafusal motor supply to the sternomastoid and trapezius. The branches from the cervical plexus are proprioceptive in function to the sternomastoid and to the craniocervical part of the trapezius. The thoracic part of the trapezius, which arises from the spines of all the thoracic vertebrae, receives its proprioceptive innervation from the posterior rami of the thoracic spinal nerves. Some of the afferents supplying muscle spindles in the thoracic trapezius do not meet up with the fusimotor supply before reaching the spindles. This is the only instance, *in any muscle known*, where the fusimotor and afferent fibers to some spindles travel by completely independent routes.

GLOSSOPHARYNGEAL, VAGUS, AND CRANIAL ACCESSORY NERVES

Especially relevant to nerves IX, X, and cranial XI are the solitary nucleus and the nucleus ambiguus. The solitary nucleus extends from the lower border of the pons to the level of the gracile nucleus. Its lower end merges with its opposite number in the midline; hence the term **commissural nucleus** for the lower part of the solitary nucleus.

Anatomically, the nucleus is divisible into eight parts. Functionally, four *regions* have been clarified (*Figure 15.4*):

1 The uppermost region is the **gustatory nucleus**, which receives primary afferents supplying taste buds in the tongue and palate.

2 The lateral midregion is the **dorsal respiratory nucleus** (see Ch. 19).

3 The medial midregion is the **baroreceptor nucleus**, which receives the primary afferents supplying blood pressure detectors in the carotid sinus and aortic arch.

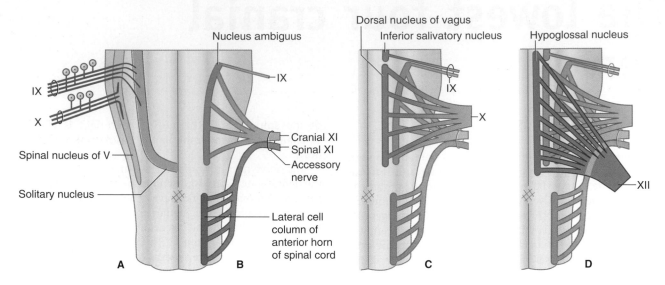

Figure 15.1 (A) Sensory nuclei (left) and motor nuclei (right) serving cranial nerves IX–XII. **(B)** shows the special visceral efferent cell column giving a contribution to the glossopharyngeal nerve and forming the cranial accessory nerve. **(C)** shows the general visceral efferent cell column contributing to the glossopharyngeal and vagus nerves. **(D)** shows the somatic efferent cell column giving rise to the hypoglossal nerve.

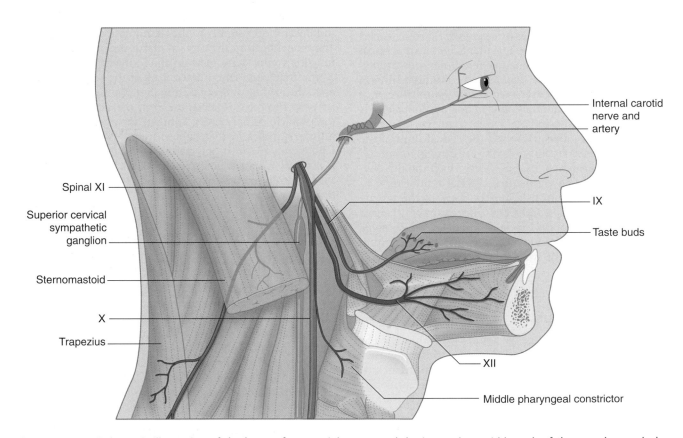

Figure 15.2 Semischematic illustration of the lowest four cranial nerves and the internal carotid branch of the superior cervical ganglion. ICA, internal carotid artery.

4 The most caudal region, including the commissural nucleus, is the major **visceral afferent nucleus** of the brainstem. It receives primary afferents supplying the alimentary tract and respiratory tract.

From the nucleus ambiguus, *special visceral efferent* fibers supply the constrictor muscles of the pharynx, stylopharyngeus, levator palati, intrinsic muscles of the larynx, and (via the recurrent laryngeal nerve) the

Clinical Panel 15.3   Infranuclear lesions of the lowest four cranial nerves

Jugular foramen syndrome

The last four cranial nerves, and the internal carotid (sympathetic) nerve nearby, are at risk of entrapment by a tumor spreading along the base of the skull. The tumor may be a primary one in the nasopharynx, or a metastatic one within lymph nodes of the upper cervical chain. In the second case, the primary tumor may be in an air sinus or in the tongue, larynx, or pharynx. In either case, a mass can usually be felt behind the ramus of the mandible. The symptomatology varies with the number of nerves caught up in the tumor, and the degree to which they are compromised.

Symptoms

- Pain in or behind the ear, attributable to irritation of the auricular branches of the IX and X nerves. *Whenever an adult complains of constant pain in one ear, without evidence of middle ear disease, a cancer of the pharynx must be suspected.*

- Headache, from irritation of the meningeal branch of the vagus.

- Hoarseness, owing to paralysis of laryngomotor fibers.

- Dysphagia (difficulty in swallowing) owing to paralysis of pharyngomotor fibers.

Signs   (Figure CP 15.3.1)

- Horner's syndrome (ptosis of the upper eyelid, with some pupillary constriction) from interruption of the sympathetic internal carotid nerve.

- Infranuclear paralysis of the hypoglossal nerve, with wasting of the affected side of the tongue and deviation of the tongue to the affected side on protrusion.

- When the patient is asked to say 'Aahh', the uvula is pulled away from the affected side by the unopposed healthy levator palati.

- Sensory loss in the oropharynx on the affected side.

- On laryngoscopic examination, inability to adduct the vocal cord to the midline.

- Interruption of the spinal accessory nerve produces weakness and wasting of the sternomastoid and trapezius.

A jugular foramen syndrome may also be caused by invasion of the jugular foramen from above, for instance by a tumor extending from the cerebellopontine angle (Ch. 17). In this case, the sympathetic and spinal accessory nerves will be out of reach, and unaffected.

Isolated lesion of the spinal accessory nerve

The surface marking for the spinal accessory nerve in the posterior triangle of the neck is a line drawn from the posterior border of the sternomastoid one-third of the way down to the anterior border of the trapezius two-thirds of the way down. It may be injured in this part of its course by a stab wound, or during a surgical procedure for removal of cancerous lymph nodes. The trapezius is selectively paralyzed, whereupon the scapula and clavicle sag noticeably because trapezius normally helps to carry the upper limb. Shrugging of the shoulder is weakened because the levator scapulae must work alone. Progressive atrophy of the muscle leads to characteristic scalloping of the contour of the neck (*Figure CP 15.3.2*).

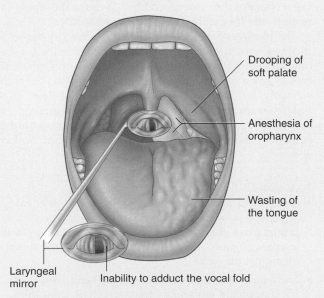

Drooping of soft palate

Anesthesia of oropharynx

Wasting of the tongue

Laryngeal mirror

Inability to adduct the vocal fold

Figure CP 15.3.1 Left-sided jugular foramen syndrome. A laryngeal mirror is being used to inspect the vocal folds during an attempt to cough.

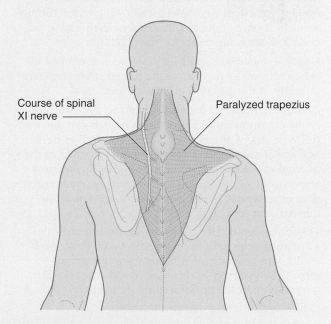

Course of spinal XI nerve

Paralyzed trapezius

Figure CP 15.3.2 Visible effects of right-sided spinal XI paralysis: scalloping of the neck and drooping of the shoulder.

Core Information

Hypoglossal nerve

XII contains somatic efferent neurons supplying extrinsic and intrinsic muscles of the tongue. Its nucleus is close to midline and is innervated by reticular neurons for automatic/reflex movements and by (mainly crossed) corticonuclear neurons for speech articulation. XII emerges beside the pyramid, exits the hypoglossal canal and descends on the carotid sheath where it collects cervical proprioceptive fibers for the supply of lingual muscle spindles. Supranuclear paralysis of XII is characterized by temporary deviation to the paralyzed side on protrusion. Nuclear/infranuclear paralysis is characterized by wasting and fasciculation as well as deviation.

Spinal accessory nerve

Spinal XI is purely motor. From motor neurons of spinal segments C1–C5, the axons enter the foramen magnum and exit the jugular foramen; they pierce and supply sternomastoid, then pass deep to trapezius and supply it. Proprioceptive connections are received from cervical and thoracic spinal nerves. Supranuclear lesions are characterized by weakness of the contralateral trapezius and contralateral head rotators; nuclear/infranuclear lesions by ipsilateral wasting of the two muscles and drooping of the scapula.

Glossopharyngeal nerve

IX emerges behind the olive and exits the jugular foramen where it shows two unipolar-cell ganglia and gives off a tympanic branch which is partly sensory to the middle ear, partly parasympathetic to the parotid gland via the otic ganglion. IX then passes between superior and middle constrictors to gain the oropharynx, where it supplies sensation to that mucous membrane including the posterior third of tongue (hence the name), and taste fibers to the circumvallate papillae. A carotid branch supplies the carotid sinus and carotid body.

Vagus and cranial accessory nerves

X and cranial XI rootlets emerge behind the olive and unite in the jugular foramen. Cranial XI fibers arise in nucleus ambiguus and utilize laryngeal and pharyngeal branches of X to supply the intrinsic muscles of larynx and pharynx, and levator palati.

Preganglionic fibers from the dorsal nucleus of X travel to intramural ganglia in the walls of heart, bronchi, and alimentary tract. Visceral afferents from these regions, and from larynx and pharynx, have unipolar cell bodies in the nodose ganglion and project to the commissural nucleus.

---

accompanying nausea. To test the integrity of the IX nerve, it is usually sufficient to test sensation on the pharyngeal wall.) Generalized stimulation of the oropharynx elicits a complete swallowing reflex, through a linkage between the commissural nucleus and a specific swallowing center nearby (Ch. 21).

- Gustatory neurons supply the taste buds contained in the circumvallate papillae of the tongue; they terminate centrally in the gustatory nucleus (*Figure 15.4*).

- An important *carotid branch* descends to the bifurcation of the common carotid artery. This branch contains two different sets of afferent fibers. One set ramifies in the wall of the carotid sinus (at the commencement of the internal carotid artery), terminating in *stretch receptors* responsive to systolic blood pressure; these *baroreceptor neurons* terminate centrally in the medial part of the nucleus solitarius (*Figure 15.4*).

- The second set of afferents in the carotid branch supplies glomus cells in the carotid body. These nerve endings are *chemoreceptors* monitoring the carbon dioxide and oxygen levels in the blood. The central terminals enter the dorsal respiratory nucleus (*Figure 15.4*).

Vagus and cranial accessory nerves

The vagus is the main parasympathetic nerve. Its preganglionic component has a huge territory which includes the heart, the lungs, and the alimentary tract from esophagus through transverse colon (Ch. 10). At the same time, the vagus is the largest visceral afferent nerve; afferents outnumber parasympathetic motor fibers by four to one. Overall, the vagus contains the same seven fiber classes as the glossopharyngeal, and they will be listed in the same order.

The rootlets of the vagus and cranial accessory nerves are in series with the glossopharyngeal, and the three nerves travel together into the jugular foramen. At this point, the cranial accessory nerve shares a dural sheath with the spinal accessory, but there is no exchange of fibers (*Figure 15.3*). Just below the foramen, the cranial accessory is incorporated into the vagus. The vagus itself shows a small, jugular (superior) and a large, nodose (inferior) ganglion; both are sensory.

Functional divisions and branches

- An *auricular branch* supplies skin lining the outer ear canal, and a *meningeal branch* ramifies in the posterior cranial fossa. Both branches have their cell bodies in the jugular ganglion; the central processes enter the spinal trigeminal nucleus.

- The parasympathetic neurons for the heart, and respiratory and alimentary tracts originate from the dorsal nucleus of the vagus. (Some cardiac neurons are probably embedded in the nucleus ambiguus.)

- Special visceral efferent neurons of the nucleus ambiguus constitute the motor elements in the pharyngeal and laryngeal branches of the vagus. They supply the pharyngeal and laryngeal muscles already noted, and levator palati. They also supply the striated musculature of the upper third of the esophagus.

- General visceral afferent fibers from the heart, and from the respiratory and alimentary tracts have their cell bodies in the nodose ganglion and synapse centrally in the commissural nucleus. They serve important reflexes including the *Bainbridge reflex* (cardiac acceleration brought about by distension of the right atrium); the *cough reflex* (stimulation of a coughing center (Ch. 21) by irritation of the tracheobronchial tree); and the *Hering–Breuer reflex* (inhibition of the dorsal respiratory center by pulmonary stretch receptors). In addition, afferent information from the stomach (in particular) is forwarded to the hypothalamus and influences feeding behavior (Ch. 23).

- A few taste buds on the epiglottis report to the gustatory nucleus.
- *Baroreceptors* in the aortic arch are supplied.
- *Chemoreceptors* in the tiny aortic bodies are supplied; these supplement the corresponding receptors at the carotid bifurcation.

Supranuclear, nuclear, and infranuclear lesions of the IX, X, and XI nerves are described in the *Clinical Panels*.

REFERENCES

Andresen, M.C. (1994) Nucleus tractus solitarii – gateway to neural circulatory control. *Ann. Rev. Physiol.* **56**: 93–116.

Dampney, R.A.L. (1994) Functional organization of the central pathways regulating the cardiovascular system. *Physiol. Rev.* **74**: 323–364.

FitzGerald, M.J.T. (2000) Sternomastoid paradox. Clin. Anat. 14: 330–331.

FitzGerald, M.J.T. and Sachithanandan, S.R. (1979) The structure and source of lingual proprioceptors in the monkey. *J. Anat.* **128**: 523–552.

FitzGerald, M.J.T., Comerford, P.T. and Tuffery, A.R. (1982) Sources of innervation of the neuromuscular spindles in sternomastoid and trapezius. *J. Anat.* **134**: 174–190.

Mtui, E.P., Anwar, M., Reis, D.J. and Ruggiero, D.A. (1995) Medullary visceral reflex circuits: local afferents to nucleus tractus solitarii synthesize catecholamines and project to thoracic spinal cord. *J. Comp. Neur.* **351**: 5–26.

Saxina, P.R. (1995) Serotonin receptors: subtypes, functional responses and therapeutic relevance. *Pharmacol. Therap.* **66**: 339–368.

Thompson, P.D., Thickbroom, G.W. and Mastaglia, F.L. (1997) Corticomotor representation of the sternocleidomastoid muscle. *Brain* **120**: 245–255.

Urban, P.P., Hopf, H.C., Fleischer, S., Zorowka, P.G. and Muller-Forell, W. (1997) Impaired corticobulbar tract function in dysarthria due to hemispheric stroke. *Brain* **120**: 1077–1084.

Vestibular nerve

INTRODUCTION

The **vestibulocochlear nerve** is primarily composed of the centrally directed axons of bipolar neurons housed in the petrous temporal bone (*Figure 16.1*). The peripheral processes are applied to neuroepithelial cells in the vestibular labyrinth and cochlea. The nerve enters the brainstem at the junctional region of pons and medulla oblongata. The functional anatomy of the vestibular division of the nerve is described in this chapter.

VESTIBULAR SYSTEM

The **bony labyrinth** of the inner ear is a very dense shell containing **perilymph**, which resembles extracellular fluid in general. The perilymph provides a water jacket for the **membranous labyrinth**, which encloses the sense organs of balance and of hearing. The sense organs are bathed in **endolymph**. The endolymph resembles intracellular fluid, being potassium-rich and sodium-poor.

The vestibular labyrinth comprises the **utricle**, the **saccule**, and three **semicircular ducts** (*Figure 16.2*). The utricle and saccule each contain a $3 \times 2\,mm^2$ **macula**. Each semicircular duct contains an **ampulla** at one end, and the ampulla houses a **crista**. (It should be pointed out that clinicians commonly speak of 'canals' where 'ducts' would be strictly more appropriate.)

The two maculae are the sensory end organs of the *static labyrinth*, which signals head position. The three cristae are the end organs of the *kinetic* or *dynamic labyrinth*, which signals head movement.

The bipolar cells of the **vestibular ganglion** occupy the internal acoustic meatus. Their peripheral processes are applied to the five sensory end organs. Their central processes, which constitute the **vestibular nerve**, cross the subarachnoid space and synapse in the vestibular nucleus previously seen in *Figures 14.14 and 14.15*.

Static labyrinth: anatomy and actions

The position and structure of the maculae are shown in *Figure 16.3*. The **utricular macula** is relatively horizontal, the **saccular macula** is relatively vertical. The cuboidal cells lining the membranous labyrinth become columnar **supporting cells** in the maculae. Among the supporting cells are so-called **hair cells**, to which vestibular nerve endings are applied. Some hair cells are almost completely enclosed by large nerve endings whereas others (phylogenetically older) receive only small contacts. At the cell bases are **ribbon synapses**, the synaptic vesicles being lined up along synaptic bars. Projecting from the free surface of each hair cell are about 100 **stereocilia** and, close to the cell margin, a single, long **kinocilium**. The hair cells discharge continuously, the resting rate being about 100 Hz.

The cilia are embedded in a gelatinous matrix containing protein-bound calcium carbonate crystals called **otoconia** ('ear sand'). (The term 'otoliths', when used, refers to the

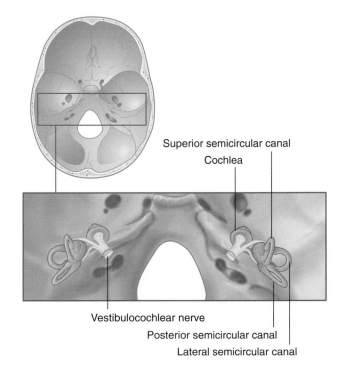

Figure 16.1 Bony labyrinth, viewed from above.

Superior semicircular canal
Cochlea
Vestibulocochlear nerve
Posterior semicircular canal
Lateral semicircular canal

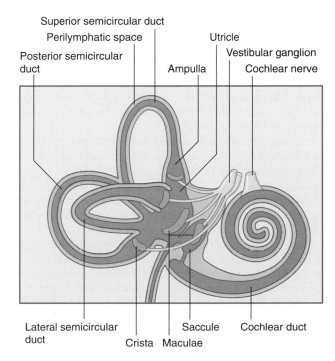

Figure 16.2 Locations of the five vestibular sense organs.

Superior semicircular duct
Perilymphatic space
Posterior semicircular duct
Ampulla
Utricle
Vestibular ganglion
Cochlear nerve
Lateral semicircular duct
Crista Maculae
Saccule Cochlear duct

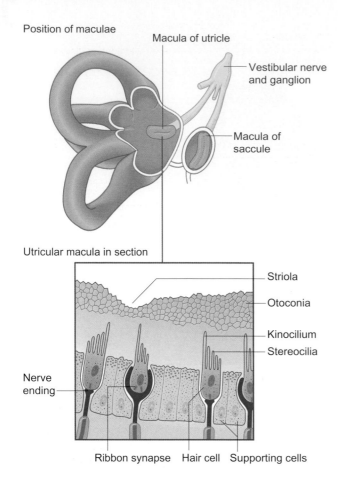

Position of maculae

Macula of utricle

Vestibular nerve and ganglion

Macula of saccule

Utricular macula in section

Striola

Otoconia

Kinocilium

Stereocilia

Nerve ending

Ribbon synapse　Hair cell　Supporting cells

Figure 16.3 Static labyrinth.

larger, 'ear stones' of reptiles.) The otoconia exert gravitational drag on the hair cells. Whenever kinocilia are dragged away from stereocilia, depolarization is facilitated. The macula has a central groove (**striola**) and the hair cell orientations have a mirror arrangement in relation to the groove. Electrical activity of hair cells is facilitated on one side of the groove by a given gravitational vector, and disfacilitated on the other side.

The maculae also respond to linear acceleration of the head in the horizontal plane (e.g. during walking) or in the vertical (gravitational) plane. Also, when the tilted head is stationary in a flexed or extended position, the facilitated half of the utricular macula discharges intensely in both ears. The saccular ones are more responsive when the head is held to the side.

The primary function of the static labyrinth is to signal the position of the head relative to the trunk. In response to this signal, the vestibular nucleus initiates compensatory movements, with the effect of maintaining the center of gravity between the feet (in standing) or just in front of the feet (during locomotion), and of keeping the head horizontal. These effects are mediated by the vestibulospinal tracts.

The **lateral vestibulospinal tract**, seen earlier in sections of medulla oblongata in Chapter 14, arises from large neurons in the **lateral vestibular nucleus** (of *Deiters*). The fibers descend in the anterior funiculus on the same side of the spinal cord and synapse upon extensor (antigravity) motoneurons. Both α and γ motoneurons are excited, and a

significant part of the increased muscle tone is exerted by way of the gamma loop (Ch. 13). During standing, the tract is tonically active on both sides of the spinal cord. During walking, activity is selective for the quadriceps motoneurons of the leading leg; this commences following heel strike and continues during the stance phase (when the other leg is off the ground). Deiters' nucleus is somatotopically organized, and the functionally appropriate neurons are selected by the flocculonodular lobe of the cerebellum. The flocculonodular lobe (Ch. 22) has two-way connections with all four vestibular nuclei.

Antigravity action is triggered mainly from the horizontal macula of the utricle. The vertical macula of the saccule, on the other hand, is maximally activated by a *free fall*. The shearing effect produces powerful extensor thrust in anticipation of a hard landing.

A small, **medial vestibulospinal tract** arises in the medial and inferior vestibular nuclei (*Figure 14.8*). It descends bilaterally in the medial longitudinal fasciculus and terminates upon excitatory and inhibitory internuncials in the cervical part of the cord. It operates *head-righting reflexes*, which serve to keep the head – and the gaze – horizontal when the body is craned forward or to one side. Good examples of head-righting reflexes are to be seen around pool tables and in bowling alleys. An added twist can be provided, if required, by torsion of the eyeballs (up to 10°) within the orbital sockets. This eye-righting reflex is mediated by axons *ascending* the medial longitudinal fasciculus from the *lateral* vestibular nucleus to reach nuclei controlling the extraocular muscles. Evidence derived from unilateral vestibular destruction (*Clinical Panel 16.1*) indicates that the horizontal position of the eyes when the head is upright is the result of a canceling effect of bilateral tonic activity in these Deitero-ocular pathways.

The medial vestibulospinal tract is also activated by the kinetic labyrinth.

The static labyrinth contributes to the sense of position. The sense of position of the body in space is normally provided by three sensory systems: the visual system, the conscious proprioceptive system, and the vestibular system. Deprived of one of the three, the individual can stand and walk by using information provided by the other two. Following loss of vision, for example, the subject can get about, although the constraints imposed by blindness are known to all. Following loss of conscious proprioception instead, the subject uses vision as a substitute for proprioceptive sense, and is disabled by closure of the eyes (sensory ataxia, Ch. 12). If the static labyrinths alone are inactive, closure of the eyes may lead to a heavy fall.

Kinetic labyrinth: anatomy and action

Basic features of macular epithelium are repeated in the three cristae. Again there are supporting cells, and hair cells to which vestibular nerve endings are applied. The kinocilia of the hair cells are long, penetrating into a gelatinous projection called the **cupula** (*Figure 16.4*). The cupula is bonded to the opposite wall of the ampulla.

The cristae are sensitive to angular acceleration of the labyrinths. Angular acceleration occurs during rotary 'yes' and 'no' movements of the head. The endolymph tends to lag behind because of its inertia, and the cupula balloons

A

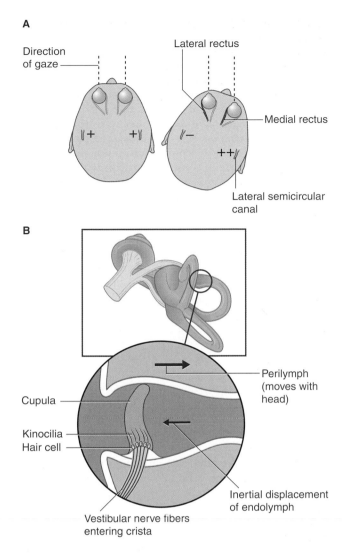

Direction of gaze

Lateral rectus

Medial rectus

Lateral semicircular canal

B

Cupula

Kinocilia
Hair cell

Vestibular nerve fibers entering crista

Perilymph (moves with head)

Inertial displacement of endolymph

Figure 16.4 (A) A rightward head turn activates nerve endings in the right lateral semicircular canal, resulting in contraction of the left lateral and right medial rectus muscles. **(B)** The nerve endings in the cupula are excited by passive displacement of the cupula toward the ampulla. Impulse traffic increases along parent unipolar neurons whose central fibers excite the medial and superior vestibular nuclei.

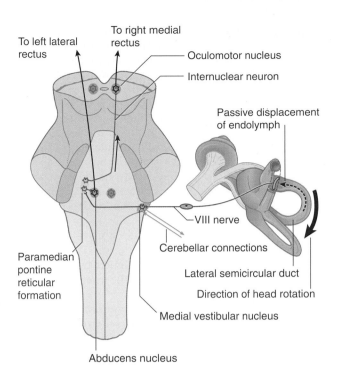

To left lateral rectus

To right medial rectus

Oculomotor nucleus

Internuclear neuron

Passive displacement of endolymph

VIII nerve

Cerebellar connections

Lateral semicircular duct

Direction of head rotation

Medial vestibular nucleus

Paramedian pontine reticular formation

Abducens nucleus

Figure 16.5 Under cerebellar guidance, the right medial vestibular nucleus responds to a rightward head turn by sending impulses to the contralateral paramedian reticular formation (PPRF, *Figure 14.15*). The PPRF selects abducens motor neurons supplying the left lateral rectus, and sends internuclear fibers up the right medial longitudinal fasciculus to the right oculomotor nucleus, where they seek out motor neurons serving the right medial rectus.

Not shown is the superior vestibular nucleus, which sends ipsilateral fibers having the function of inhibiting motor neurons to the two antagonist recti.

like a sail when thrust against it. The disposition of the kinocilia is uniform across each crista, and is such that the *lateral* ampullary crista is facilitated by cupular displacement *toward* the utricle; the *superior* and *posterior* cristae are facilitated by cupular displacement *away from* the utricle. In practical terms, the right lateral ampulla is activated by turning the head to the right; both superior ampullae are activated by flexion of the head; and both posterior ampullae by extension of the head.

Afferents from the cristae terminate in the medial and superior vestibular nuclei. As with the macular afferents, there are two-way connections with the flocculonodular lobe of the cerebellum.

The function of the kinetic labyrinth is to provide information for compensatory movements of the eyes in response to movement of the head. *Vestibulo-ocular reflexes* operate to

maintain the gaze on a selected target. A simple example is our ability to gaze at the period (full stop) at the end of a sentence, while moving the head about. The two eyes move *conjugately*, i.e. in parallel.

The horizontal vestibulo-ocular reflex response to a rightward turn of the head is depicted in *Figures 16.4 and 16.5*, and described in their captions.

Appropriate point-to-point connections also exist between the vestibular nuclei and gaze centers in the midbrain for similar reflexes in the vertical plane.

In order to control the vestibulo-ocular reflexes, the cerebellum is informed about the initial position of the head in relation to the trunk. This information is provided by a great wealth of muscle spindles in the deep muscles surrounding the cervical vertebral column. The spindle afferents enter the rostral spinocerebellar tract and relay in the accessory cuneate nucleus (*Figure 14.12*).

Nystagmus

A horizontal vestibulo-ocular reflex can be elicited artificially by warming or cooling the endolymph in the semicircular canals. In routine tests of vestibular function, advantage is taken of the proximity of the lateral semicircular canal to the middle ear. The canal is angled at 30° to the horizontal plane. Tilting the head back by 60° brings the canal into the vertical plane, with the ampulla uppermost. In the *warm caloric test*, water at 44°C is then instilled into the ear. The air in the middle ear is heated, and heat transfer to the lateral canal produces convection currents within the endolymph. Whether through displacement of the cupula or by some other mechanism, the crista of the warmer lateral ampulla becomes more active than its opposite number. The result is a slow drift of the eyes away from the stimulated side. *It is as if the head had been turned to the side being tested.* The drift is followed by a recovery phase in which the eyes snap back to the resting position. Slow and fast phases are repeated several times per second. This is *vestibular nystagmus*. The direction of the nystagmus is named in accordance with the fast phase because of the obvious 'beat'. A warm caloric test applied to the right ear should produce a right-beating nystagmus ('nystagmus to the right').

Subjectively, nystagmus is accompanied by vertigo – a sense of rotation of self in relation to the external world, or vice versa.

Unilateral and bilateral vestibular syndromes are considered in *Clinical Panel 16.1*. A vascular syndrome involving the vestibular system in the medulla oblongata is described in *Clinical Panel 16.2*.

Vestibulocortical connections

Second-order sensory neurons project from the vestibular nucleus to the contralateral thalamus. The fibers terminate in company with trigeminothalamic fibers in the ventral posterior nucleus. The main cortical area in receipt of third-order vestibular fibers has been perceived as a patch immediately behind the face representation on the somatic sensory cortex, because in conscious patients with the cortex exposed at operation, a mild electrical stimulus to this patch may elicit a sensation of vertigo. However, positron emission tomography (PET) reveals that the caloric test (in volunteers) activates other areas including insula and temporoparietal cortex. It is still uncertain which is the primary vestibular cortex. (By analogy, PET studies of tactile sensation show activity throughout most of the parietal lobe, but we know from other sources that the postcentral gyrus is the primary area, being the take-off point for analysis in the posterior parietal cortex.)

Clinical Panel 16.1   Vestibular disorders

Unilateral vestibular disease

Acute failure of one vestibular labyrinth may follow spread of disease from the middle ear or thrombosis of the labyrinthine artery. A common cause of unilateral vestibular symptoms in the elderly is a *transient ischemic attack* involving the vertebrobasilar arterial system. Transient ischemic attacks usually last 15 minutes or less and leave no residual neurological deficit.

The effects of unilateral vestibular disease are well demonstrated when the vestibular system is inactivated surgically, either during removal of an acoustic neuroma (Ch. 19) or as a last resort in treating paroxysmal attacks of vertigo. During the immediate postoperative period, the patient shows triple effects of loss of tonic input from the static labyrinth:

- Loss of function in the Deitero-ocular pathway on one side leads to about 10° of torsion of both eyeballs toward that side. The patient's perception of the horizontal shows a corresponding tilt, so that reaching movements become inaccurate.

- The head tilts to the same side, matching the gaze with the tilted horizon.

- The patient tends to fall to the same side, because the Deiterospinal tract no longer compensates for tilting of the head.

Because function continues in the normal lateral semicircular canal, there is a nystagmus to the normal side.

Bilateral vestibular disease

Following total loss of static labyrinthine function, visual guidance becomes important, and the patient dare not walk out-of-doors after twilight. By day, any distraction causing the patient to look overhead may result in a heavy fall. Loss of kinetic labyrinthine function makes it impossible to fix the gaze on an object while the head is moving. During walking, the scene bobs up and down as if it were being viewed through a hand-held camera.

Clinical Panel 16.2   Lateral medullary syndrome

Thrombosis of the vertebral or posterior inferior cerebellar artery may produce an infarct (area of necrosis) in the lateral part of the medulla. The clinical picture depends on the extent to which the various nuclei and pathways are damaged. Brainstem pathology must always be suspected when a cranial nerve lesion on one side is accompanied by 'upper motoneuron signs' on the other side – so-called *alternating* or *crossed hemiplegia*.

Lateral medullary syndrome   (Figure CP 16.2.1)

1 Damage to the vestibular nucleus leads to vertigo (often with initial vomiting), together with the symptoms of unilateral disconnection of the labyrinth described in *Clinical Panel 16.1*.

2 Interruption of posterior and rostral spinocerebellar fibers may produce signs of cerebellar ataxia in the ipsilateral limbs. Cerebellar ataxia is a prominent feature if blood flow is interrupted in the posterior inferior cerebellar artery.

3 Damage to the spinal tract of the trigeminal nerve interrupts fine primary afferent fibers descending the brainstem from the trigeminal ganglion (Ch. 17). These fibers are functionally equivalent to those of Lissauer's tract in the spinal cord (Ch. 12). The result of interruption is loss of pain and thermal senses from the face on the same side.

4 Interruption of the central sympathetic pathway to the spinal cord produces a complete Horner's syndrome (ptosis, miosis, anhidrosis).

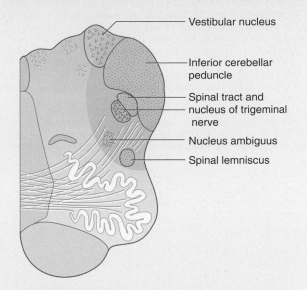

Figure CP 16.2.1 Lateral medullary infarct (shaded).

Vestibular nucleus

Inferior cerebellar peduncle

Spinal tract and nucleus of trigeminal nerve

Nucleus ambiguus

Spinal lemniscus

5 Damage to the nucleus ambiguus causes hoarseness, and sometimes difficulty in swallowing.

6 The only *contralateral* sign is loss of pain and temperature sense in the trunk and limbs, resulting from damage to the lateral spinothalamic tract. There is no motor weakness because the corticospinal tract is spared.

Core Information

The static labyrinth comprises the maculae in the utricle and the saccule. The dynamic labyrinth comprises the semicircular ducts and their cristae. Vestibular bipolar neurons supply all five and synapse in the vestibular nucleus, which is controlled by the flocculonodular lobe of cerebellum. The static labyrinth functions to control balance, via the lateral vestibulospinal tract, by increasing antigravity tone on the side to which the head is tilted. This system is in partnership with proprioceptors and retina in maintaining upright posture. In the absence of good vision, a fall is likely if the system has been compromised.

The dynamic labyrinth operates vestibulo-ocular reflexes so as to keep the gaze on target during rotatory movements of the head. For sideways rotation, the main projection is from medial vestibular nucleus to contralateral PPRF which activates VI neurons supplying the lateral rectus muscle and internuclear neurons projecting via the MLF to the contralateral medial rectus. Clinically, this pathway can be activated by the caloric test, which normally elicits nystagmus.

REFERENCES

Anniko, M. (1988) Functional morphology of the vestibular system. In *Physiology of the Ear* (Jahn, A.F. and Santos-Sacchi, J., eds), pp. 457–475. New York: Raven Press.

Brandt, T. and Dieterich, M. (1996) Postural imbalance in peripheral and central vestibular disorders. In *Clinical Disorders of Posture and Gait* (Bronstein, A.M., Brandt, T. and Woollacott, M., eds), pp. 131–146. London: Arnold.

Elliott, L.L. (1994) Functional brain imaging and hearing. *J. Acoust. Soc. Am.* **96**: 1397–1408.

Fitzpatrick, R. and McCloskey, D.I. (1994) Proprioceptive, visual and vestibular thresholds for the perception of sway during standing in humans. *J. Physiol.* **478**: 173–186.

Hart, C.W., McKinley, P.A. and Peterson, B.W. (1987) Compensation following acute unilateral total loss of peripheral vestibular function. In *The Vestibular System: Neurologic and Clinical Research* (Graham, M.D. and Kemink, J.L., eds), pp. 187–192. New York: Raven Press.

Markham, C.H. (1987) Vestibular control of muscular tone and posture. *Can. J. Neurol. Sci.* **14**: 493–496.

Paulesu, E., Frackowiak, R.S.J. and Bottini, G. (1997) Maps of somatosensory systems. In *Human Brain Function* (Frackowiak, R.S.J., Friston, K.J., Frith, C.D. and Mazziota, J.C. eds.), pp. 218–231. San Diego: Academic Press.

Spoendlin, H. (1988) Neural anatomy of the inner ear. In *Physiology of the Ear* (Jahn, A.F. and Santos-Sacchi, J., eds), pp. 201–219. New York: Raven Press.

Cochlear nerve

AUDITORY SYSTEM

The auditory system comprises the cochlea, the cochlear nerve, and the central auditory pathway from the cochlear nucleus in the brainstem to the cortex of the temporal lobe. The central auditory pathway is more elaborate than the somatosensory or visual pathway. This is because the same sounds are detected by both ears. In order to signal the location of a sound, a very complex neuronal network is in place, with numerous connections (mainly inhibitory) between the two central pathways in order to magnify minute differences in intensity and timing of sounds that exist during normal, binaural hearing.

The cochlea

The main features of cochlear structure are seen in *Figures 17.1* and *17.2*. The cochlea is pictured as though it were upright, but in life it lies on its side, as shown in *Figure 16.1*. The central bony pillar of the cochlea (the **modiolus**) is in the axis of the internal acoustic meatus. Projecting from the modiolus, like the flange of a screw, is the **osseous spiral lamina**. The **basilar membrane** is attached to the tip of this lamina; it reaches across the cavity of the bony cochlea to become attached to the **spiral ligament** on the outer wall. The osseous spiral lamina and spiral ligament become progressively smaller as one ascends the two and one half turns of the cochlea, and the fibers of the basal lamina become progressively longer.

The basal lamina and its attachments divide the cochlear chamber into upper and lower compartments. These are the **scala vestibuli** and the **scala tympani**, respectively, and

they are filled with perilymph. They communicate at the apex of the cochlea, through the **helicotrema**. A third compartment, the **scala media (cochlear duct)**, lies above the basilar membrane and is filled with endolymph. It is separated from the scala vestibuli by the delicate **vestibular membrane**.

Sitting on the basilar membrane is the **spiral organ** *(organ of Corti)*. The principal sensory receptor epithelium consists of a single row of **inner hair cells**, each one having up to 20 large afferent nerve endings applied to it. The hair cells rest upon **supporting cells**, and there are ancillary cells as well. The organ of Corti contains a central tunnel, filled with perilymph diffusing through the basilar membrane. On the outer side of the tunnel are several rows of **outer hair cells**, attended by supporting and ancillary cells.

All of the hair cells are surmounted by **stereocilia**. Unlike the vestibular hair cells, they have no kinocilium in the adult state. The stereocilia of the outer hair cells are embedded in the overlying tectorial membrane. Those of the inner hair cells lie immediately below the membrane.

The outer hair cells are contractile (in tissue culture), and they have substantial efferent nerve endings *(Figure 17.2)*. In theory at least, oscillatory movements of outer hair cells could influence the sensitivity of the inner hair cells through effects on the tectorial or basilar membrane.

Sound transduction

The vibrations of the tympanic membrane in response to sound waves are transmitted along the ossicular chain. The footplate of the stapes fits snugly into the oval window, and vibrations of the stapes are converted to pressure waves in the scala vestibuli. The pressure waves are transmitted through the vestibular membrane to reach the basilar membrane. High-frequency pressure waves, created by high-pitched sounds, cause the short fibers of the basilar membrane in the basal turn of the cochlea to resonate and absorb their energy. Low-frequency waves produce resonance in the apical turn where the fibers are longest. The basilar membrane is therefore *tonotopic* in its fiber sequence. Not surprisingly, the inner hair cells have a similar tonotopic sequence. In response to local resonance, the cells become depolarized and liberate excitatory transmitter substance from synaptic ribbons *(Figure 17.2)*.

The nerve fibers supplying the hair cells are the peripheral processes of the bipolar spiral ganglion cells lodged in the base of the osseous spiral lamina.

Cochlear nerve

The bulk of the cochlear nerve consists of the myelinated central processes of some 30 000 large bipolar neurons of the spiral ganglion. Unmyelinated fibers come from small ganglion cells supplying dendrites to the outer hair cells. (Motor fibers do not travel in the cochlear nerve trunk.) The nerve traverses the subarachnoid space in company with the vestibular and facial nerves, and it enters the brainstem at the pontomedullary junction.

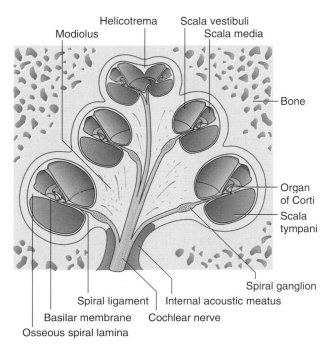

Helicotrema   Scala vestibuli
Modiolus   Scala media

Bone

Organ of Corti

Scala tympani

Spiral ganglion

Spiral ligament   Internal acoustic meatus
Basilar membrane   Cochlear nerve
Osseous spiral lamina

Figure 17.1 The cochlea in section.

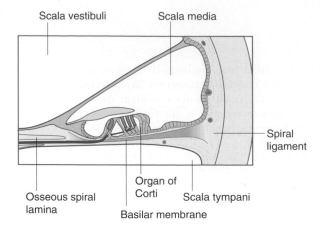

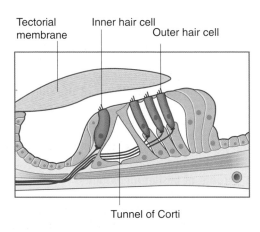

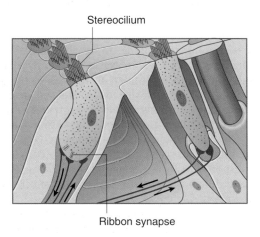

Figure 17.2 Organ of Corti at three levels of magnification. Arrows indicate directions of impulse traffic.

Central auditory pathways

The general plan of the central auditory pathway from the left cochlear nerve to the cerebral cortex is shown in *Figure 17.3*. The first cell station is the **cochlear nucleus**, where all cochlear nerve fibers terminate upon entry to the brainstem. From here, some second-order fibers project all the way to

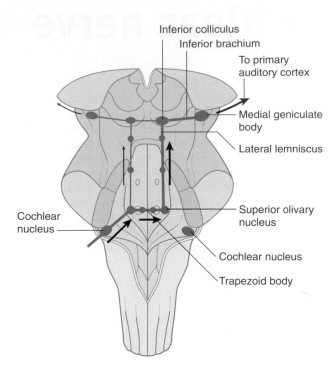

Figure 17.3 Dorsal view of brainstem showing basic plan of central auditory pathways.

the opposite **inferior colliculus** by way of the **trapezoid body** and **lateral lemniscus**. The **inferior brachium** links the inferior colliculus to the **medial geniculate body**, which projects to the **primary auditory cortex** in the temporal lobe.

A small but important purely ipsilateral relay passes from the superior olivary nucleus to the higher auditory centers.

Functional anatomy (Figure 17.4)

Cochlear nucleus

The cochlear nucleus comprises dorsal and ventral nuclei, on the surface of the inferior cerebellar peduncle as was shown in *Figure 14.12*. Many incoming fibers of the cochlear nerve bifurcate and enter both nuclei. The cells in both are tonotopically arranged.

Responses of many cells in the ventral nucleus are called primary-like, because their frequency (firing rate) resembles that of primary afferents. Most of the output neurons project to the nearby superior olivary nucleus.

The cells of the dorsal nucleus are heterogeneous. At least six different cell types have been characterized by their morphology and electrical behavior. Most of the output neurons project to the contralateral inferior colliculus. Individually, they exhibit an extremely narrow range of tonal responses, being 'focused' by collateral inhibition.

Superior olivary nucleus

The superior olivary complex of nuclei is relatively small in the human brain. It contains *binaural neurons* affected by inputs from both ears. Ipsilateral inputs are excitatory to the binaural neurons whereas contralateral inputs are inhibitory.

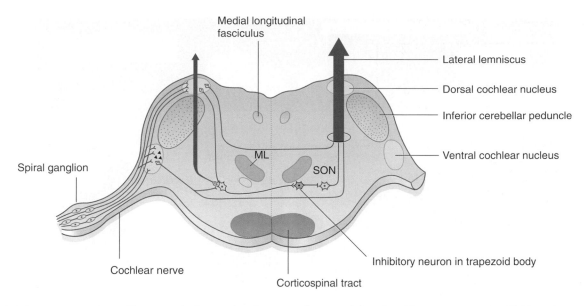

Figure 17.4 Transverse section of lower end of pons showing central connections of cochlear nerve. ML, medial lemniscus; SON, superior olivary nucleus.

The inhibitory effect is mediated by internuncial neurons in the **nucleus of the trapezoid body**.

The superior olivary nucleus is responsive to differences in intensity and timing between sounds entering both ears simultaneously. On the side ipsilateral to a sound, stimulation of the cochlea, and of the nucleus, is earlier and more intense than on the contralateral side. By exaggerating these differences through crossed inhibition, the superior olivary nucleus helps to indicate the spatial direction of incoming sounds. At the same time, the excited nucleus projects to the inferior colliculus of both sides, giving rise to binaural responses in the neurons of the inferior colliculus and beyond.

Lateral lemniscus

Fibers of the lateral lemniscus arise from the dorsal and ventral cochlear nuclei and from the superior olivary nuclei – in each case, mainly contralaterally. The tract terminates in the **central nucleus of the inferior colliculus**. Nuclei within the lateral lemniscus participate in reflex arcs (see later).

Inferior colliculus

Spatial information from the superior olivary nucleus, intensity information from the ventral cochlear nucleus, and pitch information from the dorsal cochlear nucleus are integrated in the inferior colliculus. The main (central) part of the nucleus is laminated in a tonotopic manner. Within each tonal lamina, cells differ in their responses: some have a characteristic 'tuning curve' (they respond only to a particular tone); some fire spontaneously but are inhibited by sound; and some respond only to a moving source of sound.

In addition to projecting to the medial geniculate nucleus, the inferior colliculus exerts inhibitory effects on its opposite number through the **collicular commissure** (*Figure 17.3*). It also contributes to the tectospinal tract.

Medial geniculate body

The medial geniculate body is the specific thalamic nucleus for hearing. The main (ventral) nucleus is laminated and tonotopic, and the large (magnocellular) principal neurons project as the **auditory radiation** to the primary auditory cortex (*Figure 17.5*).

Primary auditory cortex

The upper surface of the temporal lobe shows two or more **transverse temporal gyri**. The anterior one (the **gyrus of Heschl**) contains the **primary auditory cortex** (*Figure 17.6*). Tonotopic arrangement is preserved in Heschl's gyrus, its posterior part being responsive to high tones and its anterior part to low tones. The cortex responds to auditory stimuli within the *contralateral sound field*. In cats, destruction of a patch of primary cortex on one side produces a *sigoma* or 'deaf spot' in the contralateral sound field. In humans, ablation of the superior temporal gyrus (in the course of tumor removal) does not cause deafness, but it significantly reduces ability to judge the direction and distance of a source of sound.

Brainstem acoustic reflexes

Collateral branches emerging from the lateral lemniscus form the internuncial linkage for certain reflex arcs:

* Fibers entering the motor nuclei of the trigeminal and facial nerves link up with motor neurons supplying the tensor tympani and stapedius, respectively. These muscles exert a damping action on the ossicles of the middle ear. The tensor tympani is activated by the subject's own voice, the stapedius by external sounds.

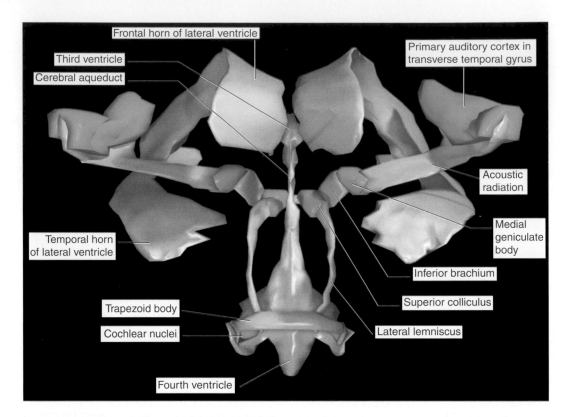

Figure 17.5 Graphic reconstruction of the central auditory pathways from a postmortem brain. (Reproduced from Kretschmann, H-J. and Weinrich, W. (1998) *Neurofunctional Systems: 3D Reconstructions with Correlated Neuroimaging: Text and CD-ROM*. New York: Thieme, with kind permission of the authors and the publisher.)

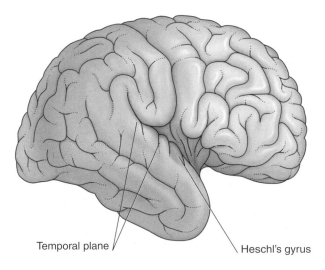

Figure 17.6 Tilted view of the right cerebral hemisphere; the frontal and parietal opercula of the insula have been removed to show the anterior temporal gyrus of Heschl (*blue*).

- Fibers entering the reticular formation have an important arousal effect, as exemplified by the alarm clock. Sudden loud sounds cause the subject to flinch; this is the 'startle response', mediated by outputs from the reticular formation to the spinal cord and to the motor nucleus of the facial nerve.

Descending auditory pathways

A cascade of descending fibers runs from the primary auditory cortex to the medial geniculate nucleus and inferior colliculus, and from the inferior colliculus to the superior olivary nucleus. The **olivocochlear bundle** emerges in the vestibular nerve and carries efferent, cholinergic fibers to the cochlea, with some for the vestibular labyrinth. The cochlear fibers apply large synaptic boutons to outer hair cells, and small boutons to the afferent nerve endings on inner hair cells.

The function of the olivocochlear bundle is uncertain. Experimental evidence indicates an involvement in enhancing detection of faint sounds.

Deafness

Deafness is a widespread problem in the community. About 10% of adults suffer from it in some degree. The cause may lie in the outer, middle, or inner ear, or in the cochlear neural pathway. The two fundamental types of deafness are described in *Clinical Panel 17.1*.

Box 17.1   Brainstem auditory evoked potentials

Remarkably, it is possible to follow the sequence of electrical events in the auditory pathway, step by step from cochlea to primary auditory cortex. Following placement of scalp electrodes for detection of electrical activity, a thousand or more 0.1 msec clicksounds are quickly presented to each ear in turn. A computer separates the responses along the auditory pathway from the background 'noise' of neighboring electric traffic (see Example below).

A sequence of seven averaged-out waves is detected within 10 msec after the collective click. Explanations are as shown.

Pathology anywhere along the auditory pathway results in reduction or abolition of the wave above that level. The technique is used for suspected lesions at the cerebellopontine angle (Ch. 19) or at higher levels of the auditory pathway. It is also used in the medicolegal domain, in assessment of claims of deafness from environmental noise in industry.

Example
Consider brainstem cranial nerve traffic alone, in a subject looking straight ahead.
We have:

- III, IV and VI maintaining the steady gaze
- VIII preventing sagging of the jaw
- VII keeping the lips together
- VIII upgoing MLF fibers busy with vestibulo-ocular reflexes; medial vestibulospinal MLF fibers operating head-righting reflexes

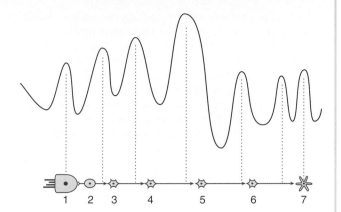

Figure Box 17.1.1 Brainstem auditory-evoked potentials. **1** Cochlear hair cells; **2** Cochlear nerve; **3** From cochlear nucleus; **4** From superior olivary nucleus; **5** From inferior colliculus; **6** From medial geniculate body; **7** Primary auditory cortex.

- IX monitoring blood pressure, arterial and CSF pH
- X discussing heart rate with the vasomotor center
- XIc keeping the vocal cords apart
- XIs twitching sternomastoid now and then, to keep the head straight
- XII tonic to genioglossus, to keep the airway clear.

Clinical Panel 17.1   Two kinds of deafness

All forms of deafness can be grouped into two categories. *Conductive deafness* is caused by disease in the outer ear canal or in the middle ear. *Sensorineural deafness* is caused by disease in the cochlea or in the neural pathway from cochlea to brain.

Common causes of conductive deafness include accumulation of cerumen (wax) in the outer ear, and *otitis media* (inflammation in the middle ear). *Otosclerosis* is a disorder of the oval window in which the capsule of the synovial joint between the footplate of the stapes and the vestibule of the bony labyrinth is progressively replaced by bone. The stapes becomes immobilized, with severe impairment of hearing throughout the full tonal range. Replacement of the stapes by a prosthesis (artificial substitute) often restores normal hearing.

Sensorineural deafness usually originates within the cochlea. The commonest form is the high-frequency hearing loss of the elderly, resulting from deterioration of the organ of Corti in the basal turn. As a result, the

elderly have difficulty in distinguishing among high-frequency consonants (d, s, t); vowels, which are low frequency, are quite audible. Therefore the elderly should be addressed distinctly rather than loudly.

Occupational deafness arises from a noisy environment at work. A persistent noise, especially indoors, may eventually lead to degeneration of the organ of Corti in the region corresponding to the particular frequency.

Ototoxic deafness may follow administration of drugs, including streptomycin, neomycin, and quinine.

Infectious deafness may follow more or less complete destruction of the cochlea by the virus of mumps or congenital rubella (German measles).

An important cause of sensorineural deafness in adults is an *acoustic neuroma*. Because the trigeminal and facial nerves may be affected as well as the cochlear and vestibular, this tumor is described in Chapter 19.

Core Information

The bipolar cochlear neurons occupy the osseous spiral lamina of the modiolus. Their peripheral processes supply hair cells in the organ of Corti. Their central processes end in the cochlear nucleus; from here, a polyneuronal pathway leads mainly through the trapezoid body and lateral lemniscus to the inferior colliculus, but there is a significant ipsilateral pathway too. From the inferior colliculus, fibers run to the medial geniculate body, and from there to the primary auditory cortex on the upper surface of the temporal lobe of the brain.

Clinically, deafness is of two kinds: conductive, involving disease in the outer or middle ear; and sensorineural, involving disease of the cochlea (usually) or of central auditory pathways. Hearing is seldom significantly compromised by central pathway lesions because of the bilateral projections to the inferior colliculus and beyond.

REFERENCES

Adams, J.C. (1986) Neuronal morphology in the human cochlear nucleus. *Arch. Otolaryngol. Head Neck Surg.* **112**: 1253–1261.

Aitkin, L.M. (1989) The auditory system. In *Handbook of Chemical Neuroanatomy*, Vol. 7: Integrated Systems of the CNS, Part II (Bjorklund, A., Hokfeld, T. and Swanson, L.W., eds), pp. 165–218. New York: Elsevier.

Corwin J.T. and Warchol, M.E. (1991) Auditory hair cells: structure, function, development, and regeneration. *Ann. Rev. Neurosci.* **14**: 301–333.

Phillips, D.P. (1988) Introduction to anatomy and physiology of the central auditory nervous system. In *Physiology of the Ear* (Jahn, A.F. and Santos-Sacchi, J., eds), pp. 407–427. New York: Raven Press.

Trigeminal nerve

TRIGEMINAL NERVE

The trigeminal nerve has a very large sensory territory which includes the skin of the face, the oronasal mucous membranes and the teeth, the dura mater, and major intracranial blood vessels. The nerve is also both motor and sensory to the muscles of mastication. The **motor root** lies medial to the large **sensory root** at the site of attachment to the pons (*Figure 14.16*). The **trigeminal** (*Gasserian*) **ganglion**, near the apex of the petrous temporal bone, gives rise to the sensory root and consists of unipolar neurons.

Details of the distribution of the ophthalmic, maxillary, and mandibular divisions are available in gross anatomy textbooks. Accurate appreciation of their respective territories on the face is essential if trigeminal neuralgia is to be distinguished from other sources of facial pain (*Clinical Panel 18.1*).

Motor nucleus   (Figures 14.16, 18.1)

The motor nucleus is the special visceral nucleus supplying the muscles derived from the embryonic mandibular arch. These comprise the masticatory muscles attached to each half of the mandible (*Figure 18.2*), along with the tensor tympani and tensor palati. The nucleus occupies the lateral pontine tegmentum. Embedded in its upper pole is a node of the reticular formation, the **supratrigeminal nucleus**, which acts as a pattern generator for masticatory rhythm.

Voluntary control is provided by corticonuclear projections from each motor cortex to both motor nuclei, but mainly the contralateral one (*Figure 14.3*).

Sensory nuclei

Three sensory nuclei are associated with the trigeminal nerve: **mesencephalic**, **pontine** (*principal*), and **spinal**.

Clinical Panel 18.1   Trigeminal neuralgia

Trigeminal neuralgia is an important condition, characterized by attacks of excruciating pain in the territory of one or more divisions of the trigeminal nerve (usually II or III). The patient (who is usually more than 60 years old) is able to map out the affected division(s) accurately. Because it must be distinguished from many other causes of facial pain, the clinician should be able to mark out a trigeminal sensory map (*Figure CP 18.1.1*). Sometimes there is an underlying osteitis of the petrous temporal bone, or compression of the sensory root by an arterial loop, but usually no explanation is found.

Most patients respond well to drug therapy. For those who do not, surgery is indicated. A procedure of historic interest is *medullary tractotomy*, whereby the spinal root was sectioned through the dorsolateral surface of the medulla. In successful cases, pain and temperature sensitivity was lost from the face but touch (mediated by the pontine nucleus) was preserved. This procedure has been abandoned owing to a high mortality rate associated with compromise of underlying respiratory and cardiovascular centers.

A procedure which can be performed under local anesthesia is electrocoagulation of the affected division, through a needle electrode inserted through the foramen ovale from below. The intention is to heat the nerve sufficiently to destroy only the finest fibers, in which case analgesia is produced but touch (including the corneal reflex) is preserved.

Another option is to *decompress* the afflicted nerve

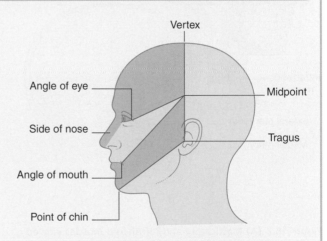

Figure CP 18.1.1 Trigeminal nerve sensory map.

root through an intracranial approach whereby neighboring small vessels are lifted away from it; the notion being that chronic compression causes local demyelination with *ephaptic* (*Gr.* touching) spread of nerve impulses from an active denuded axon to its denuded neighbors. This concept is bolstered by the fact that trigeminal neuralgia may be a presenting symptom in patients undergoing the demyelination process of multiple sclerosis. An alternative suggestion concerning the beneficial effect of this and other local manipulations is that they may alter gene transcription in the nuclei of the related somas.

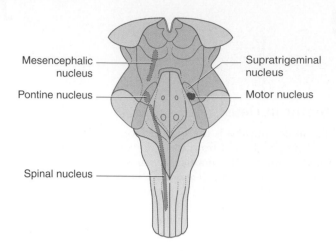

Figure 18.1 Trigeminal nuclei. *Left*: sensory nuclei; *right*: motor nucleus, supratrigeminal nucleus.

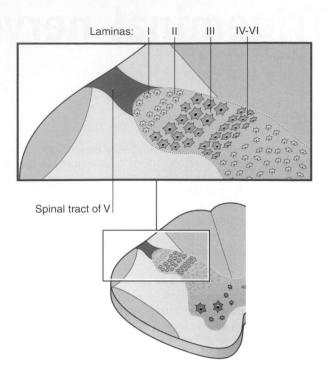

Figure 18.3 Spinal tract and nucleus of trigeminal nerve, at level of spinomedullary junction.

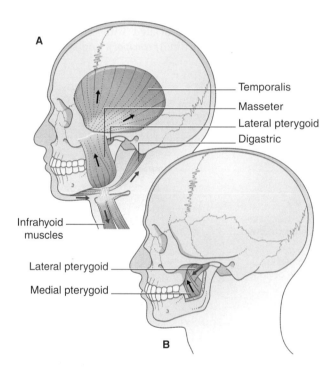

Figure 18.2 (A) Masticatory and infrahyoid muscles viewed from the left side. **(B)** Medial view of the pterygoid muscles of the right side. Red arrows indicate directions of pull of jaw-closing muscles. Black arrows indicate directions of pull of jaw openers.

Mesencephalic nucleus

The mesencephalic nucleus is unique in being the only nucleus in the CNS which contains the cell bodies of primary sensory neurons. Their peripheral processes enter the sensory root via the mesencephalic tract of the trigeminal. Some travel in the mandibular division to supply stretch receptors (neuromuscular spindles) in the masticatory muscles. Others travel in the maxillary and mandibular divisions to supply stretch receptors (Ruffini endings) in the suspensory, periodontal ligaments of the teeth.

The central processes of the mesencephalic afferent neurons descend through the pontine tegmentum in the small *tract of Probst*. Most fibers of this tract terminate in the supratrigeminal nucleus; others end in the motor nucleus or in the pontine sensory nucleus; a few travel as far as the dorsal nucleus of the vagus.

Pontine nucleus

The pontine (principal sensory) nucleus (*Figure 14.11*) is homologous with the posterior column nuclei (gracile and cuneate). It processes discriminative tactile information from the face and oronasal cavity.

Spinal nucleus

The spinal nucleus extends from the lower part of the pons to the third cervical segment of the spinal cord (hence the term 'spinal'). Two minor nuclei in its upper part (called **pars oralis** and **pars interpolaris**) receive afferents from the mouth. The main spinal nucleus (**pars caudalis**) receives nociceptive and thermal information from the entire trigeminal area, and even beyond.

In section, the main spinal nucleus is seen to be an expanded continuation of the outer laminae (I–III) of the posterior horn of the cord (*Figure 18.3*). The inner three laminae (IV–VI) are relatively compressed. Laminae III and IV are referred to as the magnocellular part of the nucleus. In animals, nociceptive-specific internuncials are found in lamina I. 'Polymodal' neurons are in the magnocellular nucleus and correspond to lamina V neurons lower down; they respond to tactile stimuli applied to the trigeminal skin area; also to noxious mechanical stimuli (e.g. pinching the skin with a forceps). Whereas the nociceptive-specific neurons have small receptive fields confined to one territory

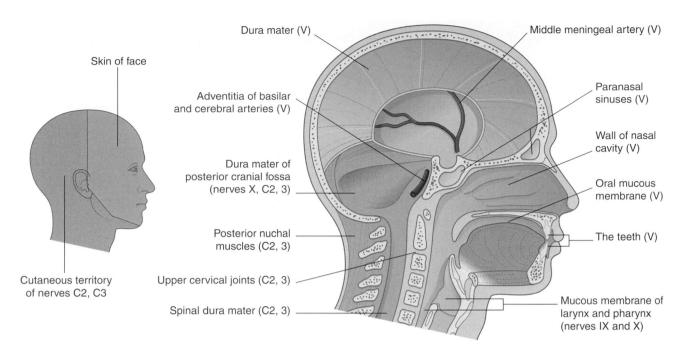

Figure 18.4 Diagram to indicate the extensive nociceptive territory of the spinal trigeminal nucleus. Structures labeled (V) are supplied by the trigeminal nerve. The remainder are supplied by other nerves having central nociceptive projections to the spinal trigeminal nucleus.

(a patch of skin or mucous membrane), many of the polymodal neurons show the phenomenon of *convergence* to a marked degree. In anesthetized animals, a single neuron may be responsive to noxious stimuli applied to a tooth, or to facial skin, or to the temporomandibular joint. This finding provides a plausible basis of explanation for erroneous localization of pain by patients. Examples are given in *Clinical Panel 18.2*.

Arrangements for pain modulation appear to be the same as for the spinal cord (Ch. 21). They include the presence of enkephalinergic and GABAergic internuncials in the substantia gelatinosa, and serotonininergic projections from the raphe magnus nucleus.

Afferents to the spinal nucleus come from three sources (*Figure 18.4*):

1 *Trigeminal afferents* are the central processes of trigeminal ganglion cells. The peripheral processes terminate in tactile and nociceptive endings in the territory of the three divisions of the nerve. Most often involved clinically are the nociceptive terminals in (a) the teeth, (b) the cornea, (c) the temporomandibular joint, and (d) the dura mater of the anterior and middle cranial fossae. In Chapter 4, it was noted that tension of the supratentorial dura gives rise to frontal or parietal headache.

Topographic representation of the trigeminal territory is onion-like (*Figure 18.5*); central fibers terminate in the rostral part of the nucleus, intermediate fibers in the midregion, and the peripheral fibers caudally.

2 *Glossopharyngeal* and *vagal afferents* enter from the mucous membranes of the pharyngotympanic tube, middle ear, pharynx, and larynx. These afferents are often involved in acute inflammatory processes during

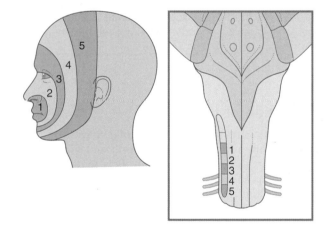

Figure 18.5 Representation of the face in the spinal trigeminal nucleus.

wintertime. Their cell bodies occupy the inferior sensory ganglia of the glossopharyngeal and vagus nerves.

3 *Cervical afferents* come from the territory of the first three cervical posterior nerve roots. (The first posterior nerve root is either small or absent.) Most often involved clinically are nociceptive fibers supplying (a) the intervertebral joints and spinal dura mater, and (b) the dura mater of the posterior cranial fossa, reached by cervical fibers ascending through the hypoglossal canal. In Chapter 4, it was noted that infratentorial meningitis is associated with severe occipital headache, and with reflex head retraction because the suboccipital muscles are supplied by the upper three cervical anterior nerve roots.

Clinical Panel 18.2   Referred pain in diseases of the head and neck

Cervicogenic headache

Experiments on healthy volunteers have demonstrated that noxious stimulation of tissues supplied by the upper cervical nerves may induce pain referred to the head. Tissues tested include the ligaments of the upper cervical joints, the suboccipital muscles, and the sternomastoid and trapezius muscles. The unilateral pain is primarily occipital, as would be expected from the cutaneous distribution of the greater occipital nerve given off by the posterior ramus of nerve C2, but it may radiate to the forehead. Diagnostic features include intensification of the pain by head movement, and temporary abolition by ipsilateral local anesthetic blockade of the greater occipital nerve. A common source of cervicogenic headache in the elderly is spondylosis, a degenerative arthritis in which bony excrescences compress the emerging spinal nerves (Ch. 11). Another source appears to be myofascial disease of the sternomastoid–trapezius continuum close to the base of the skull. *Trigger points* – tender nodules within the muscles which give rise to occipital pain when compressed – are often detected by physical therapists during palpation of these muscles.

Earache

Earache is most often due to an acute infection of the outer ear canal or middle ear. However, pain may be referred to a perfectly healthy ear from a variety of sources. The outer ear skin receives small sensory branches from the mandibular, facial, vagus, and upper cervical nerves; the middle ear epithelium is supplied by the glossopharyngeal and vagus. Earache may be a leading symptom of disease in the territory of one of these nerves. Important examples:

- Cancer of the pharynx – perhaps concealed in the piriform fossa beside the larynx, or near the tonsil.
- An impacted wisdom tooth in the mandible.
- Temporomandibular joint disease.
- Spondylosis of the upper cervical spine.

Pain in the face

Important causes of pain referred to the face below the eye include:

- Dental caries or an impacted maxillary wisdom tooth.
- Cancer in a mucous membrane supplied by the maxillary nerve: maxillary air sinus, nasal cavity, nasopharynx.
- Acute maxillary sinusitis.
- Trigeminal neuralgia affecting the maxillary nerve.

Innervation of the teeth

From the superior and inferior alveolar nerves, Aδ and C fibers enter the root canals of the teeth and form a dense plexus within the pulp. Individual fibers terminate in the pulp, in the predentin, and in dentinal tubules. Most dentinal tubules underlying the occlusal surfaces of the teeth contain single nerve fibers; however, the fibers are restricted to the inner ends of the tubules whereas pain can be elicited from the outer surface of dentin after removal of the enamel. Hydrodynamic and chemical factors have been invoked to fill the gap, also possible participation of odontoblasts as intermediaries.

The periodontal ligaments are richly innervated by the nerves supplying the oral epithelium including the gums. Some of the nerve endings are a potential source of pain during dental extraction or periodontal disease. Others function as tension receptors comparable to Ruffini endings found in joint capsules; tension receptors would be anticipated because the periodontal ligaments are arranged like hammocks around the roots of the teeth.

Innervation of cerebral arteries

The ophthalmic division of the trigeminal nerve comes close to the internal carotid artery in the cavernous sinus. Here it gives off afferent fibers which accompany the artery to its point of bifurcation into anterior and middle cerebral branches. The nerve fibers accompany these, and also reach the posterior cerebral artery via branches accompanying the vertebral. Several peptide substances have been detected in these axons; they include substance P, the peptide particularly associated with nociceptive transmission.

The function of the *trigeminovascular neurons* (as they are called) is the subject of speculation. Their presence accounts well for the *frontal headache* associated with distortion of the cerebral arteries by space-occupying lesions.

Trigeminothalamic tract and trigeminal lemniscus   (Figure 18.6)

The lower part of the **trigeminothalamic tract** commences in the spinal trigeminal nucleus. Nearly all of these fibers cross the midline before ascending into the pons. This component has features in common with the spinal lemniscus which accompanies it in the brainstem (*Figures 14.15–14.18*), mediating tactile, nociceptive, and thermal sensations. In the pons, it is joined by fibers crossing from the principal sensory nucleus, thus completing the **trigeminal lemniscus** which terminates in the ventral posterior medial nucleus of thalamus (Ch. 24). From the thalamus, third-order afferents project to the large area of facial representation in the lower half of the somatic sensory cortex.

Trigeminoreticular fibers synapse in the parvocellular reticular formation on both sides of the brainstem. They are coun-

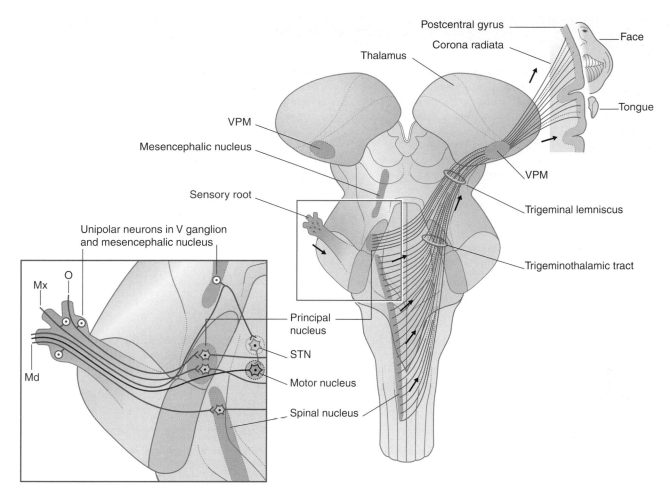

Figure 18.6 Primary, secondary, and tertiary trigeminal (V) afferents. O, Md, Mx, ophthalmic, mandibular maxillary divisions of trigeminal nerve; STN, supratrigeminal nucleus; VPM, ventral posterior medial nucleus of thalamus.

terparts of the spinoreticular tract, and they mediate the arousal effect of stroking or slapping the face, and of old-fashioned 'smelling salts' (the ammonia irritates trigeminal afferents in the nose).

Mastication

Mastication is a complex activity requiring orchestration of the nuclear groups supplying the muscles that move the mandible, tongue, cheeks, and hyoid bone. The chief controlling center seems to be an area of the premotor cortex directly in front of the face representation on the motor cortex. Stimulation of this area produces masticatory cycles.

Brainstem control of mandibular activity resides in the **supratrigeminal nucleus**, which functions as a pattern generator. The supratrigeminal nucleus receives proprioceptive information from the spindle-rich, jaw-closing muscles (masseter, temporalis, medial pterygoid) and from the periodontal ligaments. The supratrigeminal nucleus also receives tactile information (food in the mouth) from the pontine nucleus, and nociceptive information from the spinal nucleus. It gives rise to an ipsilateral trigeminocerebellar projection and a contralateral trigeminothalamic projection,

both containing proprioceptive information. It controls mastication directly by means of excitatory and inhibitory inputs to the trigeminal motor nucleus.

The *jaw-closing reflex* is initiated by contact of food with the oral mucous membrane. The response of the pattern generator is to activate the jaw-closing motorneurons so that the teeth are brought into occlusion.

The *jaw-opening reflex* is initiated by periodontal stretch afferents activated by dental occlusion. The pattern generator responds by inhibiting the closure motorneurons and activating the jaw openers. Muscle spindles are especially numerous in the anterior part of the masseter, and when stretch reaches a critical level the pattern generator is switched to a jaw-closing mode.

The jaw jerk

The jaw jerk is a tendon reflex elicited by tapping the chin with a downward stroke. The normal response is a twitch of the jaw-closing muscles, because muscle spindle afferents make some direct synaptic contacts upon trigeminal motor neurons. Supranuclear lesions of the motor nucleus (e.g. *pseudobulbar palsy*, Ch. 15) may be accompanied by an exaggerated (abnormally brisk) jaw jerk.

Core Information

The motor root of V enters the mandibular division to supply the six muscles of mastication and tensor tympani and tensor palati. Automatic control is by the supratrigeminal nucleus, and voluntary control from the motor cortex (mainly contralaterally).

The V ganglion (unipolar cells) sends peripheral processes into all three divisions, providing sensory endings in face, oronasal mucous membranes, teeth, meninges, and intracranial blood vessels. Central processes synapse in the pontine (principal sensory) and spinal nuclei.

Peripheral processes proprioceptive to masticatory muscles and periodontal ligaments belong to the unipolar-celled mesencephalic nucleus. The main target of the central processes of these cells is the supratrigeminal nucleus, which is the masticatory generator.

The pontine nucleus processes tactile information from the face and oronasal mucous membranes. The spinal nucleus receives nociceptive signals from the entire trigeminal sensory field; from the oropharynx via the glossopharyngeal; from laryngopharynx and larynx via the vagus; and from the posterior rami of upper cervical nerves.

The pontine and spinal nuclei project fibers into the reticular formation (serving arousal) and to the contralateral thalamus via the trigeminothalamic tract.

The supratrigeminal nucleus is seldom dormant. In the erect posture, it activates the jaw closers to keep the mandible elevated. During sleep, it activates the lateral pterygoid so that the pharynx is not occluded by the tongue. (The root of the tongue is anchored to the mandible.) However, *the nucleus is inactivated by general anesthesia*, in which circumstance the ramus of the mandible must be held forward constantly in order to prevent choking.

REFERENCES

Lambert, G.A. (1993) Pathways for headache. In *Science and Practice in Clinical Neurology* (Gandevia, S.C., Burke, D. and Anthony, M., eds), pp. 284–302. Cambridge: Cambridge University Press.

Pollmann, W., Keidel, M. and Pfaffenrath, V. (1997) Headache and the cervical spine: a critical review. *Cephalalgia* 17: 801–816.

Rappaport, Z.H. (1994) Trigeminal neuralgia: the role of self-sustaining discharge in the trigeminal ganglion. *Pain* 56: 127–138.

Sessle, B.J. (1990) Anatomy, physiology and pathophysiology of orofacial pain. In *Headache and Facial Pain* (Jacobson, A.L. and Donlon, W.C., eds), pp. 1–24. New York: Raven Press.

Tenser, R.B. (1998) Trigeminal neuralgia. *Neurology* 51: 17–19.

Yokota, T. (1988) Anatomy and physiology of intra- and extracranial nociceptive afferents and their central projections. In *Basic Mechanisms of Headache* (Olesen, J. and Edvinsson, L., eds), pp. 117–128. Amsterdam: Elsevier.

Facial nerve

FACIAL NERVE

The **facial nerve** supplies the muscles derived from the second branchial arch. These include the muscles of facial expression, and four minor ones to be mentioned. It is accompanied during part of its course by the **nervus intermedius** which supplies secretomotor fibers to glands in the eye, nose and mouth, also gustatory fibers to the tongue and palate.

The facial nerve arises from the branchial (special visceral) efferent cell column caudal to the motor nucleus of the trigeminal nerve (*Figure 14.2*). The **facial nucleus** occupies the lateral region of the tegmentum in the caudal part of the pons (*Figures 14.15, 19.1*). Before emerging from the brainstem, it loops, as the **internal genu**, around the abducens nucleus, creating the **facial colliculus** in the floor of the fourth ventricle.

The nerve emerges at the lower border of the pons together with the nervus intermedius. Both nerves cross the subarachnoid space in company with the vestibulocochlear nerve, to the internal acoustic meatus. Above the vestibule of the labyrinth, it enters a 7-shaped bony canal having a backward bend at the **external genu** of the facial nerve. Prior to escaping the canal at the stylomastoid foramen, it supplies the stapedius muscle. Upon escape, it supplies the posterior belly of the occipitofrontalis, the stylohyoid, and the posterior belly of the digastric. It then turns forward within the substance of the parotid gland while breaking up into the five named branches to the muscles of facial expression (*Figure 19.2*).

Supranuclear connections

All of the cells of the motor nucleus receive a corticonuclear supply from the 'face' area of the contralateral motor cortex. In addition, those to the muscles of the upper face (occipitofrontalis and orbicularis oculi) receive an equal supply from the *ipsilateral* motor cortex. The bilateral supply for the upper facial muscles is reflected in their habitual paired activities in wrinkling the forehead, blinking, and squeezing the eyes closed. The muscles around the mouth, on the other hand, are often activated unilaterally for some expressive purpose. The partial bilateral supply to the facial muscles helps to distinguish a supranuclear from a nuclear or infranuclear lesion of the nerve (*Clinical Panel 19.1*).

More than any other muscle group, the muscles of facial expression are responsive to emotional states. A limbic contribution to the supranuclear supply is to be expected, and its source is the **nucleus accumbens** at the base of the forebrain. The nucleus accumbens is a ventral part of the basal ganglia, which in turn influence the motor cortex. That circuit is compromised in Parkinson's disease, which is characterized by a mask-like physiognomy (Ch. 28).

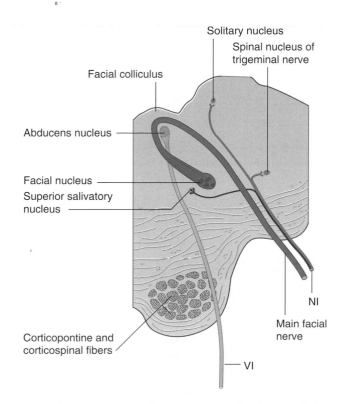

Figure 19.1 Transverse section of the pons showing the facial nerve and the nervus intermedius (NI).

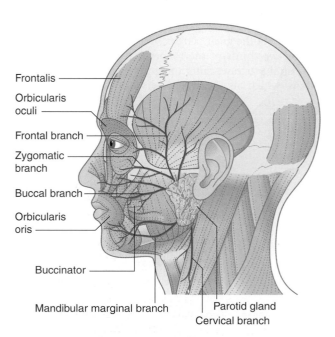

Figure 19.2 Principal extracranial branches of the facial nerve.

Nuclear connections

Five reflex arcs engaging the facial nucleus are listed in *Table 19.1*. Most important clinically is the corneal reflex.

Corneal reflex

The usual test is to touch the cornea with a cotton wisp. This should elicit a bilateral blink response. The afferent limb of the reflex is the ophthalmic division of the trigeminal nerve (nasociliary branch). The efferent limb is the facial nerve (branch to palpebral element of orbicularis oculi). Because the reflex can still be elicited following section of the spinal tract of the trigeminal nerve (*tractotomy*, Ch. 18), the ophthalmic afferents evidently synapse in the principal (pontine) nucleus of the trigeminal. Internuncials projecting from each principal nucleus to both facial nuclei complete the reflex arc.

The corneal reflex may be lost following a lesion of either the ophthalmic or facial nerves. A gradual compression of ophthalmic fibers in the sensory root of the trigeminal nerve may damage corneal neurons selectively. For this reason, the corneal reflex must be tested in patients under suspicion of an acoustic neuroma (*Clinical Panel 19.2*).

Nervus intermedius

Nervus intermedius aligns with the facial nerve distal to the internal genu. It comprises two sets of parasympathetic and two sets of special sense fibers (*Figure 19.3*).

The *parasympathetic root* of the nerve arises from the **superior salivatory nucleus** in the pons. This is the motor component of the **greater petrosal** and **chorda tympani** nerves. The greater petrosal synapses in the **pterygopalatine ganglion** ('the ganglion of hay fever') whose postganglionic fibers stimulate the lacrimal and nasal glands. The motor component of chorda tympani synapses in the **submandibular ganglion** whose postganglionic fibers stimulate the submandibular and sublingual glands.

The *special sense root* of this nerve has unipolar cell bodies in the **geniculate ganglion** of the facial nerve. The peripheral processes of these ganglion cells supply taste buds in the palate via the great petrosal nerve, and taste buds in the anterior two-thirds of the tongue via the chorda tympani. The central processes enter the gustatory part of the solitary nucleus, which also receives fibers from the glossopharyn-geal nerve (Ch. 15). From here, second-order neurons project to the thalamus on the *same* side, for relay to the anterior parts of insula and cingulate cortex.

A few cells of the geniculate ganglion supply skin in and around the external acoustic meatus (*Clinical Panel 19.1*).

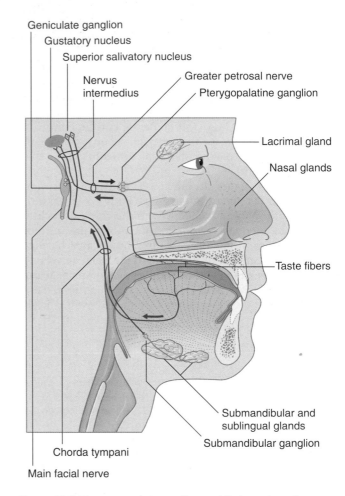

Figure 19.3 The nervus intermedius and its branches. Arrows indicate direction of impulse traffic.

Table 19.1 Brainstem reflexes involving the facial nerve

	Corneal reflex	Sucking reflex	Blinking to light	Blinking to noise	Sound attenuation
Receptor	Cornea	Lips	Retina	Cochlea	Cochlea
Afferent	Ophthalmic nerve	Mandibular nerve	Optic nerve	Cochlear nucleus	Cochlear nucleus
First synapse	Spinal nucleus of trigeminal	Pontine nucleus of trigeminal	Superior colliculus	Inferior colliculus	Superior olivary nucleus
Second synapse	Facial nucleus	Facial nucleus	Facial nucleus	Facial nucleus	Facial nucleus
Muscle	Orbicularis oculi	Orbicularis oris	Orbicularis oculi	Orbicularis oculi	Stapedius

Clinical Panel 19.1 Lesions of the facial nerve

Supranuclear lesions

Much the commonest cause of a supranuclear lesion of the seventh nerve is a vascular stroke, in which corticonuclear and corticospinal fibers are interrupted at or above the level of the internal capsule. The usual effect of a stroke is to produce a contralateral motor weakness of the lower part of the face and of the limbs. The upper face escapes because of the bilateral supranuclear supply to the upper part of the facial nucleus.

Nuclear lesions

The main motor nucleus may be involved in thrombosis of one of the pontine branches of the basilar artery. As might be anticipated from the relationships depicted in *Figure 19.1*, the usual result of such a lesion is an *alternating (crossed) hemiplegia*: complete paralysis of the facial and/or abducens nerve on one side combined with motor weakness of the limbs on the opposite side owing to concomitant involvement of the corticospinal tract.

Infranuclear lesions

Bell's palsy is a common disorder caused by a neuritis (possibly viral in origin) of the facial nerve. The inflammation causes the nerve to swell, and conduction is compromised by the close fit of the nerve in its bony canal in the interval between geniculate ganglion and stylomastoid foramen. There may be some initial pain in the ear, but the condition is otherwise painless.

Facial paralysis is usually complete. On the affected side, the patient is unable to raise the eyebrow, close the eye, or retract the lip. Tears may spill from the lax lower eyelid, and saliva may drool from the corner of the mouth. The patient may experience *hyperacusis*: ordinary sounds may be unpleasantly loud owing to loss of the damping action of the stapedius muscle.

The tight-fit segment is usually compromised. Tests may reveal blockage of nervus intermedius fibers, with reduced lacrimal and salivary secretions and loss of taste from the anterior part of the tongue.

Four out of five patients recover completely within a few weeks because the nerve has only suffered a conduction block (*neuropraxia*). In the remainder, the nerve undergoes Wallerian degeneration (Ch. 7); recovery takes about 3 months and is often incomplete. During regeneration, some preganglionic fibers of the nervus intermedius may enter the greater petrosal nerve instead of the chorda tympani, with the result

that the lacrimal gland becomes active at mealtimes (so-called 'crocodile tears').

Other causes of infranuclear palsy include a patch of demyelination within the pons in the course of multiple sclerosis, tumors in the cerebellopontine angle (*Clinical Panel 19.2*), middle ear disease, and tumors of the parotid gland. *Herpes zoster oticus* is a rare but well-recognized viral infection of the geniculate ganglion. Severe pain in one ear precedes a vesicular rash in and around the external acoustic meatus. Swelling of the geniculate ganglion may result in a complete facial palsy (*Ramsay Hunt syndrome*).

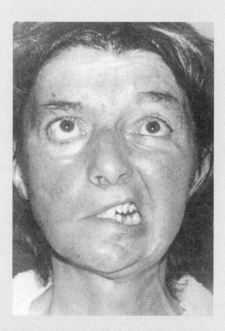

Figure CP 19.1.1 Complete facial nerve paralysis, patient's right side. The patient has been asked to show her teeth and to look upward. To compare the two sides, cover the left and right halves of the photograph alternately with a card. On the paralyzed side, note (paralyzed muscles in parentheses): inability to raise the eyebrow (frontalis muscle); drooping of the lower eyelid (orbicularis oculi); inability to retract the mouth (buccinator); no webbing of the neck (platysma). The patient was also unable to abduct the right eye (abducens nerve paralysis, Ch. 20). Together with a history of other disturbances, the clinical picture was suggestive of multiple sclerosis with a current patch of demyelination deep to the facial colliculus, affecting the emerging fibers of the facial and abducens nerves (cf. *Figure 14.15*). (Photograph reproduced from Parsons, M. (1987) *Diagnostic Picture Test in Clinical Neurology.* London: Wolfe Medical, with the kind permission of author and publisher.)

Clinical Panel 19.2   Syndromes of the cerebellopontine angle

The *cerebellopontine angle* is the recess between the hemisphere of the cerebellum and the lower border of the pons. The petrous temporal bone, laterally, completes a triangle having the V nerve at its upper corner and IX and X at its lower corner, and bisected by VII and VIII.

Several kinds of space-occupying lesions may compromise one or more of the nerves. The most frequent is an *acoustic neuroma*, a slow-growing, benign tumor of Schwann cells (*neurolemmoma*). The tumor originates on the vestibular nerve within the internal acoustic meatus, but the initial symptoms are more often cochlear than vestibular. *An acoustic neuroma must be suspected in every middle-aged or elderly patient presenting with auditory or vestibular symptoms.* Early diagnosis is important because of the difficulty of removing a large neuroma extending into the posterior cranial fossa; also because the cumulative motor and sensory disturbances may not show significant improvement after surgery.

The following is a fairly typical sequence of symptoms and signs in a case escaping early detection:

- *Tinnitus* is experienced on the affected side, in the form of a high-pitched ringing or fizzing sound.
- *Deafness* on the affected side is slowly progressive over a period of months or years.
- *Vertigo* occurs episodically. Severe vertigo with nystagmus signifies compression of the brainstem.
- *Loss of the corneal reflex* is an early sign of distortion of the V nerve by a tumor emerging from the internal acoustic meatus into the posterior cranial fossa.
- *Weakness of the masticatory muscles* is a later sign of V nerve involvement. The jaw deviates toward the affected side when the mouth is opened, because the normal lateral pterygoid is unopposed. Wasting of the masseter may be detected by palpation.
- *Weakness of the facial musculature* develops as the VII nerve becomes stretched.

- *Anesthesia of the oropharynx* signifies involvement of the IX nerve.
- *Ipsilateral 'cerebellar signs'* in the arm and leg appear when the cerebellum is compressed.
- *'Upper motor neuron signs'* in the limbs signify compression of the brainstem.
- *Signs of raised intracranial pressure* (headache, drowsiness, papilledema) signify obstruction of cerebrospinal fluid circulation either inside or around the brainstem.

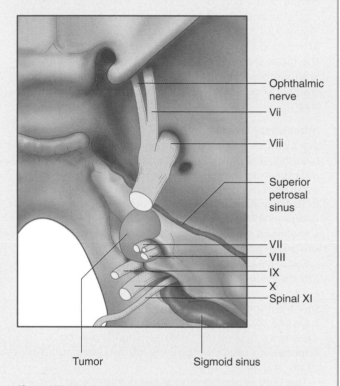

Figure CP 19.2.1 An acoustic neuroma invading the right posterior cranial fossa. XIs, spinal accessory nerve.

Core Information

Upon leaving its nucleus, the facial nerve whirls around the facial colliculus, emerges at the lower border of pons, and at the internal auditory meatus enters a long bony canal opening at the stylomastoid foramen. It supplies the muscles of facial expression, the occipital portion of occipitofrontalis, the stapedius, and the posterior digastric. The upper half of the facial nucleus receives a bilateral supranuclear supply from the motor cortex, the lower half receives only a contralateral supply.

The nervus intermedius travels in part with VII. The superior salivatory nucleus provides the motor components of greater petrosal (for lacrimal and nasal glands by the pterygopalatine ganglion) and chorda tympani (for submandibular and sublingual glands via the submandibular ganglion). The geniculate ganglion of VII has unipolar neurons receiving taste from the palate via greater petrosal nerve and tongue via chorda tympani. A few unipolar neurons supply skin in and around the external acoustic meatus.

REFERENCES

Lang, J. (1984) Clinical anatomy of the cerebellopontine angle and internal acoustic meatus. *Adv. Oto-Rhino-Laryng.* **34**: 8–24.

Manni, J.J. and Stennert, E. (1984) Diagnostic methods in facial nerve pathology. *Adv. Oto-Rhino-Laryng.* **34**: 202–213.

Parnes, S.M. (1988) The facial nerve. In *Physiology of the Ear* (Jahn, A.F. and Santos-Sacchi, J., eds), pp. 125–142. New York: Raven Press.

Ocular motor nerves

INTRODUCTORY NOTE

Because of the immense diagnostic and therapeutic importance of ocular innervation, and because of its inherent complexity, neuro-ophthalmology has become a branch of medicine in its own right.

It is especially important to note that premotor centers are able to operate bilaterally in order to keep the gaze on target, even when the head is moving.

THE NERVES

The ocular motor nerves comprise the **oculomotor** (III cranial), **trochlear** (IV cranial), and **abducens** (VI cranial) **nerves**. They provide the motor nerve supply to the four recti and two oblique muscles controlling movements of the eyeball on each side (*Figure 20.1*). The oculomotor nerve contains two additional sets of neurons: one to supply the levator of the upper eyelid, the other to control the sphincter of the pupil and the ciliary muscle.

The nuclei serving the extraocular muscles (extrinsic muscles of the eye) belong to the somatic efferent cell column of the brainstem, in line with the nucleus of the hypoglossal nerve. The oculomotor nucleus has an additional, parasympathetic nucleus which belongs to the general visceral efferent cell column.

Oculomotor nerve

The nucleus of the third nerve is at the level of the superior colliculi. It is partly embedded in the peri-aqueductal gray matter (*Figure 20.2A*). It is composed of five individual nuclei for the supply of striated muscles, and one parasympathetic nucleus.

The nerve passes through the tegmentum of the midbrain and emerges into the interpeduncular fossa (arachnoid cistern). It crosses the apex of the petrous temporal bone, pierces the dural roof of the cavernous sinus, runs in the lateral wall of the sinus, and breaks into upper and lower divisions within the superior orbital fissure. The upper division supplies the superior rectus and the levator palpebrae superioris; the lower division supplies the inferior and medial recti and the inferior oblique.

The parasympathetic fibers originate in the **Edinger–Westphal nucleus**. They accompany the main nerve as far as the orbit, then leave the branch to the inferior oblique and synapse in the **ciliary ganglion**. Postganglionic fibers emerge from the ganglion in the **short ciliary nerves**, which pierce the *lamina cribrosa* ('sieve-like layer') of the sclera and supply the *ciliaris* and *sphincter pupillae* muscles.

Trochlear nerve

The nucleus of the fourth nerve is at the level of the inferior colliculus. The nerve itself is unique in two respects (*Figure 20.2B*): it is the only nerve to emerge from the back of the brainstem; and it decussates with its opposite number.

The IV nerve winds around the crus of the midbrain and travels through the cavernous sinus in company with the III nerve (*Figure 20.3*). It passes through the superior orbital fissure and supplies the *superior oblique* muscle.

Abducens nerve

The nucleus of the sixth nerve, in the floor of the fourth ventricle, is at the level of the facial colliculus, in the middle of the pons (*Figure 20.2C*). The nerve descends, to emerge at the lower border of the pons, and runs up the pontine subarachnoid cistern beside the basilar artery. It angles over the apex of the petrous temporal bone and passes through the cavernous sinus beside the internal carotid artery (*Figure 20.3*). It enters the orbit through the superior orbital fissure and supplies the *lateral rectus* muscle, which abducts the eye.

NERVE ENDINGS

Motor endings

All of the ocular motor units are small, containing 5 to 10 muscle fibers apiece (compared with 1000 or more in the tibialis anterior).

Type A fibers produce the fast twitches required for saccadic movements. *Type B* are slow-twitch and may be used for smooth pursuit. *Type C* show only local contractions beneath the individual plates. Type C fibers may be involved in keeping the visual axes of the two eyes parallel with one another. Since the visual axes diverge following administration of muscle relaxants, keeping them parallel must require continuous muscle action, even during sleep.

Sensory endings

In addition to neuromuscular spindles of standard type, numerous *palisade endings* exist in the form of nerve spirals around individual muscle fibers.

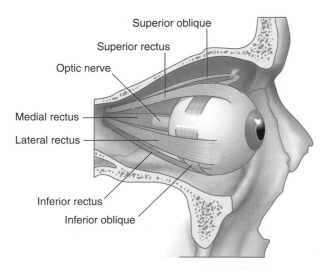

Superior oblique
Superior rectus
Optic nerve
Medial rectus
Lateral rectus
Inferior rectus
Inferior oblique

Figure 20.1 Extrinsic ocular muscles.

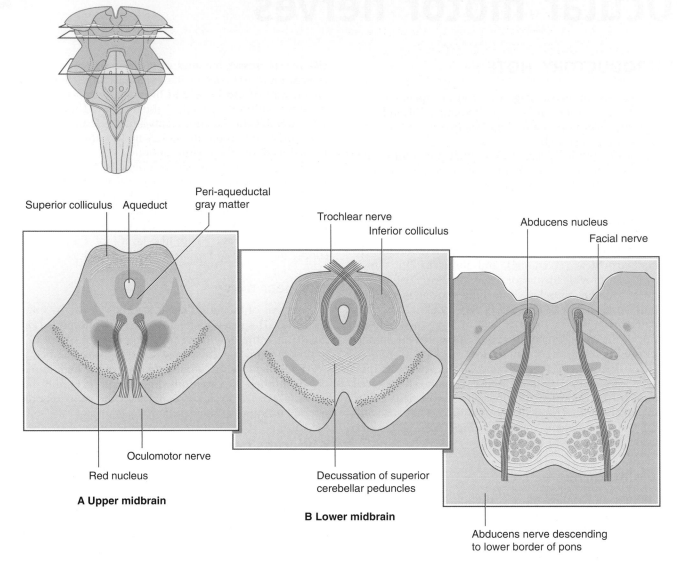

Superior colliculus   Aqueduct

Peri-aqueductal
gray matter

Trochlear nerve
Inferior colliculus

Abducens nucleus
Facial nerve

Red nucleus

Oculomotor nerve

A Upper midbrain

Decussation of superior
cerebellar peduncles

B Lower midbrain

Abducens nerve descending
to lower border of pons

C Middle of pons

Figure 20.2A–C Transverse sections of the brainstem showing the origins of the ocular motor nerves.

The extraocular muscle proprioceptors are the peripheral terminals of neurons in the mesencephalic nucleus of the trigeminal nerve. In monkeys, some of the central processes of these neurons reach as far caudally as the accessory cuneate nucleus in the medulla oblongata. This nucleus also receives proprioceptive terminals from the neck muscles, and it projects both to the ipsilateral cerebellum and to the contralateral superior colliculus. The conjunction of ocular and cervical proprioceptive information presumably assists in the co-ordination of simultaneous movements of the eyes and head.

PUPILLARY LIGHT REFLEX (Figure 20.4)

Constriction of the pupils in response to light involves four sets of neurons, as follows:

1 The afferent limb commences in the ganglionic layer of the retina, which gives rise to the optic nerve. Fibers leaving the chiasma enter both optic tracts and terminate in the **pretectal nuclei,** situated just rostral to the superior colliculus on each side (*Figure 14.19*).

2 Each pretectal nucleus is linked by internuncial neurons to both Edinger–Westphal (parasympathetic) nuclei; the contralateral nucleus is reached by way of the **posterior commissure**.

3 Preganglionic parasympathetic fibers enter the oculomotor nerve, leave the branch to the inferior oblique, and synapse in the ciliary ganglion.

4 Postganglionic fibers run in the short ciliary nerves and enter the iris to supply the sphincter pupillae.

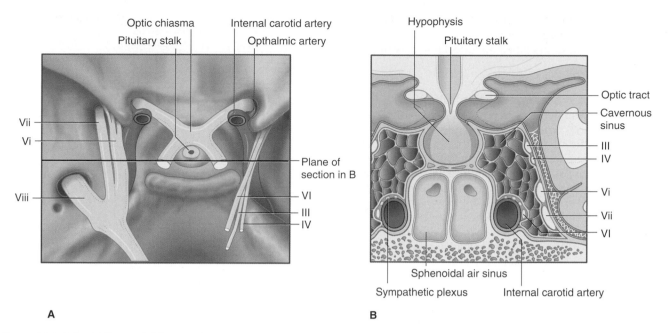

Figure 20.3 (A) Middle cranial fossa with cavernous sinuses removed. (B) Coronal section in the plane of the hypophysis with the cavernous sinuses in place. III, oculomotor nerve; IV, trochlear nerve; VI, abducens nerve; Vi, Vii, Viii ophthalmic, maxillary, mandibular divisions of trigeminal nerve.

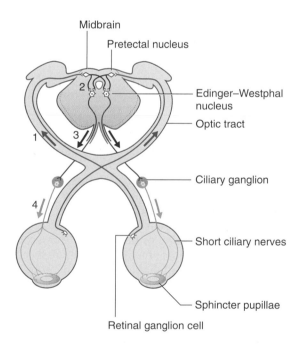

Figure 20.4 Pupillary light reflex. For numbers, see text.

Figure 20.5 Intrinsic muscles of the eye.

ACCOMMODATION

The near response

When the eyes view an object close up, the ciliary muscle contracts reflexly, thereby relaxing the suspensory ligament of the lens (*Figure 20.5*). Since the lens at rest is somewhat compressed (flattened) by tension exerted on the lens capsule by the suspensory ligament, the lens bulges passively when the ciliary muscle contracts. The thicker lens has the greater refractive power required to bring close-up objects into focus on the retina. The response of the lens is one of *accommodation*.

The *accommodation reflex*, as understood clinically, involves two additional features. The sphincter pupillae contracts in order to eliminate passage of light through the peripheral, thinner part of the lens. At the same time, the visual axes of the two eyes converge, as a result of increased tone in the medial rectus muscles.

The three features described are also known as the *near response*.

Pathway for the accommodation reflex

In order to execute the near response, a stereoscopic analysis of the object is carried out at the level of the visual association cortex. The afferent limb of the reflex passes from the retina to the occipital lobe via the lateral geniculate body. The efferent limb passes from the occipital lobe to the midbrain, where some fibers activate the Edinger–Westphal nucleus and others activate *vergence* (convergence) cells in the reticular formation. The vergence cells activate the nuclear groups serving the medial recti, with the effect of *fixating* the object onto the fovea centalis of each eye. The (con)vergence response is called the *fixation reflex*.

The far response

Just as the state of the pupil depends upon the balance of sympathetic and parasympathetic activity, so does the state of the lens. At rest, both are in midposition. The resting focal length of the lens averages 1 meter (with considerable variation between individuals). This is because the ciliary muscle is tonically active. In order to bring a distant object into focus, the ciliary muscle must be inhibited, so that the suspensory ligament becomes taut and the lens flat. The sphincter of the pupil is inhibited as well.

The sympathetic system innervates all of the intrinsic muscles. It has a dual mode of action. It causes contraction of the dilator pupillae by way of *alpha* receptors on the muscle fibers; and it causes *relaxation* of the ciliary muscle and pupillary sphincter, by way of *beta* receptors. This dual effect constitutes the *far response*, and it is used to focus the eyes upon objects at a distance. (*Note*: The unqualified use of *alpha* and *beta* receptors signifies α_1 and β_2, respectively.)

In stressed individuals, heightened sympathetic activity may interfere with the normal process of accommodation. For example, students taking an important written test may have difficulty in bringing the questions into proper focus.

NOTES ON THE SYMPATHETIC PATHWAY TO THE EYE

The great length of the sympathetic pathway to the eye is indicated in *Figure 20.6*.

1 *Central fibers* descending from the hypothalamus cross to the other side in the midbrain. In the pons and medulla, they are joined by ipsilateral fibers descending from the reticular formation.

2 *Preganglionic fibers* emerge in the first thoracic ventral nerve root, and run up in the sympathetic chain to the superior cervical ganglion.

3 *Postganglionic fibers* run along the external and internal carotid arteries and their branches.

The *external* carotid sympathetic fibers accompany all of the branches of the external carotid artery. Those accom-

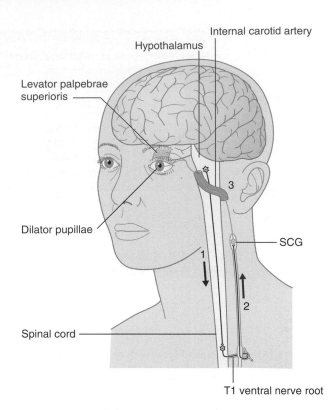

Figure 20.6 Three neuron pathways from the hypothalamus to the eye. Arrows indicate directions of impulse conduction. SCG, superior cervical ganglion. For numbers, see text.

panying the facial artery supply the arterioles of the cheek and lips and are particularly responsive to emotional states. Those accompanying the maxillary artery supply the cavernous tissue covering the nasal conchae (turbinate bones).

Two sets of sympathetic fibers accompany the *internal* carotid artery. One set leaves it to join the ophthalmic division of the V nerve in the cavernous sinus, then leaves this in the long and short ciliary nerves to supply the vessels and smooth muscles of the eyeball. The second set forms a plexus around the internal carotid artery and its branches including the ophthalmic artery. The ophthalmic artery gives off supratrochlear and supraorbital branches which carry sympathetic fibers to the skin of the forehead and scalp.

Interruption of the postganglionic fibers at the jugular foramen (see *jugular foramen syndrome*, Ch. 15), or in the cavernous sinus, produces anhidrosis (loss of sweating) on the forehead and scalp.

OCULAR PALSIES

The effects of paralysis of the motor nerves to the eye are described in *Clinical Panel 20.1*.

Clinical Panel 20.1 Ocular palsies

One or more of the three ocular motor nerves may be paralyzed by disease within the brainstem (e.g. multiple sclerosis, vascular occlusion), in the subarachnoid space (e.g. meningitis, aneurysm in the circle of Willis, distortion by an expanding intracranial lesion), or in the cavernous sinus (e.g. thrombosis of the sinus, aneurysm of the internal carotid artery).

Oculomotor nerve

Complete III nerve palsy

Characteristic signs of complete third nerve paralysis are shown in *Figure CP 20.1.1A*. They are:

1 complete ptosis of the eyelid (unopposed orbicularis oculi)

2 a fully dilated, non-reactive pupil (unopposed dilator pupilae)

3 a fully abducted eye (unopposed lateral rectus), which is also depressed (unopposed superior oblique).

Partial III nerve palsy

The pupils are *always* monitored when cases of head injury come to medical attention. Rapidly increasing intracranial pressure, resulting from an acute extradural or subdural hematoma (Ch. 4), often compresses the third nerve against the crest of the petrous temporal bone. The parasympathetic fibers are superficially placed and are the first to suffer, and the pupil dilates progressively on the affected side. *Pupillary dilatation is an urgent indication for surgical decompression of the brain.*

Trochlear nerve

The IV nerve is rarely paralyzed alone. The cardinal symptom is diplopia (double vision) on looking down, e.g. when going down stairs. This happens because the superior oblique normally assists the inferior rectus in pulling the eye downward, especially when the eye is in a medial position.

Abducens nerve

The effect of a *complete* VI nerve paralysis is shown in *Figure CP 20.1.1B*. The eye is fully abducted by the unopposed pull of the medial rectus.

The abducens has the longest course in the subarachnoid space of any cranial nerve. It also bends sharply over the crest of the petrous temporal bone. A space-occupying lesion affecting *either* cerebral hemisphere may cause compression and paralysis of one abducens nerve.

'Spontaneous' paralysis of the VI nerve may be caused by an arterial aneurysm at the base of the brain or by hardening (atherosclerosis) of the internal carotid artery in the cavernous sinus.

Ocular sympathetic supply

Any one of the three sequential sets of neurons depicted in *Figure 20.6* may be interrupted by local pathology.

1 The *central* set may be interrupted by a vascular lesion of the pons or medulla oblongata. The usual picture is one of Horner's syndrome (ptosis and miosis, as described in Ch. 10) and cranial nerve involvement on one side, together with motor weakness and/or sensory loss in the limbs on the contralateral side. The Horner's syndrome is associated with anhidrosis – absence of sweating – in the face and scalp on the same side, together with congestion of the nose (engorged turbinates).

2 The *preganglionic* set is most often interrupted by stony, cancerous deep cervical lymph nodes in the lower part of the neck. A Horner's syndrome is associated with anhidrosis of the face and scalp (and nasal congestion) on the same side.

3 The *postganglionic* set accompanying the *external* carotid artery is rarely damaged directly. The set accompanying the internal carotid artery may be interrupted as part of a jugular foramen syndrome (Ch. 15), or by pathology in the cavernous sinus. Horner's syndrome is accompanied by anhidrosis of the forehead and anterior scalp (territory of the supraorbital and supratrochlear arteries).

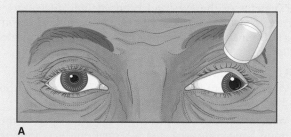

A

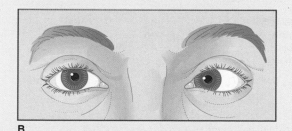

B

Figure CP 20.1.1 (A) Complete left III nerve paralysis. The closed eyelid has been raised by the examiner's finger. **(B)** Complete left VI nerve paralysis.

CONTROL OF EYE MOVEMENTS

The eyes normally move as a pair. This *conjugate* movement is of three fundamentally different kinds, as follows:

1 *Scanning.* The eyes flick from one visual target to another, in high-speed movements called *saccades*.

2 *Tracking.* In tracking, or *smooth pursuit*, the eyes follow an object of interest across the visual field.

3 *Compensation.* The gaze can be held on an object of interest during movements of the head. This is the *vestibulo-ocular* or *fixation reflex*, which depends upon displacement of endolymph in the kinetic labyrinth (Ch. 16).

Scanning

Four separate *gaze centers* in the brainstem pick out motor neurons appropriate to the direction of movement: leftward, rightward, upward, or downward. The centers are small nodes in the reticular formation. They contain *burst cells*, which discharge at 1000 Hz (impulses/sec) and entrain the appropriate motor neurons momentarily at this rate.

The paired centers (left and right) for horizontal saccades are in the paramedian pontine reticular formation (PPRF) (*Figure 14.15*). Each pulls the eyes to its own side (*Figure 20.7*). The midbrain contains a bilateral center for upward

saccades located in the rostral end of the medial longitudinal fasciculus (MLF), at the level of the pretectal nucleus. It is called the **rostral interstitial nucleus** (riMLF). At the same level but a little ventral to this is a bilateral center for downward gaze (*Figure 14.19*).

Automatic scanning movements are activated by the superior colliculus, on receipt of visual information from the retina through the medial root of the optic tract. Examples of automatic scanning include the sideward glance toward an object attracting attention in the peripheral visual field, and the saccadic movements used in reading. The tectoreticular projections concerned cross the midline before engaging the gaze centers. Saccadic accuracy is controlled by the midregion (vermis) of the cerebellum, which receives afferents from the superior colliculi and projects to the vestibular nucleus.

Voluntary scanning movements are initiated in the *frontal eye fields*, located at the junction of motor and premotor cortex (Ch. 26). From each frontal eye field, a projection descends in the anterior limb of the internal capsule. Most of the fibers cross over before terminating in the gaze centers.

As explained in Chapter 26, the ipsilateral superior colliculus is activated at the same time, to reinforce the excitation of the appropriate gaze center.

The projection from the frontal eye field is interrupted in about one-third of patients who suffer a stroke involving the internal capsule. The result is *paralysis of contraversive horizontal gaze.* 'Contraversive' refers to an inability to make a voluntary saccade away from the side of the lesion. The gaze paralysis vanishes within a week, even if the hemiplegia remains profound – presumably because of takeover by uncrossed fibers.

The best-known afferents to the frontal eye field come from the parietal cortex, from cells concerned with *visual attention.* In monkeys, some cells in the posterior parietal cortex become active when an object of interest is seen. These cells project to the frontal eye field and are thought to facilitate eye movement in the direction of the object. In humans, neglect of the contralateral visual field is a well-known feature of damage to the posterior parietal lobe, especially on the right side (Ch. 27).

Tracking

The neural mechanisms for tracking must be complex because of the following basic requirements: (a) intact visual pathways to monitor the position of the object throughout the movement; (b) neurons to signal the rate of movement of the object (velocity detectors); (c) neurons to co-ordinate movements of the eyes and head (neural integrator); and (d) a system to monitor smooth execution of the tracking movement. Monkey and cat experiments indicate the following:

- Object position information is forwarded from the visual cortex to the posterior parietal cortex, and from there to the reticular formation of the pons.
- Velocity detectors are present in the upper part of the pons, apparently receiving information direct from the retina via the medial root of the optic tract.
- Head movement is signaled by the dynamic labyrinth, and is integrated with spatial and velocity information

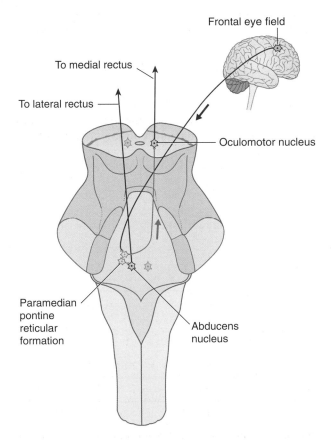

Frontal eye field

To medial rectus

To lateral rectus

Oculomotor nucleus

Paramedian pontine reticular formation

Abducens nucleus

Figure 20.7 Principal pathways involved in a voluntary ocular saccade to the left.

Core Information

Oculomotor nerve
Somatic efferent fibers of III arise from the main nucleus at superior collicular level. The nerve passes intact through the cavernous sinus and in two divisions through the superior orbital fissure. The upper division supplies superior rectus and levator palpebrae superioris; the lower division supplies inferior and medial recti and inferior oblique.

Parasympathetic fibers emerge from the Edinger–Westphal nucleus, travel with the main nerve, and synapse in the ciliary ganglion for supply of sphincter pupillae and ciliaris.

Paralysis of III is shown by a dilated pupil, followed by ptosis, and later by a divergent squint in addition.

Trochlear nerve
The nucleus of IV is at inferior collicular level. The fibers cross the midline before emerging below the inferior colliculi. IV passes through the cavernous sinus to supply superior oblique.

Paralysis of IV is characterized by diplopia on looking down.

Abducens nerve
The nucleus of VI is at the level of the facial colliculus in pons. The nerve runs in the subarachnoid space from lower border of pons to apex of petrous temporal bone, and passes through cavernous sinus and superior orbital fissure and supplies lateral rectus.

Paralysis of VI is characterized by convergent squint with inability to abduct the affected eye.

Sympathetic
Muscles stimulated (via α receptors) are dilator pupillae and levator palpebrae superioris. Paralysis is characterized by ptosis with a constricted pupil (Horner's syndrome). Muscles inhibited (via β receptors) are sphincter pupillae and ciliaris.

Parasympathetic
Muscles stimulated are the sphincter pupillae and the ciliaris.

Reflex pathways
For the pupillary light reflex: from retina to pretectal nucleus to both Edinger–Westphal nuclei to ciliary ganglion to sphincter pupillae.

For the accommodation reflex: from retina to lateral geniculate body to occipital cortex to Edinger–Westphal nucleus to ciliary ganglion to ciliaris.

Oculomotor controls
Scanning (saccading) is locally activated by six gaze centers. Clinically most important is the PPRF which operates to pull ipsilateral lateral rectus and contralateral medial rectus conjugately to its own side. Automatic scanning is controlled by the superior colliculi, and voluntary scanning by the frontal eye fields.

Tracking is complex and involves occipital cortex, dynamic labyrinth, cerebellum, superior colliculus, and reticular formation.

---

in the **nucleus prepositus hypoglossi** – a node of the reticular formation which is in fact closer to the abducens nucleus than to the hypoglossal nucleus. The nucleus prepositus projects to the PPRF, which controls conjugate eye movements. The pathway to the neck muscles (for turning the head) may involve the superior colliculus.

- Smooth execution of tracking movements is monitored by the flocculus of the cerebellum, which has two-way connections to the vestibular nucleus and pontine reticular formation.

The dynamic labyrinth and cerebellum co-operate to keep the eyes on target during movement of the head, as described in Chapter 16.

REFERENCES

American Academy of Ophthalmology (1995) *Principles of Ophthalmology.* San Francisco.

Anderson, T.J., Jenkins, I.H., Brooks, D.J., Hawken, M.B., Frackowiak, R.S.J. and Kennard, C. (1994) Cortical control of saccades and fixation in man. *Brain* 117: 1073–1084.

Dean, P., Mayhew, J.E.W. and Langdon, P. (1994) Learning and maintaining saccadic accuracy: a model of brain stem-cerebellar interactions. *J. Cog. Neurosci.* 6: 117–138.

Fukushima, K. (1991) The interstitial nucleus of Cajal in the midbrain reticular formation and vertical eye movement. *Neurosci. Res.* 10: 159–187.

Keller, E.L. and Heinen, S.J. (1991) Generation of smooth pursuit eye movements: neuronal mechanisms and pathways. *Neurosci. Res.* 11: 79–107.

Kommerell, G. (1984) Supranuclear and nuclear disorders of eye movement. In *Neuro-ophthalmology, vol. 3* (Lessell, S. and van Dalen, J.T.W., eds), pp. 277–289. Amsterdam: Elsevier.

Moschovakis, A.K. (1997) The neural integrators of the mammalian saccadic system. *Front. Biosci.* 15: D552–D557.

Miyazaki, S. (1985) Location of motoneurons in the oculomotor nucleus and the course of their axons in the oculomotor nerve. *Brain Res.* 348: 57–63.

Oda, K. (1986) Motor innervation and acetylcholine receptor distribution of human extraocular muscle fibers. *J. Neurol. Sci.* 74: 125–133.

Parkinson, D. (1988) Further observations on the sympathetic pathways to the pupil. *Anat. Rec.* 220: 108–109.

Petit, L., Clark, V.P., Ingeholm, J., et al. (1997) Dissociation of saccade-related and pursuit-related activation in human frontal eye fields as revealed by fMRI. *J. Neurophysiol.* 77: 3386–3390.

Wilhelm, H. (1998) Neuro-ophthalmology of pupillary function. *J. Neurol.* 245: 573–583.

Reticular formation

INTRODUCTION

The reticular formation is phylogenetically a very old neural network, being a prominent feature of the reptilian brainstem. It originated as a slowly conducting, polysynaptic pathway intimately connected with olfactory and limbic regions. The progressive dominance of vision and hearing over olfaction led to lateralization of sensory and motor functions within the tectum of the midbrain. Direct spinotectal and tectospinal tracts bypassed the reticular formation, which was largely relegated to automatic functions. In mammals, the tectum in turn has been relegated to minor status with the emergence of very fast pathways linking the cerebral cortex with the peripheral sensory and motor apparatus.

In the human brain, the reticular formation continues to be of importance in automatic and reflex activities, and it has retained its linkages to the limbic system.

ORGANIZATION

The term *reticular formation* refers only to the polysynaptic network in the brainstem, although the network continues rostrally into the thalamus and hypothalamus, and caudally into the propriospinal network of the spinal cord.

The ground plan is shown in *Figure 21.1A*. In the midline, the *median reticular formation* comprises a series of *raphe nuclei* (*pron.* 'raffay' and derived from the Greek word for seam). The raphe nuclei are the major source of serotoninergic projections throughout the neuraxis (see next section).

Next to this is the *paramedian reticular formation*. This part of the network contains *magnocellular* neurons throughout; in the lower pons and upper medulla, some *gigantocellular* neurons also appear, before the network blends with the *central reticular nucleus* of the medulla oblongata.

Outermost is the *lateral, parvocellular* (small-celled) *reticular formation*. Parvocellular dendrites are long and they branch at regular intervals. They have a predominantly transverse orientation and their interstices are penetrated by long pathways running to the thalamus. The lateral network is mainly afferent in nature. It receives fibers from all of the sensory pathways, including the special senses:

- Olfactory fibers are received through the median forebrain bundle, which passes alongside the hypothalamus.
- Visual pathway fibers are received from the superior colliculus.
- Auditory pathway fibers are received from the superior olivary nucleus.
- Vestibular fibers are received from the medial vestibular nucleus.

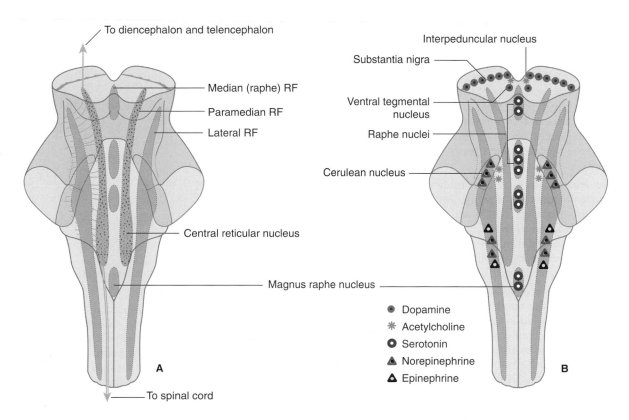

Figure 21.1 Reticular formation (RF). **(A)** Subdivisions. **(B)** Aminergic and cholinergic cell groups.

Table 21.1 Aminergic neurons of the reticular formation

Transmitter	Location
Serotonin	Raphe nuclei of midbrain, pons, medulla
Dopamine	Tegmentum of midbrain
Norepinephrine	Midbrain, pons, medulla
Epinephrine	Medulla

- Somatic sensory fibers are received from the spinoreticular tracts and from the spinal and principal (pontine) nuclei of the trigeminal nerve.

Most parvocellular axons ramify extensively among the dendrites of the paramedian reticular formation. However, some synapse within the nuclei of cranial nerves and act as pattern generators (see later).

The paramedian reticular formation is a predominantly *efferent* system. The axons are relatively long. Some ascend to synapse in the midbrain reticular formation or in the thalamus. Others have both ascending and descending branches contributing to the polysynaptic network. The magnocellular component receives corticoreticular fibers from the premotor cortex and gives rise to the pontine and medullary reticulospinal tracts.

Aminergic neurons of the brainstem

Embedded in the reticular formation are sets of aminergic neurons (*Figure 21.1B*). They include one set producing *serotonin* (5-hydroxytryptamine) and three sets producing *catecholamines*, as listed in *Table 21.1*.

- The *serotoninergic neurons* have the largest territorial distribution of any set of CNS neurons. In general terms, those of the midbrain project rostrally into the cerebral hemispheres; those of the pons ramify in the brainstem and cerebellum; and those of the medulla supply the spinal cord (*Figure 21.2*). All parts of the CNS gray matter are permeated by serotonin-secreting axonal varicosities. Clinically, enhancement of serotonin activity is part of the treatment for a prevalent condition known as major depression (Ch. 23).

- The *dopaminergic neurons* of the midbrain fall into two groups. At the junction of tegmentum and crus are those of the substantia nigra, which will be considered in Chapter 28. Medial to these, dopaminergic neurons in the **ventral tegmental nuclei** (*Figure 21.3*) project *mesocortical* fibers to the frontal lobe and *mesolimbic* fibers to the nucleus accumbens in particular (Ch. 29).

- The *noradrenergic neurons* are only marginally less prodigious than the serotoninergic ones. About 90% of the somas are pooled in the **cerulean nucleus** (*locus ceruleus*), a 'violet spot' in the floor of the fourth ventricle at the upper end of the pons (*Figure 21.5*). Neurons of the cerulean nucleus project in *all* directions, as indicated in *Figure 21.4*.

- *Epinephrine-secreting neurons* are relatively scarce and are confined to the medulla oblongata. Some project rostrally to the hypothalamus, others project caudally to

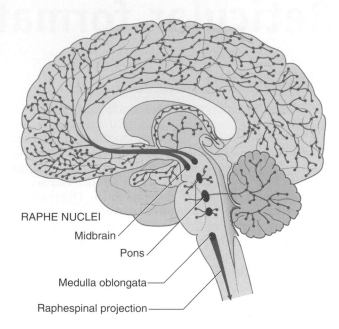

RAPHE NUCLEI
Midbrain
Pons
Medulla oblongata
Raphespinal projection

Figure 21.2 Serotoninergic projections from the brainstem midline (raphe).

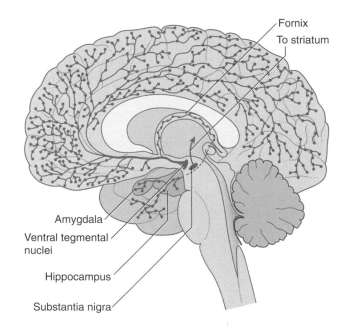

Fornix
To striatum
Amygdala
Ventral tegmental nuclei
Hippocampus
Substantia nigra

Figure 21.3 Dopaminergic projections from the midbrain.

synapse upon preganglionic sympathetic neurons in the spinal cord.

In the cerebral cortex, the ionic and electrical effects of aminergic neuronal activity are quite variable. First, more than one kind of postsynaptic receptor exists for each of the amines. Second, some aminergic neurons liberate a peptide substance also, capable of modulating the transmitter action – usually by prolonging it. Third, the larger cortical neurons receive many thousands of excitatory and inhibitory synapses from local circuit neurons and they have numerous different receptors. Activation of a single kind of aminergic

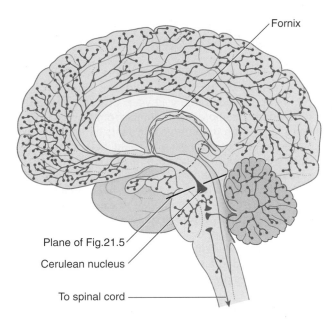

Fornix

Plane of Fig.21.5

Cerulean nucleus

To spinal cord

Figure 21.4 Noradrenergic projections from the pons and medulla oblongata.

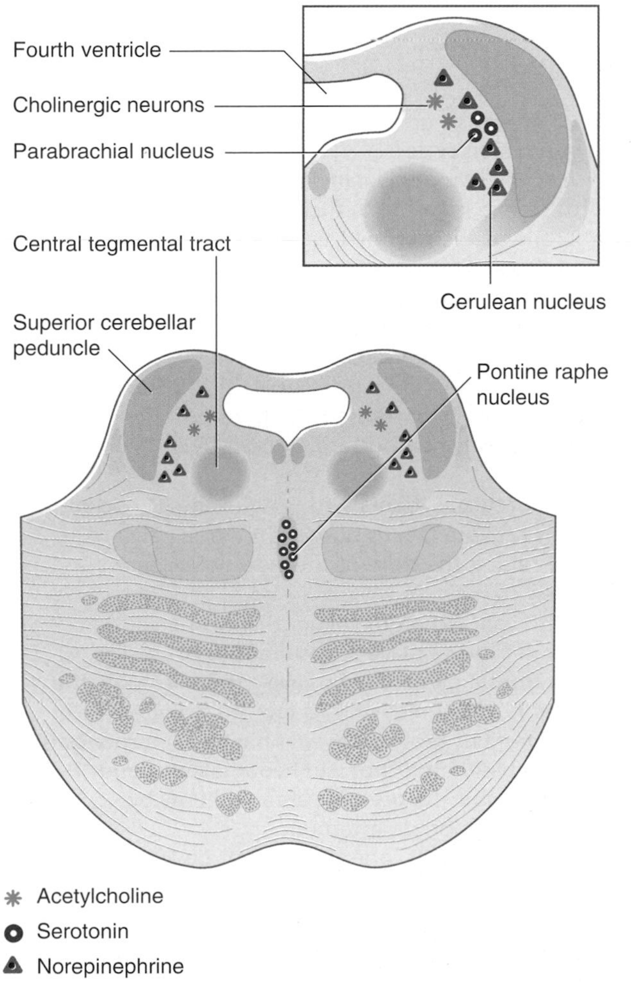

Fourth ventricle

Cholinergic neurons

Parabrachial nucleus

Central tegmental tract

Superior cerebellar peduncle

Cerulean nucleus

Pontine raphe nucleus

✳ Acetylcholine

◉ Serotonin

▲ Norepinephrine

Figure 21.5 Part of a transverse section through the upper part of the pons, showing elements of the reticular formation.

receptor may have a large or small effect depending on the existing excitatory state.

Although our understanding of the physiology and pharmacology of the monoamines is far from complete, no-one disputes their relevance to a wide range of behavioral functions.

FUNCTIONAL ANATOMY

The range of functions served by different parts of the reticular formation is indicated in *Table 21.2*.

Pattern generators

Patterned activities involving cranial nerves include:

- Conjugate (in parallel) movements of the eyes locally controlled by premotor nodal points (*gaze centers*) in the midbrain and pons linked to the nuclei of the ocular motor nerves (Ch. 20).
- Rhythmical chewing movements controlled by the supratrigeminal premotor nucleus in the pons (Ch. 18).
- Swallowing, vomiting, coughing, and sneezing, controlled by separate premotor nodal points in the medulla linked to the appropriate cranial nerves and to the respiratory centers.

Locomotor pattern generators are described in *Box 21.1*.

The salivatory nuclei belong to the parvocellular reticular formation of pons and medulla. They contribute preganglionic parasympathetic fibers to the facial and glossopharyngeal nerves.

Respiratory control

The respiratory cycle is largely regulated by *dorsal* and *ventral respiratory nuclei* located at the upper end of the medulla

Table 21.2 Elements of the reticular formation and their perceived functions

Reticular formation element	Function
Premotor cranial nerve nuclei	Patterned cranial nerve activities
Pontine locomotor center	Pattern generation
Magnocellular nuclei	Posture, locomotion
Salivatory nucleus	Salivary secretion, lacrimation
Pontine micturition center	Bladder control
Medial parabrachial nucleus	Respiratory rhythm
Central reticular nucleus of medulla oblongata	Vital centers (circulation, respiration)
Lateral medullary nucleus	Convey somatic and visceral information to the cerebellum
Aminergic neurons	Sleeping and waking, attention and mood, sensory modulation, blood pressure control
Ascending reticular activating system (ARAS)	Arousal

Box 21.1 Locomotor pattern generators

From animal experiments, it has long been agreed that lower vertebrates and lower mammals possess *locomotor pattern generators* in the spinal cord, within the gray matter neurologically connected to each of the four limbs. These *spinal generators* comprise electrically oscillating circuits delivering rhythmically entrained signals to flexor and extensor muscle groups. Spinal generator activity is subject to supraspinal commands from a *mesencephalic locomotor area* which in turn obeys commands from motor areas of the cerebral cortex and corpus striatum.

The human *locomotor center* comprises cells of the **pedunculopontine nucleus** (*Figure 14.14*) and the mesencephalic part of the cerulean nucleus. These nuclei send fibers down the central tegmental tract to the oral and caudal pontine nuclei serving extensor motor neurons and to medullary magnocellular neurons serving flexor motor neurons.

The existence of spinal generators under brainstem command in humans has received support from the first-ever case of *involuntary stepping*. This patient was the victim of a football injury 17 years previously, when he suffered an *incomplete* cord injury from fracture of vertebra C5. During the intervening years he had recovered some motor power and could walk some distance with support. Then, possibly as a consequence of increased sensory input to the gray matter from a recently inflamed hip joint, and from a heightened regimen of physiotherapy, he began to experience involuntary, rhythmic, vigorous stepping movements at nighttime when he lay on his back. The movements were physically demanding and led to high pulse and respiration rates and a sense of exhaustion. But he could terminate a given attack by turning onto one side.

Treatment of the hip infection, and reduction of physiotherapy, were sufficient to terminate these episodes.

Box 21.2 Higher level bladder controls*

The *micturition control center* is in the paramedian pontine reticular formation on each side, with interconnections across the midline. Magnocellular neurons project from here all the way to micturition-related parasympathetic neurons in segments S2–S4 of the spinal cord.

In cats, stimulation of the micturition control center produces not only a rise in intravesical pressure, but also relaxation of the external urethral sphincter brought about by simultaneous excitation of GABAergic internuncials synapsing in Onuf's nucleus in sacral segments of the spinal cord (Ch. 10).

More laterally in the pons is the 'L' (lateral) center projecting to Onuf's nucleus. In this context, the micturition control center is referred to as the 'M' (medial) center.

At higher levels, cells in the lateral part of the *right peri-aqueductal gray matter* (PAG) receive fibers ascending from the sacral posterior gray horn and project excitatory fibers to the 'M' center. The lateral PAG also receives an excitatory input from the *right* **preoptic nucleus** in the anterior hypothalamus.

Some spinoreticular projections from the sacral cord excite the 'L' center. Others relay via the thalamus to cells in a part of the *right* **anterior cingulate cortex** (ACCx) known to be active during tasks requiring attention.

This right-sided bias is thought to be related to emotional aspects of micturition.

The micturition cycle
1. When the bladder is half-full, vesical afferents from stretch receptors in the detrusor and in the mucous membrane of the trigone relay this information along spinoreticular fibers reaching pons, midbrain, and thalamus. The right 'L' center, lateral PAG, and ACCx respond by 'glowing' on PET scans.

2. As described in Chapter 10, activity in the sympathetic system is stepped up so that *bladder compliance* can be increased (via β_2 receptors); parasympathetic neurons are silenced by α_2 neuronal interaction.

3. Spinoreticular fibers synapsing in the 'L' nucleus of the pons activate Onuf's nucleus in the sacral cord, thereby raising the tone of the external urinary sphincter.

4. With completion of filling, there is perception of urgency. If time or place is unsuitable, part of the inferior frontal gyrus 'comes alive'. This area puts the ACCx 'on hold' by reducing its level of activity via association-fiber projections to inhibitory internuncials there. Likewise, projections to hypothalamus and midbrain inhibit the preoptic area and PAG by activating appropriate internuncials.

5. A final measure, one that cannot be long sustained, is voluntary contraction of the pelvic floor. The command for this contraction is sent from the prefrontal cortex to the perineal representation on the medial side of the motor cortex in the paracentral lobule.

Box 21.2 Continued

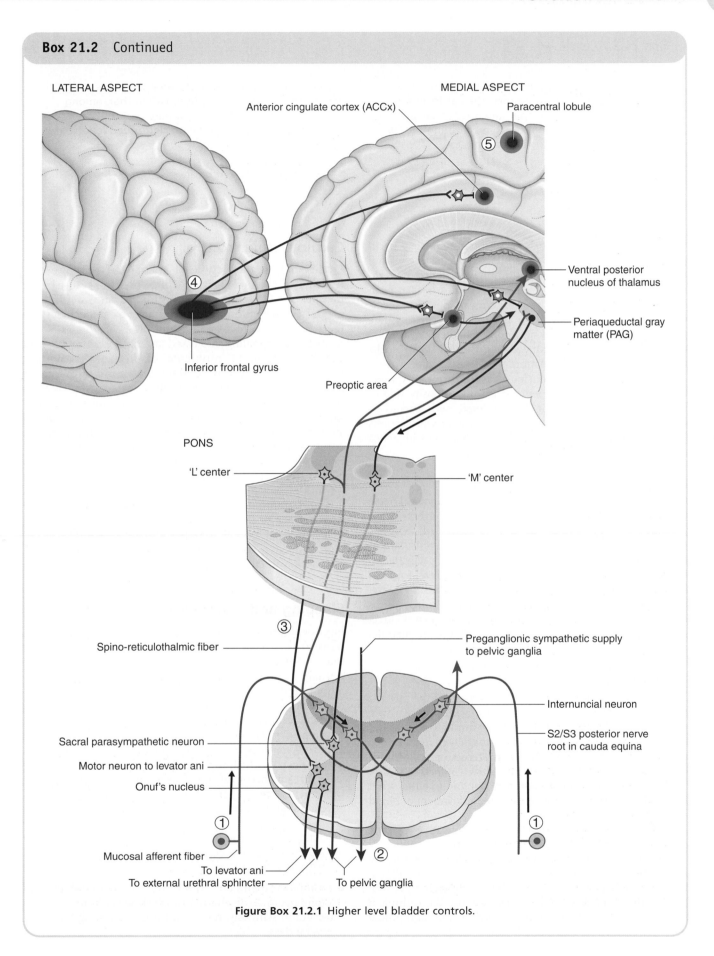

LATERAL ASPECT

MEDIAL ASPECT

Anterior cingulate cortex (ACCx)

Paracentral lobule

⑤

④

Ventral posterior
nucleus of thalamus

Periaqueductal gray
matter (PAG)

Inferior frontal gyrus

Preoptic area

PONS

'L' center

'M' center

Spino-reticulothalmic fiber

③

Preganglionic sympathetic supply
to pelvic ganglia

Internuncial neuron

S2/S3 posterior nerve
root in cauda equina

Sacral parasympathetic neuron

Motor neuron to levator ani

Onuf's nucleus

①

①

Mucosal afferent fiber

②

To levator ani

To external urethral sphincter

To pelvic ganglia

Figure Box 21.2.1 Higher level bladder controls.

Box 21.2 Continued

6. When time and place permit, the inferior frontal gyrus releases its three prisoners. The pelvic floor is allowed to sag in the manner described in Chapter 10, and the preoptic area joins PAG in activating the 'M' nucleus while inactivating 'L' via inhibitory internuncials.

The right-sided bias of micturition control is consistent with the clinical observation that, among stroke patients of either sex, urinary incontinence is more commonly associated with right-sided lesions of the brain.

* Lower level bladder controls are described in Chapter 10.

oblongata on each side. The dorsal respiratory nucleus occupies the midlateral part of the solitary nucleus. The ventral nucleus is dorsal to the nucleus ambiguus (hence the term *retroambiguus nucleus* in *Figure 14.11*). A third, *medial parabrachial nucleus*, adjacent to the cerulean nucleus, seems to have a pacemaker function governing respiratory rate (cycles per minute). As will be seen in Chapter 29, stimulation of this nucleus by the amygdala, in *anxiety states*, results in characteristic hyperventilation.

The dorsal respiratory nucleus has an inspiratory function. It projects to motor neurons on the opposite side of the spinal cord supplying diaphragm, intercostals, and accessory muscles of inspiration. It receives excitatory projections from chemoreceptors in the medullary chemosensitive area and in the carotid body.

Medullary chemosensitive area

Close to the site of attachment of the glossopharyngeal nerve to the brainstem, the choroid plexus of the fourth ventricle pouts through the lateral aperture of the fourth ventricle (*Figure 21.6*). At this location, cells of the lateral reticular formation at the medullary surface are exquisitely sensitive to the H^+ ion concentration in the neighboring cerebrospinal fluid. In effect, this *chemosensitive area* samples the PCO_2 level in the blood supplying the brain. Any increase in H^+ ions stimulates the dorsal respiratory nucleus through a direct synaptic linkage. (Several other nuclei within the medulla are also chemosensitive.)

Carotid chemoreceptors

The pinhead **carotid body**, close to the stem of the internal carotid artery (*Figure 21.6*), receives from this artery a twig which ramifies within it. Blood flow through the carotid body is so intense that the arteriovenous PO_2 changes by less than 1% during passage. The chemoreceptors are glomus cells to which branches of the sinus nerve (branch of IX) are applied. The carotid chemoreceptors respond to either a fall in PO_2 or a rise in PCO_2 and cause reflex adjustment of blood gas levels.

Chemoreceptors in the *aortic bodies* (beneath the aortic arch) are relatively insignificant in humans.

The ventral respiratory nucleus is expiratory (in the main). During quiet breathing, it functions as an oscillator, engaged in reciprocal inhibition (via GABAergic internuncials) with the inspiratory center. During forced breathing, it activates anterior horn cells supplying the abdominal muscles required to empty the lungs.

Cardiovascular control

Cardiac output and peripheral arterial resistance are controlled by the neural and endocrine systems. Because of the prevalence of essential hypertension in late middle age, major research efforts are under way to understand the mechanisms of cardiovascular control.

Afferents signaling increased arterial pressure arise in stretch receptors (a multitude of free nerve endings) in the wall of the carotid sinus and aortic arch (*Figure 21.7*). Known as *baroreceptors*, these afferents project to medially placed cells of the solitary nucleus constituting the *baroreceptor center*. Afferents from the carotid sinus travel in the glossopharyngeal nerve; those from the aortic arch travel in the vagus nerve. The baroreceptor nerves are known as 'buffer nerves' because they act to correct any deviation of the arterial blood pressure from the norm.

Cardiac output and peripheral arterial resistance depend on a balance in the activity of sympathetic and parasympathetic efferents. Two major reflexes, barovagal and barosympathetic, help to lower a raised blood pressure as detailed in the caption to *Figure 21.7*.

Sleeping and wakefulness

Electroencephalography (EEG) reveals characteristic patterns in the electrical activity of cerebral cortical neurons that accompany various states of consciousness. The normal waking state is characterized by rapid, low-amplitude waves. The onset of sleep is accompanied by slow, high-amplitude waves, the higher amplitude being due to the synchronized activity of larger numbers of neurons. This type of sleep is called S (synchronized) sleep. It lasts for about 90 minutes before being replaced by D (desynchronized) sleep in which the EEG pattern resembles the waking state. Dreams occur during D sleep and there are rapid eye movements (hence the more usual term, 'REM sleep'). Several S and D phases occur during a normal night's sleep.

Details of brainstem involvement in sleep phenomena are available in psychology texts. Some salient experimental evidence is summarized:

- In animal experiments, destruction of the midbrain raphe neurons, or pharmacological prevention of serotonin synthesis, results in insomnia lasting for several days.

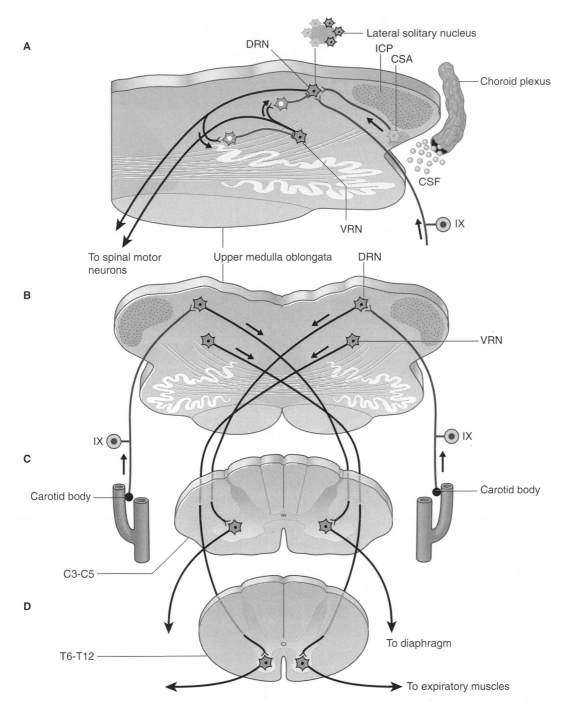

Figure 21.6 Respiratory control systems. All sections are viewed from below and behind. (A) is an enlargement taken from (B).
(A) Inhibitory interaction between dorsal and ventral respiratory nuclei (DRN, VRN). Chorodial capillaries discharge cerebrospinal fluid (CSF) close to the medullary chemosensitive area (CSA) whence neurons project to DRN.
(B) The glossopharyngeal nerve (IX) contains chemoreceptive neurons reaching from carotid body to DRN.
(C) Phrenic motor neurons are activated by the contralateral DRN.
(D) Muscles of the abdominal wall are activated by the contralateral VRN to produce forced expiration.

- Serotonin and norepinephrine neuronal activities fluctuate in parallel. Both are most active during attentive wakefulness, sluggish during S sleep, and virtually silent during REM sleep.

- Brainstem serotonin neurons form numerous surface varicosities on the walls of the third ventricle. Serotonin liberated into the cerebrospinal fluid seems to be metabolized by hypothalamic neurons to form a sleep-inducing substance.

- Cholinergic neurons close to the cerulean nucleus are active during REM sleep and they appear to cause the rapid eye movements by playing upon the ocular motor nuclei.

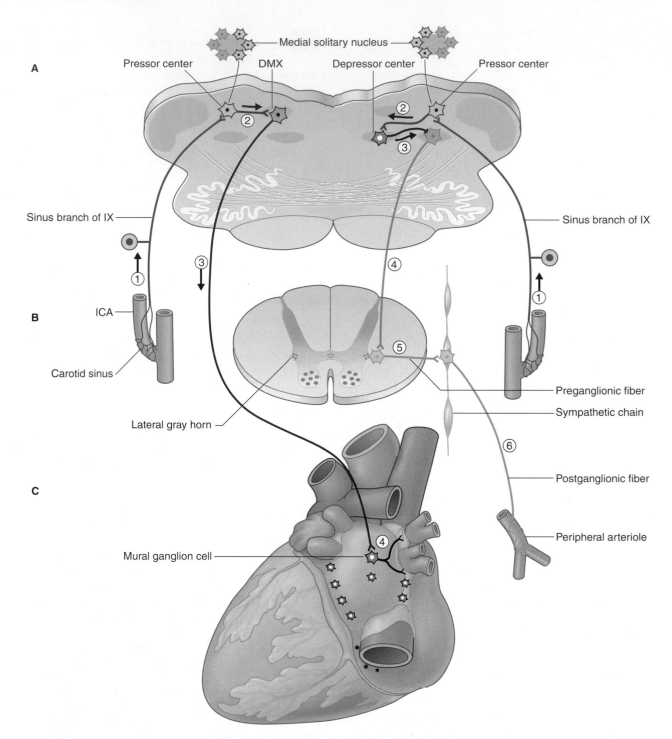

Figure 21.7 (A) Upper medulla oblongata; **(B)** Spinal cord segments T1–L3; **(C)** Posterior wall of heart.

Barovagal reflex (left)

1 Stretch receptors in the carotid sinus excite fibers in the sinus branch of the glossopharyngeal nerve. ICA, internal carotid artery.
2 Baroreceptor neurons of the solitary nucleus respond by stimulating cardioinhibitory neurons in the dorsal (motor) nucleus of the vagus (DMX).
3 Preganglionic, cholinergic parasympathetic vagal fibers synapse upon mural ganglion cells on the posterior wall of the heart.
4 Postganglionic, cholinergic parasympathetic fibers reduce pacemaker activity, thus reducing the heart rate.

Barosympathetic reflex (right).

1 Carotid sinus stretch receptor afferents excite baroreceptor medial neurons of the solitary nucleus.
2 Baroreceptor neurons respond by exciting the inhibitory neurons of the vasomotor depressor center in the central reticular nucleus of the medulla.
3 Adrenalinergic and noradrenalinergic neurons of the pressor center in the lateral reticular nucleus (rostral ventrolateral medulla) are inhibited.
4 Tonic excitation of the lateral gray horn is reduced.
5 and 6 Preganglionic and postganglionic sympathetic tone to peripheral arterioles is reduced, thus lowering the peripheral arterial resistance.

Ascending reticular activating system

This term refers to the participation of reticular formation neurons in activation of the cerebral cortex, as shown by a change in EEG records from high-amplitude, slow waves to low-amplitude, fast waves during spontaneous arousal from sleep. The strongest candidates for such a role are sets of cholinergic neurons close to the cerulean nucleus (*Figure 21.3*). In addition to supplying the above-mentioned fibers to the ocular motor nuclei, these neurons project to almost all thalamic nuclei, and they have an excitatory effect upon thalamic neurons projecting to the cerebral cortex.

The **hypothalamus** is an important control center for various body rhythms, including sleep and wakefulness. A second candidate for cortical activation has been found in the hypothalamus, namely the **tuberomammillary nucleus**. This nucleus contains histaminergic neurons having widespread projections to the cerebral cortex (Ch. 22).

Following arousal, the waking-state EEG pattern seems to be sustained by the continuing discharge of the brainstem and hypothalamic neurons mentioned; also by a third set of neurons, embedded in the basal forebrain immediately above the optic chiasm. The third set occupies the **basal nucleus of Meynert** (Ch. 28) projecting cholinergic axons to most parts of the cerebral cortex.

Sensory modulation: gate control

Sensory transmission from primary to secondary afferent neurons (at the levels of the posterior gray horn and posterior column nuclei) and from secondary to tertiary (at the level of the thalamus) is subject to *gating*. The term *gating* refers to the degree of freedom of synaptic transmission from one set of neurons to the next.

Tactile sensory transmission is gated at the level of the posterior column nuclei. Corticospinal neurons projecting from the postcentral gyrus may facilitate or inhibit sensory transmission at this level, as mentioned in Chapter 13.

Nociceptive transmission from the trunk and limbs is gated in the posterior gray horn of the spinal cord. From the head and upper part of the neck, it is gated in the spinal trigeminal nucleus. A key structure in both areas of gray matter is the substantia gelatinosa, which is packed with small excitatory and inhibitory internuncial neurons. The excitatory transmitter is glutamate; the inhibitory one is GABA for some internuncials, enkephalin (an opiate pentapeptide) for others.

Finely myelinated (Aδ) polymodal nociceptive fibers synapse directly upon dendrites of relay neurons of the lateral spinothalamic tract and of its trigeminal equivalent. The Aδ fibers signal sharp, well-localized pain. Unmyelinated, C fiber nociceptive afferents have mainly indirect access to relay cells, via excitatory gelatinosa internuncials. The C fibers signal dull, poorly localized pain. Most of them contain substance P, which may be liberated as a cotransmitter with glutamate.

Segmental antinociception

Large (A) mechanoreceptive afferents from hair follicles synapse upon *anterior* spinothalamic relay cells (and their trigeminal equivalents). They give off collaterals to

---

Core Information

Ground plan
The reticular formation extends the entire length of the brain stem, mainly in three cell columns. The lateral, parvocellular column receives afferents from the sensory components of all cranial and spinal nerves. It projects into the paramedian magnocellular reticular formation which in turn sends long axons to the brain and spinal cord. The median reticular formation contains serotoninergic neurons.

Aminergic neurons
Serotoninergic neurons of the raphe nuclei project to all parts of the gray matter of the CNS. Dopaminergic neurons project from substantia nigra to striatum and from midbrain ventral tegmental nuclei to prefrontal cortex and nucleus accumbens. Noradrenergic neurons of the cerulean nucleus project to all parts of the CNS gray matter. Epinephrine-secreting neurons of the medulla project to hypothalamus and spinal cord.

Pattern generators
Gaze centers in midbrain and pons control conjugate eye movements; a midbrain locomotor area regulates walking; a pontine supratrigeminal nucleus regulates chewing rhythm and a pontine micturition center

controls the bladder. In the medulla oblongata are respiratory, emetic, coughing and sneezing centers, and pressor and depressor centers for cardiovascular control. In addition, the medullary chemosensitive area contains reticular formation neurons sensitive to H^+ ion levels in the cerebrospinal fluid.

Sleeping and wakefulness are influenced by serotonin and norepinephrine neurons, and by cholinergic neurons in the upper pons. The ascending reticular activating system is a physiological concept based on brainstem neuronal networks having an arousal effect on the brain as seen in EEG traces. An important component is a set of pontine cholinergic neurons having an excitatory effect on thalamocortical neurons.

Antinociception
Segmental antinociception is induced by stimulating A fibers from hair follicles. *Supraspinal antinociception* is a function of the medullary magnus raphe nucleus which is activated from hypothalamus and midbrain. Serotonin from MRN terminals in substantia gelatinosa of spinal posterior horn/trigeminal nucleus activates enkephalinergic internuncials that inhibit transmission in spinothalamic/trigeminothalamic neurons.

inhibitory (mainly GABA) gelatinosa cells which synapse in turn upon *lateral* spinothalamic relay cells (*Figure 21.8*). Some of the internuncials also exert presynaptic inhibition upon C fiber terminals, either by axo-axonic contacts (which are very difficult to find in experimental material), or by dendro-axonic contacts. Gating of the spinothalamic response to C fiber activity can be induced by stimulating the mechanoreceptive afferents, thereby recruiting inhibitory gelatinosa cells. This simple circuit accounts for the relief afforded by 'rubbing the sore spot'. It also provides a rationale for the use of *transcutaneous electrical nerve stimulation* (TENS) by physical therapists for pain relief in arthritis and other chronically painful conditions. The standard procedure in TENS is to apply a stimulating electrode to the skin at the same segmental level as the source of noxious C fiber activity, and to deliver a current sufficient to produce a pronounced buzzing sensation.

Supraspinal antinociception

Magnus raphe nucleus (Figure 21.8)

From the magnus raphe nucleus (MRN) in the medulla oblongata, *raphespinal fibers* descend bilaterally within Lissauer's tract and terminate in the substantia gelatinosa at all levels of the spinal cord. In animals, electrical stimulation of the MRN may produce total analgesia throughout the body, with little effect on tactile sensation. Many fibers of the raphespinal tract liberate serotonin, which excites inhibitory internuncials in the posterior gray horn and spinal trigeminal nucleus. The internuncials induce both pre- and postsynaptic inhibition on the relevant relay cells.

- *Diffuse noxious inhibitory controls.* The MRN is not somatotopically arranged, but it does receive inputs from spinoreticular and trigeminoreticular neurons responding to peripheral noxious stimulation. This anatomical connection accounts for what are called diffuse noxious inhibitory controls. *Painful stimulation of one part of the body may produce pain relief in all other parts.* The arrangement accounts well for the heterotopic relief of pain in acupuncture, where needles are used to excite nociceptive afferents in the most superficial musculature rather than in the skin.

- *Stimulus-induced analgesia.* MRN is intensely responsive to stimulation of the PAG of the midbrain. This connection has been used to advantage for patients suffering intractable pain: a fine stimulating electrode can be inserted into PAG and wired so that the patient can control the level of self-stimulation.

- *Stress-induced analgesia.* At rest, the PAG projection to the MRN is under tonic inhibition by inhibitory internuncials present within PAG. The internuncials are themselves inhibited by opioid peptides – notably by β-endorphin released from a small set of hypothalamic neurons projecting to PAG. In life-threatening situations, where injury may be the price to be paid for escape, PAG may be released (disinhibited) by the hypothalamus. This seems to be the mechanism whereby a bullet wound may be scarcely noticed in the heat of battle. (As will be seen in Ch. 29, excitatory neurons in the PAG may also be stimulated directly by

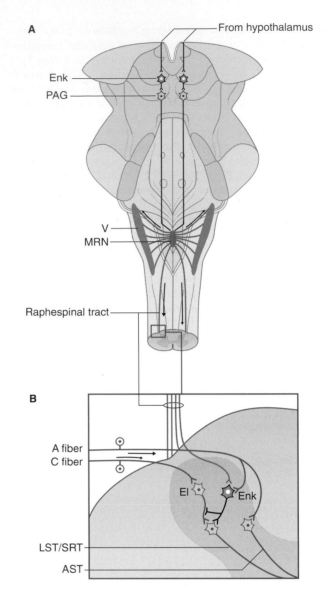

Figure 21.8 Antinociceptive pathways. **(A)** Posterior view of brainstem. **(B)** Right posterior gray horn of spinal cord, viewed from above. The peri-aqueductal gray matter (PAG) contains an excitatory projection to the midbrain raphe nucleus (MRN), and enkephalinergic internuncials (ENK) which exert tonic inhibition upon the projection cells. Inhibitory fibers from the hypothalamus release (*disinhibit*) the excitatory neurons, and MRN responds in turn.

The effects within the spinal nucleus of trigeminal (V) and posterior gray horn are the same: serotonin liberated by MRN neurons excites enkephalinergic internuncials which inhibit nociceptive projection cells.

The nociceptive pathway at cord level is represented by the C fiber input to an excitatory internuncial (EI) which in turn excites the lateral spinothalamic or spinoreticular projection cell (LST/SRT) unless this is being inhibited by the enkephalinergic internuncial. 'Rubbing the sore spot' sends impulse trains along A fibers inducing the ENK cell to exert presynaptic inhibition on the EI terminal, and postsynaptic inhibition on the LST/SRT projection cell. Passage of purely tactile information into the anterior spinothalamic tract (AST) is not impeded.

the amygdala (in the anterior temporal lobe) in fearful situations.)

In addition to the segmental and supraspinal controls of nociceptive transmission from primary to secondary afferents, gating occurs within the thalamus (see Ch. 24).

Furthermore, perception of the aversive (unpleasant) quality of pain seems to require participation of the anterior cingulate cortex (Ch. 29), which is rich in opiate receptors.

REFERENCES

Bentivoglio, M. and Steriade, M. (1990) Brainstem-diencephalic circuits as a structural substrate of the ascending reticular activation concept. In *The Diencephalon and Sleep* (Mancia, M. and Marini, G., eds), pp. 7–29. New York: Raven Press.

Bianchi, A.L., Denavit-Saube, M. and Champagnet, J. (1995) Central control of breathing. *Physiol. Rev.* **75**: 1–45.

Blok, F.M. and Holstege, G. (1998) The central nervous system control of micturition in cats and humans. *Behav. Brain Res.* **92**: 121–125.

Calancie, B., Needham-Shropshire, B., Jacobs, P., Willer, K., Zych, G. and Green, B.A. (1994) Involuntary stepping after chronic spinal cord injury: evidence for a central rhythm generator for locomotion in man. *Brain* **117**: 1143–1159.

Chalmers, J. and Pilowski, P. (1991) Brainstem and bulbospinal systems in the control of blood pressure. *J. Hypertens.* **9**: 675–694.

Fowler, C.J. (1999) Neurological disorders of micturition and their treatment. *Brain* **122**: 1213–1231.

Gonzalez, C., Almaraz, L., Obeso, A. and Rigual, R. (1994) Carotid body chemoreceptors: from natural stimuli to sensory discharges. *Physiol. Rev.* **74**: 829–898.

Jordan, L.M. (1998) Initiation of locomotion in mammals. *Ann. NY Acad. Sci.* **860**: 83–93.

Rosenfeld, J.P. (1994) Interacting brain components of opiate-activated, descending, pain-inhibitory systems. *Neurosci. Behav. Rev.* **18**: 403–409.

Siddall, P.J. (1995) Pain mechanisms and management. *Clin. Exp. Pharm. Physiol.* **22**: 679–688.

Cerebellum

INTRODUCTION

Phylogenetically, the initial development of the cerebellum (in fishes) took place in relation to the vestibular labyrinth. With development of quadrupedal locomotion, the anterior lobes (in particular) became richly connected to the spinal cord. Assumption of the erect posture and achievement of a whole new range of physical skills have been accompanied by the appearance of massive linkages between the posterior lobes and the cerebral cortex. In general, cerebellar connections with the labyrinth, spinal cord, and cerebral cortex are arranged such that each cerebellar hemisphere is primarily concerned with the co-ordination of movements *on its own side*.

The gross anatomy of the cerebellum is described briefly in Chapter 3, where it may be reviewed at this time.

FUNCTIONAL ANATOMY

Phylogenetic and functional aspects can be combined (to an approximation) by dividing the cerebellum into strips, as shown in *Figure 22.1*. The median strip contains the cortex of the vermis, together with the **fastigial nucleus** in the white matter close to the nodule (*Figure 22.2*). This strip is the *vestibulocerebellum*; it has two-way connections with the vestibular nucleus. It controls the responses of that nucleus to signals from the vestibular labyrinth. The fastigial nucleus also projects to the gaze centers of the brainstem (Ch. 21).

A paramedian strip, the *spinocerebellum*, includes the paravermal cortex and the **globose** and **emboliform nuclei** (*Figure 22.2*). The two nuclei are together called the **interposed nucleus**. The spinocerebellum is rich in spino-cerebellar connections. It is involved in the control of posture and gait.

The remaining, lateral strip is much the largest and takes in the wrinkled **dentate nucleus** (*Figure 22.2*). This strip is the *pontocerebellum*, because it receives a massive input from the contralateral nuclei pontis. It is also called the **neocerebellum** because the nuclei pontis convey information from large areas of the cerebral neocortex (phylogenetically the most recent). The neocerebellum is uniquely large in the human brain.

MICROSCOPIC ANATOMY

The structure of the cerebellar cortex is uniform throughout. From within outward, the cortex comprises granular, piriform, and molecular layers (*Figure 22.3*).

The **granular layer** contains billions of **granule cells**, whose somas are only 6–8 μm in diameter. Their short dendrites receive so-called **mossy fibers** from all sources except the inferior olivary nucleus. Before reaching the cerebellar cortex, the mossy fibers, which are excitatory in nature, give off collateral branches to the central nuclei.

The axons of the granule cells penetrate to the molecular layer where they divide in a T-shaped manner to form **par-**

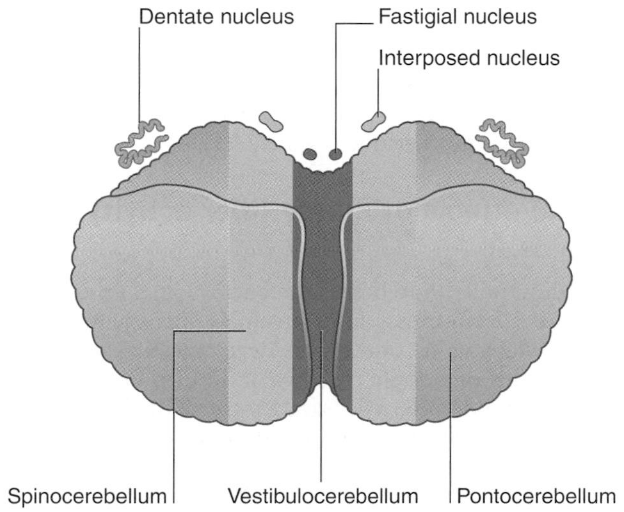

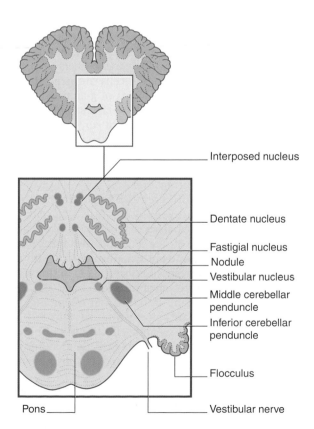

Figure 22.1 Zonation of cerebellum. The central nuclei are represented separately.

Dentate nucleus — Fastigial nucleus
Interposed nucleus

Spinocerebellum | Vestibulocerebellum | Pontocerebellum

Interposed nucleus
Dentate nucleus
Fastigial nucleus
Nodule
Vestibular nucleus
Middle cerebellar peduncle
Inferior cerebellar peduncle
Flocculus
Pons
Vestibular nerve

Figure 22.2 Transverse section of lower pons and cerebellum showing the position of the central and vestibular nuclei.

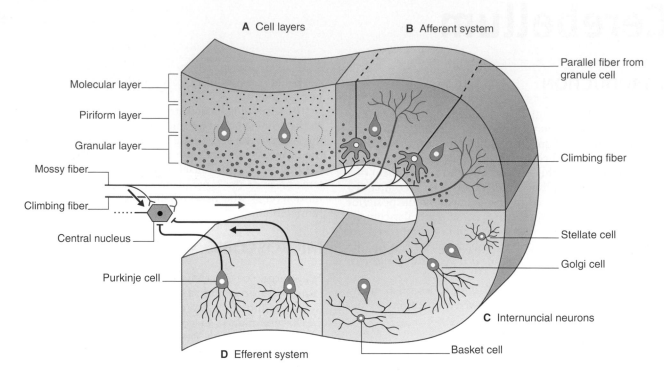

Figure 22.3 Cerebellar cortex. **(A)** Cell layers. **(B)** Afferent systems. **(C)** Internuncial neurons. **(D)** Efferent systems.

allel fibers. The parallel fibers run parallel to the axes of the folia. They make excitatory contacts with dendrites of Purkinje cells.

The granular layer also contains Golgi cells (see later).

The **piriform layer** consists of very large **Purkinje cells**. The fan-shaped dendritic trees of the Purkinje cells are the largest dendritic trees in the entire nervous system. The fans are disposed at right angles to the parallel fibers.

The dendritic trees of Purkinje cells are penetrated by huge numbers of parallel fiber axons of granule cells, each one making successive, one per cell, synapses upon dendritic spines of about 400 Purkinje cells. Not surprisingly, stimulation of small numbers of granule cells by mossy fibers has a merely facilitatory effect upon Purkinje cells. Many thousands of parallel fibers must act simultaneously to bring the membrane potential to firing level.

Each dendritic tree also receives a single **climbing fiber** from the contralateral inferior olivary nucleus. In stark contrast to the one-per-cell synapses of parallel fibers, the olivocerebellar fiber divides at the Purkinje dendritic branch points and makes thousands of synaptic contacts with dendritic spines. A single threshold pulse applied to one climbing fiber is sufficient to elicit a short burst of action potentials from the client Purkinje cell. Climbing fiber effects on Purkinje cells are so powerful that, for some time after they cease firing, the synaptic effectiveness of bundles of parallel fibers is reduced. In this sense, the Purkinje cells *remember* that they have been excited by olivocerebellar fibers.

The axons of the Purkinje cells are the only axons to emerge from the cerebellar cortex. Remarkably, they are entirely inhibitory in their effects. Their principal targets are the central nuclei. They give off collateral branches also, mainly to Golgi cells.

The **molecular layer** is almost entirely taken up with Purkinje dendrites, parallel fibers, supporting neuroglial cells, and blood vessels. However, two sets of inhibitory neurons are also found there, lying in the same plane as the Purkinje cell dendritic trees. Near the cortical surface are small, **stellate cells**, and close to the piriform layer are larger, **basket cells**. Both sets are contacted by parallel fibers, and they both synapse on Purkinje cells. The stellate cells synapse upon dendritic shafts whereas the basket cells form a 'basket' of synaptic contacts around the soma, as well as forming axo-axonic synapses upon the initial segment of the axon. A single basket cell synapses upon some 250 Purkinje cells.

The final cell type in the cortex is the **Golgi cell**, whose dendrites are contacted by parallel fibers and whose axons divide extensively before synapsing upon the short dendrites of granule cells. The synaptic ensemble that includes a mossy fiber terminal, granule cell dendrites, and Golgi cell boutons, is known as a **glomerulus** (*Figure 22.4*).

Spatial effects of mossy fiber activity

(Figure 22.5)

As already noted, cerebellar afferents other than olivocerebellar ones form mossy fiber terminals after giving off excitatory collaterals to one of the deep nuclei. The afferents excite groups of granule cells, which in turn facilitate many hundreds of Purkinje cells. Along most of the beam of excitation, known as a *microzone*, the Purkinje cells begin to fire, and to inhibit patches of cells in one of the deep nuclei. At the same time, weakly facilitated Purkinje cells along the edges of the microzone are shut off by stellate and basket cells. As a result, the beam of excitation is sharply focused. The excitation is terminated by Golgi cell inhibition of the

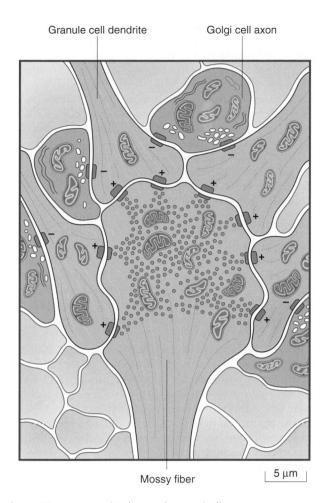

Granule cell dendrite   Golgi cell axon

Mossy fiber   5 μm

Figure 22.4 A synaptic glomerulus. +/– indicates excitation/inhibition.

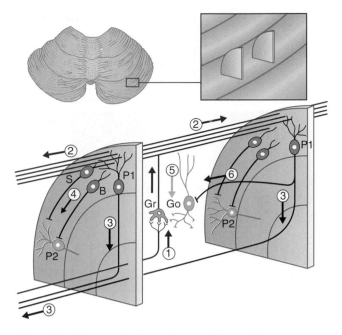

Figure 22.5 Scheme of effects of mossy fiber activity.

1 Mossy fiber stimulating a granule cell (Gr).
2 Beam of parallel fiber activity follows simultaneous activation of many granule cells.
3 Activation of on-line Purkinje cells (P1) results in selective inhibition of neurons within the appropriate central cerebellar nucleus.
4 Activation of stellate (S) and basket cells (B) inhibits off-line Purkinje cells (P2).
5 Golgi cells (Go) terminate granule cell activity.
6 Intense on-line activity can be sustained by inhibition of Golgi cells by Purkinje cells.

granule cells that initiated it. Powerful excitation will last longer because highly active Purkinje cells inhibit underlying Golgi cells through their collateral branches.

REPRESENTATION OF BODY PARTS

Representation of body parts in the human cerebellar cortex is currently under investigation by means of positron emission tomography (PET). These investigations, along with some evidence from clinical cases, indicate the presence of somatotopic maps in the anterior and posterior lobes (*Figure 22.6*).

The maps have been worked out in some detail in laboratory animals during movements. The maps for movement match up with maps of skin, eye, ear, and visceral representation worked out by stimulation of body parts. The expression, *fractionated somatotopy*, refers to the patchy nature of the representation of body parts. Simple representations like those in *Figure 22.6* are likely to be quite inaccurate in view of the vast areas of cortex buried in the fissures.

Figure 22.7, based on PET scans, shows simultaneous activation of the left motor cortex and right cerebellum during repetitive movements of the fingers of the right hand.

See also Higher Brain Functions, later.

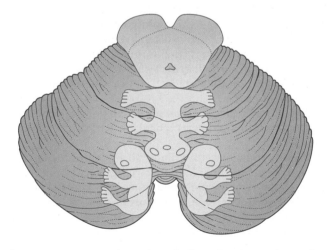

Figure 22.6 Upper surface of cerebellum showing position of somatotopic maps, based on animal experiments.

AFFERENT PATHWAYS

From the muscles and skin of the trunk and limbs, afferent information travels in the posterior spinocerebellar and the

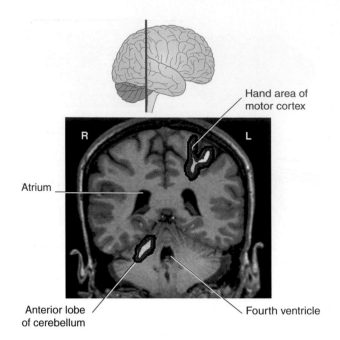

Hand area of
motor cortex

R L

Atrium

Anterior lobe
of cerebellum

Fourth ventricle

Figure 22.7 Representation of fMRI activity (viewed from behind) in a volunteer executing repetitive movement of the fingers of the right hand. (Based on a series kindly provided by Professor J. Paul Finn, Director, MRI Facility, Northwestern University School of Medicine, Chicago.)

cuneocerebellar tract and enters the inferior cerebellar peduncle on the same side. Comparable information from the territory served by the trigeminal nerve enters all three cerebellar peduncles.

Afferents from spinal reflex arcs run in the anterior spinocerebellar tract, which reaches the upper pons before looping into the superior cerebellar peduncle.

Special sense (visual, auditory, vestibular) pathways comprise tectocerebellar fibers entering the superior peduncle from the ipsilateral midbrain colliculi, and vestibulocerebellar fibers from the ipsilateral vestibular nucleus.

Two massive pathways enter from the contralateral brainstem. The pontocerebellar tract enters through the middle peduncle, and the olivocerebellar tract enters through the inferior peduncle.

Reticulocerebellar fibers enter the inferior peduncle from the paramedian and lateral reticular nuclei of the medulla oblongata.

Finally, aminergic fibers enter all three peduncles from noradrenergic and serotoninergic cell groups in the brainstem. Under experimental conditions, both kinds of neuron appear to facilitate excitatory transmission in mossy and climbing fiber terminals.

Olivocerebellar tract

The sensorimotor cortex projects, via corticospinal collaterals, in an orderly, somatotopic manner on to the ipsilateral inferior and accessory olivary nuclei. The order is preserved in the olivary projections onto the body maps in the contralateral cerebellar cortex (from principal nucleus to the posterior map, from the accessory nuclei to the anterior map). Under resting conditions in animal experiments,

groups of olivary neurons discharge synchronously at 5–10 Hz (impulses/second). The synchrony is probably due to the observed presence of electrical synapses (gap junctions) between dendrites of neighboring neurons. In the cerebellar cortex, the response of Purkinje cells takes the form of *complex spikes* (multiple action potentials in response to single pulses), because of the spatiotemporal effects of climbing fiber activity along the branches of the dendritic tree.

When a monkey has been trained to perform a motor task, increased discharge of Purkinje cells during task performance takes the form of simple spikes produced by bundles of active parallel fibers. If an unexpected obstacle is introduced into the task (e.g. momentary braking of a lever that the monkey is operating), bursts of complex spikes occur each time the obstacle is encountered. As the animal learns to overcome the obstacle so that the task is completed in the set time, the spike bursts dwindle in number and finally disappear. This is just one of several experimental indicators that the inferior olivary nucleus has a significant *teaching function* in the acquisition of new motor skills.

The olive receives direct ipsilateral projections from the premotor and motor areas of the cerebral cortex, and from the visual association cortex, providing an apparently suitable substrate for its activities. It is also in touch with the outside world through the spino-olivary tract (Ch. 12).

In theory, the red nucleus of the midbrain could function as a *novelty detector* because it receives collaterals both from cortical fibers descending to the olive and from cerebellar output fibers ascending to the thalamus. Much the largest output from the red nucleus is to the ipsilateral olive, which it appears to inhibit. Upon detection of a mismatch between a movement intended and a movement organized, the red nucleus could release the appropriate cell groups in the olive until the two are harmonized.

EFFERENT PATHWAYS (Figure 22.8)

From the *vestibulocerebellum* (fastigial nucleus), axons project to the vestibular nuclei of both sides, through the inferior cerebellar peduncle. The contralateral projection crosses over within the cerebellar white matter.

Vestibulocerebellar outputs to the medial and superior vestibular nuclei control movements of the eyes through the medial longitudinal fasciculus (Chs 14, 20). A separate output to the lateral vestibular (Deiters') nucleus of the same side controls the balancing function of the vestibulospinal tract. Some Purkinje axons skirt the fastigial nucleus and exert direct tonic inhibition on Deiters' nucleus.

From the interposed nucleus of the *spinocerebellum*, axons emerge in the superior cerebellar peduncle. They terminate mainly in the contralateral reticular formation and red nucleus. Those reaching the pontomedullary reticular formation regulate the functions of the reticulospinal tracts in relation to posture and locomotion. Those ascending to the red nucleus may be involved in motor learning.

From the *neocerebellum*, the massive **dentatorubrothalamic tract** forms the bulk of the superior cerebellar peduncle. It decussates with its opposite number in the lower midbrain and later gives collaterals to the red nucleus

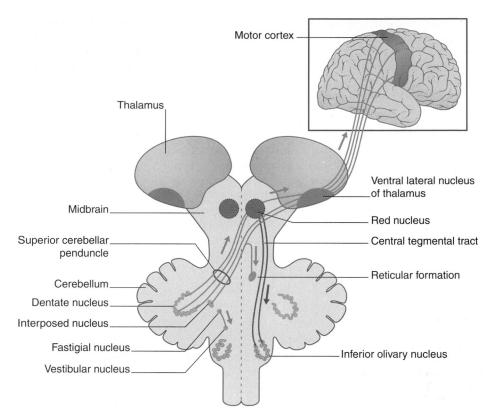

Figure 22.8 Principal cerebellar efferents. Arrows indicate directions of impulse conduction.

before synapsing in the ventral lateral nucleus of the thalamus. The onward projection from the thalamus is to the motor cortex.

ANTICIPATORY FUNCTION OF THE CEREBELLUM

The cerebellum plays a sophisticated role in *postural stabilization*, and in *postural fixation*, as indicated by the following examples.

Postural stabilization

Figure 22.9 illustrates anticipatory contraction of the gastrocnemius serving to stabilize a trunk about to receive a displacement impetus produced by contraction of the biceps brachii. In more general terms, displacement of the upper trunk away from the center of gravity by a voluntary movement of the head or upper limb, is *anticipated* by the cerebellum. Having read instructions delivered from premotor areas of the frontal lobe (Ch. 26) concerning the *intended* movement, the cerebellum ensures proportionate contractions of postural muscles in a bottom-up manner, from leg to thigh to trunk, in order to keep the center of gravity in the midline between the feet. Damage to the cerebellar vermis affects normal anticipatory activation, through the lateral vestibulospinal tract, of slow-twitch, close-to-the-bone

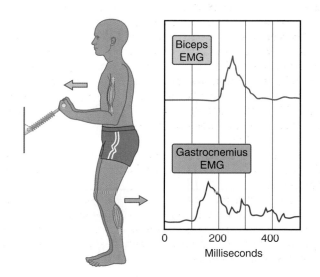

Figure 22.9 *Postural stabilization.* The subject is pulling a stiff spring attached to the wall. Flexion of the elbow during contraction of biceps brachii tends to pull the trunk forward (arrow). This movement is prevented by equivalent contraction of the gastrocnemius, exerting downward pressure on the forefoot which tends to thrust the trunk backward (arrow). Simultaneous electromyographic (EMG) recordings show that onset of (automatic) gastrocnemius contraction precedes voluntary biceps contraction by 80 msec. (Adapted from Nashner.)

muscle bundles, with consequent failure to counter the effect of gravity displacement produced by movement of any body part (see *Clinical Panel 22.1*).

Damage to the anterior lobe is associated with failure of the reticulospinal tracts to anticipate the gravitational effects produced by locomotion (see *Clinical Panel 22.2*).

Postural fixation

Figure 22.10 illustrates an experiment where the subject was instructed to execute sudden wrist extension and to maintain the extended wrist posture for 2 seconds, while electromyographic records were being taken from prime wrist extensors (extensors carpi radialis longus and brevis) and a prime antagonist (flexor carpi radialis). The readout revealed that the *antagonist* began to contract prior to completion of the movement, and that it played 'shivering ping pong' with

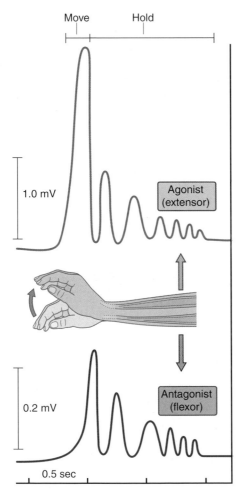

Figure 22.10 *Postural fixation.* The subject was instructed to perform sudden wrist extension and to briefly hold the extended posture. Electromyographic recordings show that wrist flexors come into action before completion of the movement. In the 'hold' position note alternation of electrical activity between agonist and antagonist. Antagonist EMG activity is much weaker, as indicated by the scale bars on the left. (Adapted from Topke et al.)

the prime mover during the fixation period. The contribution of the antagonist is to prevent spontaneous oscillatory torques (tremors) caused by viscoelastic properties of the muscles. It has been shown that this 'freeze' arrangement can be disrupted in healthy volunteers by transcranial electromagnetic stimulation aimed at the superior cerebellar peduncle, and in disease of the lateral cerebellar lobe (see *Clinical Panel 22.3*).

CLINICAL DISORDERS OF THE CEREBELLUM

Diseases involving the cerebellum usually involve more than one lobe and/or more than one of the three sagittal strips. However, characteristic clinical pictures have been described in association with lesions of the vermis (*Clinical Panel 22.1*), of the anterior lobe (*Clinical Panel 22.2*), and of the neocerebellum (*Clinical Panel 22.3*).

THE CEREBELLUM AND HIGHER BRAIN FUNCTIONS

PET provides information about regional changes in blood flow and oxygen consumption. 'Movement maps' such as those in *Figure 22.7* are derived from simple repetitive movements such as opening and closing a fist. A striking feature of movement maps is *how small* and *how medial* they are. Prior to PET, it was assumed that the lateral expansion of the human posterior lobe was necessary for manual dexterity. It now appears that the lateral expansion may be associated with cognitive functions (e.g. thinking), having an anatomical base in linkages with the lateral prefrontal cortex of the cerebral hemisphere. Lateral cerebellar activity seems to be greatest during speech, with a one-sided predominance consistent with a possible linkage (via the thalamus) with the motor speech area of the dominant frontal cortex (Ch. 24). Something more than mere motor control may be involved, because lateral cerebellar activity is greater during functional naming, e.g. 'dig', 'fly', than during object identification, e.g. 'shovel', 'airplane'.

Cerebellar cognitive affective syndrome is the summary term recently introduced to indicate cerebral functional deficits that follow sudden severe damage to the cerebellum, e.g. thrombosis of one of the three pairs of cerebellar arteries, or the unavoidable damage inflicted during removal of a cerebellar tumor. Such patients show *cognitive* defects in the form of diminished reasoning power, inattention, grammatic errors in speech, poor spatial sense, and patchy memory loss. If the vermis is included in the damage, *affective* (emotional) symptoms appear, sometimes in the form of *flatness of affect* (dulling of emotional responses), other times in the form of aberrant emotional behavior. The cognitive affective syndrome is temporary, and it is of interest that it my be associated with reduction of blood flow (on PET) in one or more of the association areas linked to the cerebellum by corticopontocerebellar fibers. Recent studies in monkeys have shown that, in addition to its well-known thalamocortical projection to the motor cortex, the cerebellum also 'drives' thalamic neurons projecting to association areas serving cognitive and affective functions.

Clinical Panel 22.1   Midline lesions: truncal ataxia

Lesions of the vermis occur most often in children, in the form of medulloblastomas in the roof of the fourth ventricle. These tumors expand rapidly and produce signs of raised intracranial pressure: headache, vomiting, drowsiness, papilledema. In the recumbent position there may be no abnormality of motor co-ordination in the limbs. A dramatic feature is an inability to stand upright without support – a state of *truncal ataxia*. This tumor, which is highly sensitive to radiotherapy, attacks the pathway from the vermis to

the nucleus of the vestibular nerve. The ataxia reflects malfunction of the lateral vestibular nucleus and consequently of the (lateral) vestibulospinal tract. Deficient antigravity function in this uncrossed pathway causes the child to fall to the more affected side on attempting to stand or walk.

Nystagmus can usually be elicited on visual tracking of the examiner's finger from side to side. Scanning movements of the eyes are also inaccurate owing to poor control of the gaze centers by the vermis.

Clinical Panel 22.2   Anterior lobe lesions: gait ataxia

Disease of the anterior lobe is most often observed in chronic alcoholics. Postmortem studies reveal pronounced shrinkage of the cortex of the anterior lobe, with up to 10% loss of granule cells, 20% loss of Purkinje cells, and 30% reduction in the thickness of the molecular layer. The lower limbs are most affected, and a staggering, drunken gait is evident even when the individual is sober. Some degree of correction may be exercised by voluntary control.

Instability of station with the feet together, and failure to 'toe the line' on walking, are present even

when the eyes are open. A head tremor at 3 Hz is usually present. As the disease progresses, a peripheral sensory neuropathy may be added, giving rise to signs of sensory ataxia (Ch. 12) in addition. Tendon reflexes may be depressed in the lower limbs owing to loss of tonic stimulation of fusimotor neurons via the pontine reticulospinal tract. Consequent reduction of monosynaptic reflex activity during walking may eventually result in stretching of soft tissues, with hyperextension of the knee joint during standing.

Clinical Panel 22.3   Neocerebellar lesions: inco-ordination of voluntary movements

Disease of the neocerebellar cortex, dentate nucleus, or superior cerebellar peduncle leads to inco-ordination of voluntary movements, particularly in the upper limb. When fine purposive movements are attempted (e.g. grasping a glass, using a key) an *intention tremor* (*action tremor*) develops: the hand and forearm quiver as the target is approached owing to faulty agonist/antagonist muscle synergies around the elbow and wrist. The hand may travel past the target ('overshoot'). Because cerebellar guidance is lost, the normal smooth trajectory of reaching movements may be replaced by stepped flexions, abductions, etc. ('decomposition of movement').

Rapid alternating movements performed under command, such as pronation/supination, become quite irregular (*dysdiadochokinesia*). The 'finger-to-nose' and 'heel-to-knee' tests are performed with equal clumsiness whether the eyes are open or closed – in

contrast to performance in posterior column disease, where performance is adequate when the eyes are open (Ch. 12).

Speech is impaired both with regard to phonation and to articulation. Phonation (production of vowel sounds) is uneven and often tremulous owing to loss of smoothness of contraction of the diaphragm and the intercostal muscles. The terms 'explosive' and 'scanning' have been applied to this feature. Articulation is slurred because of faulty co-ordination of impulses in the nerves supplying the lips, mandible, tongue, palate, and the infrahyoid muscles.

Signs of neocerebellar disorder sometimes originate in the midbrain or pons rather than in the cerebellum itself. The lesion responsible (usually vascular) interrupts one or other cerebellothalamic pathway (or both, if the lesion is at the decussation of the superior cerebellar peduncles).

Posturography

Posturography is the instrumental recording of the erect posture. The subject stands on a platform and spontaneous body sway is detected by strain gauges beneath the corners of the platform. Linkage of the strain-gauge data to a computer can yield a graphic record of anteroposterior and side-to-side sway, first with the eyes open and then with the eyes closed. This is *static posturography*, and it helps to distinguish among different causes of ataxia.

Dynamic posturography provides information on the effects of an abrupt 4° backward tilt of the supporting platform. For this phase of the examination, surface EMG electrodes are applied over the calf muscles (ankle plantarflexors) and over the tibialis anterior (an ankle dorsiflexor). The normal response to the backward tilt is threefold; (a) a monosynaptic, spinal, stretch reflex contraction of the calf muscles after 45 msec; (b) a polysynaptic stretch reflex contraction of the calf muscles after 95 msec; and (c) a long-loop, reflex contraction of the ankle dorsiflexors after 120 msec. The ascending limb of the long loop is via the tibial–sciatic nerve and the posterior column–medial lemniscal pathway to the somatosensory cortex; the descending limb is via the corticospinal tract and the sciatic–peroneal nerve. Dynamic posturography helps to distinguish among a wide variety of disorders affecting different levels of the CNS and PNS.

Core Information

The cerebellum is primarily concerned with co-ordination of movements on its own side of the body. Therefore, disease in one cerebellar hemisphere leads to inco-ordination of limb movements on that side.

The cerebellar cortex contains a thick inner layer of tiny granule cells, a piriform layer of Purkinje cells, and a molecular layer containing granule cell axons and Purkinje dendrites. Granule cells are excitatory to Purkinje cells (via parallel fibers) but Purkinje cells – the only output cells of the cortex – are inhibitory to the central nuclei, which themselves are excitatory. Inhibitory purely cortical neurons are the stellate, basket, and Golgi cells.

The two types of afferents to the cortex are (a) mossy fibers from all sources except the olive – they excite granule cells; and (b) climbing fibers from the olive which powerfully excite Purkinje cells.

The basic input–output circuit is: mossy fibers → granule cells → Purkinje cells → deep nucleus → brainstem or thalamus. Olivocerebellar neurons are most active during novel learning; they elicit poststimulus depression of the Purkinje cell response to mossy fiber activity – a feature surely related to motor learning. The red nucleus is in a position to match the intended input to the cerebellum with the output achieved after passage through the basic circuit.

Functional parts

Vestibulocerebellum comprises vermis and fastigial nuclei, having two-way connections with the vestibular nucleus. It may be affected by midline tumors, yielding nystagmus and truncal ataxia.

Spinocerebellum, next to vermis and including much of the anterior lobe, includes the interposed nucleus. It receives spinocerebellar pathways and it controls posture and gait. Lesions are characterized by ataxia of stance and gait.

Neocerebellum is largest and most lateral, receiving the corticopontocerebellar system. The dentate nucleus projects to the contralateral motor cortex via thalamus, and to the contralateral red nucleus. Lesions result in ipsilateral inco-ordination, notably of the upper limb; and to faulty phonation and articulation.

REFERENCES

Burke, D. and Gandevia, S.C. (1993) Muscle spindles, muscle tone and the fusimotor system. In *Science and Practice in Clinical Neurology* (Gandevia, S.C., Burke, D. and Anthony, M., eds), pp. 89–105. Cambridge: Cambridge University Press.

Ebner, T.J. and Bloedel, J.R. (1987) Climbing fiber afferent system: intrinsic properties and role in cerebellar information processing. In *New Concepts in Cerebellar Neurobiology* (King, J.S., ed.), pp. 371–386. New York: Alan R. Liss.

Fox, P.T., Raichle, M.E. and Thach, W.T. (1985) Functional mapping of the human cerebellum with positron emission tomography. *Proc. Natl. Acad. Sci. USA* **82**: 7462–7466.

Horne, M.K. and Butler, E.G. (1995) The role of the cerebello-thalamocortical pathway in skilled movements. *Progr. Neurobiol.* **46**: 190–213.

Houk, J.C. and Gibson, A.R. (1987) Sensorimotor processing through the cerebellum. In *New Concepts in Cerebellar Neurobiology* (King, J.S., ed.), pp. 387–416. New York: Alan R. Liss.

Kennedy, P.R. (1979) The rubro-olivo-cerebellar teaching circuit. *Med. Hypoth.* **5**: 799–807.

Leiner, H.C., Leiner, A.L. and Dow, R.S. (1991) The human cerebro-cerebellar system: its computing, cognitive, and language skills. *Behav. Brain Res.* **44**: 113–128.

Middleton, F.A. and Strick, P.L. (1997) Cerebellar output channels. In *The Cerebellum and Cognition: International Review of Neurobiology, vol 41* (Schmahmann, J.D., ed.), pp. 255–271. San Diego: Academic Press.

Nashner, L.M. (1979) Reflex control of posture and movement. *Progr. Brain Res.* **50**: 177–184.

Nitschke, M.F., Kleinschmidt, A., Wessel, K. and Frahm, J. (1996) Somatotopic motor representation in the human anterior cerebellum. *Brain* **119**: 1023–1029.

Schmahmann, J.D. and Sherman, J.C. (1998) The cerebellar cognitive affective syndrome. *Brain* **121**: 561–579.

Strata, P. and Rossi, F. Plasticity of the olivocerebellar pathway. *Trends Neurosci.* **21**: 407–412.

Topke, H., Mescheriakov, S., Boose, A., Kunz, R., Hetrich, I., Seydel, L., Dichgans, J. and Rothwell, J. (1999) A cerebellar-like terminal and postural tremor induced in normal man by transcranial magnetic stimulation. *Brain* **122**: 1551–1562.

Woogd, J. and Glickstein, M. (1998) The anatomy of the cerebellum. *Trends Neurosci.* **21**: 370–375.

Hypothalamus

INTRODUCTION

The hypothalamus develops as part of the limbic system, which is concerned with preservation of the individual and of the species. Therefore it is logical that the hypothalamus should have significant controls over basic survival strategies including reproduction, growth and metabolism, food and fluid intake, attack and defense, temperature control, the sleep–wake cycle, and aspects of memory.

Most of its functions are expressed through its control of the pituitary gland and of both divisions of the autonomic nervous system.

GROSS ANATOMY

The hypothalamus occupies the side walls and floor of the third ventricle. It is a bilateral, paired structure. Despite its small size – it weighs only 4 g – it has major functions in homeostasis and survival. Its homeostatic functions include control of the body temperature and the circulation of the blood. Its survival functions include regulation of food and water intake, the sleep–wake cycle, sexual behavior patterns, and defense mechanisms against attack.

Boundaries

The boundaries of the hypothalamus are as follows (see *Figures 23.1* and *23.2*):

- *Superior*: the **hypothalamic sulcus** separating it from the thalamus.
- *Inferior*: the **optic chiasm, tuber cinereum** and **mammillary bodies**. The tuber cinereum shows a small swelling, the **median eminence**, immediately behind the **infundibulum** ('funnel') atop the pituitary stalk.
- *Anterior*: the lamina terminalis.
- *Posterior*: the tegmentum of the midbrain.
- *Medial*: the third ventricle.
- *Lateral*: the internal capsule.

Subdivisions and nuclei

In the sagittal plane, it is customary to divide the hypothalamus into three regions: *anterior* (supraoptic), *middle* (tuberal) and posterior (mammillary). The descriptive use of 'regions' has been convenient for animal experiments involving placement of lesions. Named nuclei in the three regions are listed in *Table 23.1*.

In the coronal plane, the hypothalamus can be divided into *lateral*, *medial*, and *periventricular* regions. The full length of the lateral region is occupied by the **lateral hypothalamic nucleus**. Merging with the lateral nucleus is the **medial forebrain bundle**, carrying aminergic fibers to the hypothalamus and to the cerebral cortex.

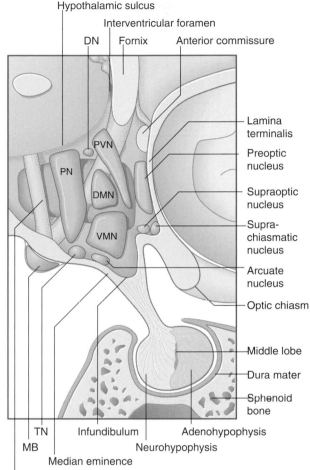

Figure 23.1 Hypothalamic nuclei and hypophysis, viewed from the right side. DN, dorsal nucleus; DMN, dorsomedial nucleus; MB, mammillary body; PN, posterior nucleus; PVN, paraventricular nucleus; TN, tuberomammillary nucleus; VMN, ventromedial nucleus. The lateral hypothalamic nucleus is shown in pink.

Table 23.1 Hypothalamic nuclei

Posterior	Middle	Anterior
Posterior Mammillary	Paraventricular	Preoptic
Tuberomammillary	Dorsomedial	Supraoptic
Dorsal	Lateral	Suprachiasmatic
	Ventromedial	
	Arcuate	

Plane of section

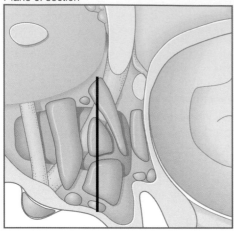

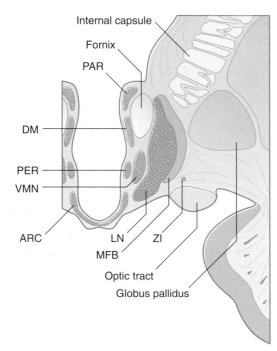

Internal capsule
Fornix
PAR

DM

PER
VMN

ARC
LN   ZI
MFB
Optic tract
Globus pallidus

Figure 23.2 Hypothalamic nuclei, and related neural pathways, in a coronal section. ARC, arcuate nucleus; DM, dorsomedial nucleus; LN, lateral nucleus; MFB, medial forebrain bundle; PAR, paraventricular nucleus; PER, periventricular nucleus; VMN, ventromedial nucleus; ZI, zona incerta.

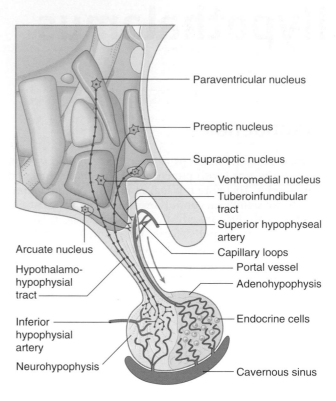

Paraventricular nucleus
Preoptic nucleus
Supraoptic nucleus
Ventromedial nucleus
Tuberoinfundibular tract
Superior hypophyseal artery
Capillary loops
Arcuate nucleus
Portal vessel
Hypothalamo-hypophysial tract
Adenohypophysis
Endocrine cells
Inferior hypophysial artery
Neurohypophysis
Cavernous sinus

Figure 23.3 Hypothalamic neuroendocrine cells. The blood supply to the hypophysis, including the endocrine cells of the adenohypophysis, is also shown (arrow indicates direction of blood flow in the portal system).

FUNCTIONS

Hypothalamic control of the pituitary gland

The arterial supply of the pituitary gland comes from hypophyseal branches of the internal carotid artery (*Figure 23.3*). One set of branches supplies a capillary bed in the wall of the infundibulum. These capillaries drain into **portal vessels** which pass into the adenohypophysis (anterior lobe). There they break up to form a second capillary bed which bathes the endocrine cells and drains into the cavernous sinus.

The neurohypophysis receives a direct supply from another set of hypophyseal arteries. The capillaries drain into

the cavernous sinus, which delivers the secretions of the anterior and posterior lobes into the general circulation.

Secretions of the pituitary gland are controlled by two sets of **neuroendocrine cells**. Neuroendocrine cells are true neurons in having dendrites and axons and in conducting nerve impulses. They are also true endocrine cells because they liberate their secretions into capillary beds (*Figure 23.4*). With one exception (mentioned below), the secretions are peptides, synthesized in clumps of granular endoplasmic reticulum and packaged in Golgi complexes. The peptides are attached to long-chain polypeptides called *neurophysins*. The capillaries concerned are outside the blood–brain barrier, and are fenestrated.

The somas of the neuroendocrine cells occupy the *hypophysiotropic area* in the lower half of the preoptic and tuberal regions. Contributory nuclei are the **preoptic**, **supraoptic**, **paraventricular**, **ventromedial**, and **arcuate** (infundibular). Two classes of neurons can be identified: **parvocellular** (small) **neurons** reaching the median eminence, and **magnocellular** (large) **neurons** reaching the posterior lobe of the pituitary gland.

The parvocellular neuroendocrine system

Parvocellular neurons of the hypophysiotropic area give rise to the **tuberoinfundibular** tract, which reaches the infundibular capillary bed. Action potentials traveling along these neurons result in calcium-dependent exocytosis of *releasing hormones* from some and *inhibiting hormones* from others, for transport to the adenohypophysis in the portal

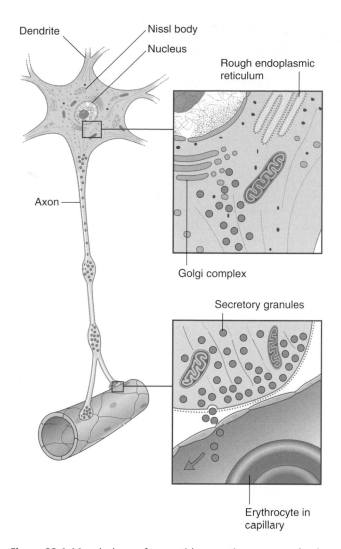

Dendrite

Nissl body

Nucleus

Rough endoplasmic reticulum

Axon

Golgi complex

Secretory granules

Erythrocyte in capillary

Figure 23.4 Morphology of a peptide-secreting neuroendocrine cell.

Table 23.2 Hypothalamic parvocellular releasing/inhibiting hormones (RH/IH)

RH/IH	Anterior lobe hormone
Corticotropin RH	ACTH
Thyrotropin RH	Thyrotropin
Growth hormone RH	Growth hormone
Growth hormone IH	Growth hormone
Prolactin RH	Prolactin
Prolactin IH	Prolactin
Gonadotropic hormone RH	FSH/LH

exerts a negative feedback effect by exciting inhibitory hypothalamic neurons having glucocorticoid receptors. In patients suffering from major depression, this feedback system fails (*Clinical Panel 23.2*).

The magnocellular neuroendocrine system

Magnocellular neurons in the supraoptic and paraventricular nuclei give rise to the **hypothalamohypophyseal tract**, which descends to the neurohypophysis (posterior lobe) (*Figure 23.3*). Minor contributions to the tract are received from opiatergic and other peptidergic neurons in the periventricular region of the hypothalamus, and from aminergic neurons of the brainstem.

Two hormones are secreted by separate neurons located in both the supraoptic and paraventricular nuclei: *antidiuretic hormone* (*vasopressin*) and *oxytocin*. Axonal swellings containing the secretory granules for these hormones make up nearly half the volume of the neurohypophysis. The largest swellings, called Herring bodies, may be as large as erythrocytes. The Herring bodies provide a local depot of granules for release by smaller, terminal swellings into the capillary bed.

Antidiuretic hormone

Antidiuretic hormone (ADH) continuously stimulates water uptake by the distal convoluted tubules and collecting ducts of the kidneys. The chief regulator of electrical activity in the ADH-secreting neurons is the osmotic pressure of the blood. A rise of as little as 1% in the osmotic pressure causes the plasma to be diluted to normal levels by means of increased water uptake. The neurons are themselves sensitive to osmolar changes, but they are facilitated by inputs from osmolar and volume detectors elsewhere, notably from the **vascular** and **subfornical circumventricular organs** (*Box 23.1*).

Some ADH neurons also synthesize *corticotropin-releasing hormone* (CRH), the two hormones being released together from collateral branches into the capillary pool of the infundibulum. It is of interest that ADH neuronal activity is increased when the body is stressed, and that the output of ACTH is boosted by the presence of ADH in the adenohypophysis.

Withdrawal of ADH secretion results in *diabetes insipidus* (*Clinical Panel 23.1*).

A prevalent disorder, *major depression*, is chemically characterized by reduced production of bioamines and excessive release of CRH (*Clinical Panel 23.2*).

vessels. The cell types of the adenohypophysis are stimulated/inhibited in accordance with *Table 23.2*. In the left-hand column, the only non-peptide parvocellular hormone is the prolactin-inhibiting hormone, which is *dopamine*, secreted from the arcuate (infundibular) nucleus.

The releasing/inhibiting hormones are not wholly specific: they have major effects on a single cell type, and minor effects on one or two others.

Multiple controls exist for parvocellular neurons of the hypophysiotropic area. The controls include: depolarization by afferents entering from the limbic system and from the reticular formation; hyperpolarization by local-circuit GABA neurons, some of which are sensitive to circulating hormones; and inhibition of transmitter release by opiate-releasing internuncials, which are numerous in the intermediate region of the hypothalamus. The picture is further complicated by the fact that opiates and other modulatory peptides may be released into the portal vessels and activate receptors on the endocrine cells of the adenohypophysis.

Stress causes increased secretion of ACTH which in turn stimulates the adrenal cortex to raise the plasma concentration of glucocorticoids including cortisol. Normally, cortisol

Clinical Panel 23.1 Hypothalamic disorders

The most dramatic disorder of hypothalamic function is *diabetes insipidus*, which is brought about by interruption of the hypothalamohypophyseal pathway – sometimes by tumors in the region, sometimes by head injury. The patient drinks upwards of 10 liters of water per day, and excretes a similar amount of urine. Historically, the term insipidus refers to the absence of taste sensation from the urine, in contrast to *diabetes mellitus*, in which the urine is sweet-tasting (mellitus) owing to its sugar content.

Hypophysectomy (surgical removal of the pituitary gland) can be performed in the treatment of other diseases, without causing more than temporary diabetes insipidus, provided the pituitary stalk is sectioned at a low level. Within a short period, sufficient ADH is secreted into the capillary bed of the median eminence to ensure adequate water conservation.

A wide variety of hypothalamic dysfunctions have been reported in the clinical literature. Causes are also varied, and include tumors, congenital malformations, and head injury. Clinical manifestations include gross obesity, disturbances of autonomic control, excessive sleepiness, and memory loss.

Clinical Panel 23.2 Major depression

Major depression is a state of depressed mood occurring without an adequate explanation in terms of external events. The condition affects about 4% of the adult population, and there is a genetic predisposition: about 20% of first-degree relatives have it too. Phases of depression may begin in childhood or adolescence.

Major depression is characterized by at least several of the following features:

- Depressed general mood, with loss of interest in normal activities and outside events.
- Diminished energy, easy fatigue, loss of appetite and of sex drive, constipation.
- Impairment of self-image, with a feeling of personal inadequacy.
- Disturbance of the sleep–wake cycle, typically shown by early morning wakefulness.
- Aches and pains. Recurrent abdominal pains may simulate organ disease.
- Periods of agitation, with restlessness and perhaps suicidal tendency.

Involvement of *monoamines* was first indicated by the chance observation that the use of reserpine in treatment of hypertension produced depression as a side effect. Reserpine depletes monoamine stores (serotonin, norepinephrine, dopamine).

The symptoms listed above are also characteristic of *chronic stress*. It is therefore not surprising to find that the suprarenal cortex is hyperactive in depressed patients. Serum cortisol levels are elevated. As already mentioned, a rising serum cortisol level normally inhibits production of CRH by the hypothalamus. In depressed patients, the central glucocorticoid receptors are relatively insensitive. This change forms the basis of the *dexamethasone suppression test*. Dexamethasone is a potent synthetic glucocorticoid which reduces ACTH secretion in healthy individuals.

Some of the CRH neurons send branches into the brain itself. In the midbrain, CRH inhibits mesocortical dopaminergic neurons, which are normally associated with positive motivational drive. In the midbrain, they also inhibit raphe serotoninergic neurons critically involved with diurnal rhythms, mainly through intense innervation of the suprachiasmatic nucleus.

The front line of therapy is dominated by drugs that enhance serotoninergic transmission. The range of antidepressants is large and their sites of action vary, e.g. some inhibit reuptake from the synaptic cleft, others inhibit degradation by monoamine oxidase (Ch. 10). They take several weeks to take effect; the latent interval is taken up with desensitizing (inhibitory) autoreceptors on serotoninergic cell membranes.

Electroconvulsive therapy (ECT) is at least as effective as the antidepressants. It seems to desensitize autoreceptors, to sensitize (excitatory) serotonin receptors on target neurons, and to depress noradrenergic transmission.

Box 23.1 Circumventricular organs

Six patches of brain tissue close to the ventricular system contain neurons and specialized glial cells abutting fenestrated capillaries. These are the **circumventricular organs** (CVOs). The **median eminence** and **neurohypophysis** are described in the main text. The **vascular organ of the lamina terminalis** and the **subfornical organ** close to the interventricular foramen send axons into the supraoptic and paraventricular nuclei of the hypothalamus and facilitate depolarization of neurons secreting ADH. In conditions of lowered blood volume, the kidney secretes renin which, on conversion to angiotensin II, stimulates these two CVOs to complete a positive feedback loop.

The **pineal gland** synthesizes *melatonin*, an amine hormone implicated in the sleep–wake cycle. Melatonin is synthesized from serotonin, the requisite enzymes being unique to this gland. Melatonin is liberated into the pineal capillary bed at night and has a sleep-inducing effect; it may have other benefits including clearance of harmful free radicals liberated from tissues during the aging process. Daytime secretion is suppressed by activity in sympathetic fibers reaching it from the superior cervical ganglia by way of the walls of the straight venous sinus. The relevant central pathway is from the paired suprachiasmatic nuclei via the posterior longitudinal fasciculus.

From the third decade onward, calcareous deposits ('pineal sand') accumulate within astrocytes in the pineal. Calcification is often detectable in plain radiographs of the head. A shift of the gland may denote a space-occupying lesion within the skull. However, a normal pineal may lie slightly to the left because the right cerebral hemisphere is usually a little wider than the left at this level.

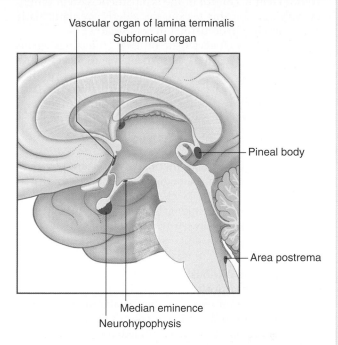

Figure Box 23.1.1 Circumventricular organs.

The **area postrema** is embedded in the roof of the fourth ventricle at the level of the obex. It is the *chemoreceptor trigger zone*, or *emetic* (vomiting) *center*. The emetic center contains neurons sensitive to a wide range of toxic substances, and it serves a protective function by reflexly eliciting emesis via connections with hypothalamus and reticular formation.

Oxytocin

The principal function of oxytocin is to participate in a *neurohumoral reflex* when an infant is suckling at the breast. The afferent limb of this reflex is provided by impulses traveling from the nipple to the hypothalamus via the spinoreticular tract. Oxytocin is liberated by magnocellular neurons in response to suckling. Having entered the general circulation, it causes the expression of milk by stimulating myoepithelial cells surrounding the lactiferous ducts of the breast.

Oxytocin also has a mild stimulating action on uterine muscle during labor. The afferent stimulus in this case originates in the genital tract once labor gets under way.

Other hypothalamic connections and functions

Autonomic centers

In animals, stimulation of the anterior hypothalamic area produces *parasympathetic effects*: slowing of the heart, con-striction of the pupil, salivary secretion, and intestinal peristalsis. On the other hand, stimulation of the posterior hypothalamic area produces *sympathetic effects*: increase in heart rate and blood pressure, pupillary dilation, and intestinal stasis. Axons from both areas project to autonomic nuclei in the brainstem and spinal cord. In the midbrain and pons, this projection occupies the dorsal longitudinal fasciculus as seen in chapter 14.

Temperature regulation

The hypothalamus contains *thermosensitive neurons* which initiate appropriate responses to changes in the core temperature of the body. Activity of these neurons is reinforced by thermal information received (via the spinoreticular tract) from thermosensitive neurons supplying the skin (Ch. 9).

A slight change in the core temperature can usually be corrected by directing blood flow into or away from the skin, as appropriate. The requisite control of the sympathetic nervous system resides in the region of the posterior nucleus of the hypothalamus, which sends axons all the way to the lateral horn of the spinal cord.

Hypothalamic control of the sympathetic system diminishes with age. For this reason, the elderly are particularly prone to develop hypothermia in cold weather.

Hyperthermia is characteristic of *fevers*. Infectious agents (bacteria, viruses, parasites) cause tissue macrophages to liberate *endogenous pyrogen*, a protein that causes the hypothalamic 'thermostat' to be reset to a higher value. The chief mechanisms used to raise the body temperature to the new set point are cutaneous vasoconstriction and shivering.

Drinking

The chief center controlling the intake of water appears to be a ribbon of cells alongside the lateral nucleus known as the **zona incerta** (*Figure 23.2*). Stimulation of this region may produce excessive drinking; lesions may result in refusal to drink, with consequent severe dehydration.

Eating

Eating habits have obvious social and cultural components, causing dietary practice to vary widely among individuals and among communities. The hypothalamus provides a baseline for caloric and nutrient intake, in the form of interplay between the lateral and ventromedial nuclei. Together, they constitute the *appestat* (appetite set point). Stimulation of a lateral hypothalamic *feeding center* causes a cat or rat to eat excessively, whereas destruction of this center results in refusal to eat. Conversely, stimulation of a ventromedial *satiety center* inhibits the urge to eat, and bilateral ventromedial lesions result in persistent overeating and gross obesity. The satiety center is normally very sensitive to glucose levels in the blood.

Of interest here is that serotonin is capable of altering the appetite set point, by inhibiting the lateral nucleus. Anorexics tend to have a raised level of serotonin production, and bulimics a reduced level.

Rage and fear

The lateral and ventromedial nuclei are concerned with *mood* as well as food. Cats that are overweight in consequence of ventromedial lesions tend to be highly aggressive. Conversely, animals rendered underweight by ventromedial stimulation tend to be unduly docile (see also the amygdala in Ch. 29).

Sleeping and waking

The tiny (0.25 mm³) **suprachiasmatic nucleus** embedded in the upper surface of the optic chiasm receives a direct input from the retina. It participates in setting the normal sleep–wake cycle, through connections with the pineal gland. For reasons unknown, this nucleus contains peptidergic (vasopressin) neurons which are twice as numerous in homosexual men than in heterosexuals of either sex.

Lesions of the posterior hypothalamic area may cause hypersomnolence or even coma. This area contains the **tuberomammillary nucleus** (*Figure 23.1*), housing hundreds of *histaminergic neurons*, which project widely to the gray matter of the brain and spinal cord. Some of the fibers run rostrally within the medial forebrain bundle, in company with aminergic fibers of brainstem origin. Histaminergic fibers destined for the cerebral cortex fan out below the genu of the corpus callosum. They branch within the superficial layers of the frontal cortex, and run back to supply the cortex of the parietal, occipital, and temporal lobes.

Core Information

The hypothalamus is a bilateral structure beside the third ventricle. In the sagittal plane, it can be divided into an anterior (supraoptic) region containing three nuclei, an intermediate (tuberal) region with five nuclei, and a posterior (mammillary) region with three. In the coronal plane, lateral, medial, and periventricular regions are described.

The pituitary gland is controlled by hypothalamic neuroendocrine cells, which are characterized by impulse transmission and hormonal secretion into capillary beds. Parvocellular neuroendocrine cells project to the median eminence. They secrete releasing/inhibiting hormones into the capillary bed there, to be taken to the adenohypophysis in a portal system of vessels. Large (magnocellular) neuroendocrine cells form the hypothalamohypophyseal tract, which liberates ADH and oxytocin into the capillary bed of the neurohypophysis.

Circumventricular organs comprise the median eminence and neurohypophysis, the vascular organ of lamina terminalis and subfornical organ (both of these involved in a feedback loop regulating plasma volume); the pineal gland which secretes melatonin; the emetic area postrema; and the subfornical organ.

Anterior and posterior regions of the hypothalamus contain neurons that activate the parasympathetic and sympathetic system, respectively. Thermoregulatory neurons maintain the body temperature set point, mainly by manipulating the sympathetic system.

Stimulation of the lateral hypothalamic area provokes an increase in food and water consumption. Destruction of this area, or stimulation of a ventromedial satiety center, results in refusal to eat.

The suprachiasmatic nucleus participates in control of the sleep–wake cycle. The medial preoptic area contains androgen-sensitive neurons and the ventromedial nucleus contains estrogen-sensitive neurons. The mammillary bodies receive inputs from the limbic system via the formix, having a function in relation to memory.

In animals, there is abundant physiological evidence in support of an *arousal function* for the histaminergic system.

In laboratory animals, electrical stimulation of these nuclei elicits appropriate sexual responses.

Sexual arousal

A subset of neurons (known as INAH3) within the medial part of the preoptic nucleus is more than twice as large in males than females. It is also rich in androgen receptors and activated by circulating testosterone. In females, estrogen-rich neurons are contained within the ventromedial nucleus.

Memory

The mammillary bodies belong to a limbic, *Papez circuit* involving the fornix, which sends fibers to it, and the mammillothalamic tract which projects to the anterior nucleus of the thalamus. This circuit has a function in relation to memory (Ch. 29).

REFERENCES

Akil, H. and Watson, S.J. (1987) Neuropeptides in brain and pituitary: overview. In *Psychopharmacology: The Third Generation of Progress* (Meltzer, H.Y., ed.), pp. 367–371. New York: Raven Press.

Gordon, C.J. (1986) Integration and central processing in temperature control. *Ann. Rev. Physiol.* **48**: 595–612.

Hatton, G.L. (1990) Emerging concepts of structure-function dynamics in adult brain: the hypothalamo-neurohypophysial system. *Prog. Neurobiol.* **34**: 337–504.

Lutten, P.G.M., ter Horst, T.J. and Steffens, A.B. (1986) The hypothalamus: intrinsic connections and outflow pathways to the endocrine system in relation to the control of feeding and metabolism. *Prog. Neurobiol.* **28**: 1–54.

Rothwell, N.J. (1994) CNS regulation of thermogenesis. *Crit. Rev. Neurobiol.* **8**: 1–10.

Sawchenko, P.E. (1998) Toward a new neurobiology of energy balance, appetite, and obesity: the anatomists weigh in. *J. Comp. Neurol.* **402**: 435–441.

Schwartz, J-C., Arrang, J-M., Garbarg, M., Pollard, H. and Ruat, M. (1991) Histaminergic transmission in the mammalian brain. *Physiol. Rev.* **71**: 1–51.

Swaab, D.F. and Hofman, M.A. (1994) Age, sex and light: variability in the human suprachiasmatic nucleus in relation to its functions. *Prog. Brain Res.* **100**: 261–265.

Weltzin, K. (1991) Serotonin activity in anorexia and bulimia. *J. Clin. Psychiat.* **52**(Suppl): 41–48.

Thalamus, epithalamus

THALAMUS

The thalamus is the largest nuclear mass in the entire nervous system. It is a prominent feature in MRI scans in each of the three planes in which slices are taken. The afferent and efferent connections of the main nuclear groups are listed in *Table 24.1*. The connections are so diverse that the thalamus cannot be said to have a unitary function.

As noted in Chapter 2, the two thalami lie at the center of the brain. Their medial surfaces are usually linked across the third ventricle and their lateral surfaces are in contact with the posterior limb of the internal capsule. The upper surface of each occupies the floor of a lateral ventricle. The under aspect receives sensory and cerebellar inputs as well as an upward continuum of the reticular formation.

Thalamic nuclei

All thalamic nuclei except one (the reticular nucleus) have reciprocal excitatory connections with the cerebral cortex. The Y-shaped **internal medullary lamina** of white matter divides the thalamus into three large cell groups: *medial dorsal*, *anterior*, and *lateral* (*Figure 24.1A*). The lateral group comprises *dorsal and ventral nuclear tiers*. At the back of the thalamus are the **medial** and **lateral geniculate bodies**. The **external medullary lamina** separates the thalamus from the shell-like **reticular nucleus**.

The thalamic nuclei are categorized into three functional groups: *specific* or *relay nuclei, association nuclei*, and *non-specific nuclei*.

Specific nuclei

The specific or relay nuclei are reciprocally connected to specific motor or sensory areas of the cerebral cortex. They comprise the nuclei of the ventral tier and the geniculate nuclei. Their afferent and efferent connections are indicated in *Figure 24.1B*.

The **anterior nucleus** receives the mammillothalamic tract and projects to the cingulate cortex. It is involved in a limbic circuit and has a function in relation to memory (Ch. 29).

The **ventral anterior nucleus** (VA) receives afferents from the globus pallidus, and it projects to the prefrontal cortex.

The anterior part of the **ventral lateral nucleus** (VL) receives afferents from the globus pallidus and projects to the supplementary motor area. The posterior part of VL is the principal target of the contralateral superior cerebellar peduncle, which originates in the dentate nucleus of the cerebellum; the posterior VL projects to the motor cortex.

The **ventral posterior nucleus** (VP) receives all of the fibers of the medial, spinal, and trigeminal lemnisci (*Figure 24.2*). It projects to the somatic sensory cortex (SI). A smaller projection is sent to the second somatic sensory area (SII) at the foot of the postcentral gyrus (see Ch. 26).

The VP is somatotopically arranged, as indicated in *Figure 24.3*. The portion of the nucleus devoted to the face and head is called the **ventral posterior medial nucleus** (VPM), that for the trunk and limbs the **ventral posterior lateral nucleus** (VPL). Modality segregation is a feature of both nuclei, with proprioceptive neurons most anterior, tactile neurons in the midregion, and nociceptive neurons at the back. The nociceptive region is sometimes called the *posterior nucleus*.

There is no evidence in the VP of an antinociceptive mechanism comparable to that found in the substantia gelatinosa region of the spinal cord and spinal trigeminal nucleus. An unexplained disorder, the *thalamic syndrome*, may follow a vascular lesion that disconnects the posterior thalamic nucleus from the somatic sensory cortex. In this condition, a period of complete sensory loss may occur on the contralateral side of the body, to be replaced by bouts of severe pain occurring either spontaneously or in response to tactile stimuli.

The **medial geniculate body** (medial geniculate nucleus) is the thalamic nucleus of the auditory pathway. It receives

Table 24.1 Thalamic nuclei and their connections

Type	Nucleus	Afferents	Efferents
Specific	Anterior	Mammillary body	Cingulate gyrus
	Ventral anterior (VA)	Globus pallidus	Prefrontal cortex
	Ventral lateral (VL)		
	anterior part	Globus pallidus	Supplementary motor area (SMA)
	posterior part	Cerebellum	Motor cortex
	Ventral posterior medial (VPM)	Somatic afferents from head region	Somatic sensory cortex (SI)
	Ventral posterior lateral (VPL)	Somatic afferents from trunk and limbs	Somatic sensory cortex
	Medial geniculate body	Inferior colliculus	Primary auditory cortex
	Lateral geniculate body	Superior colliculus, optic tract	Primary visual cortex
Association	Lateral dorsal	Parietal lobe	Cingulate cortex
	Posterior dorsal and pulvinar	Superior colliculus, parietal lobe	Visual association cortex
Non-specific	Intralaminar	Reticular formation	Cortex everywhere
	Reticular	Thalamus	Thalamus

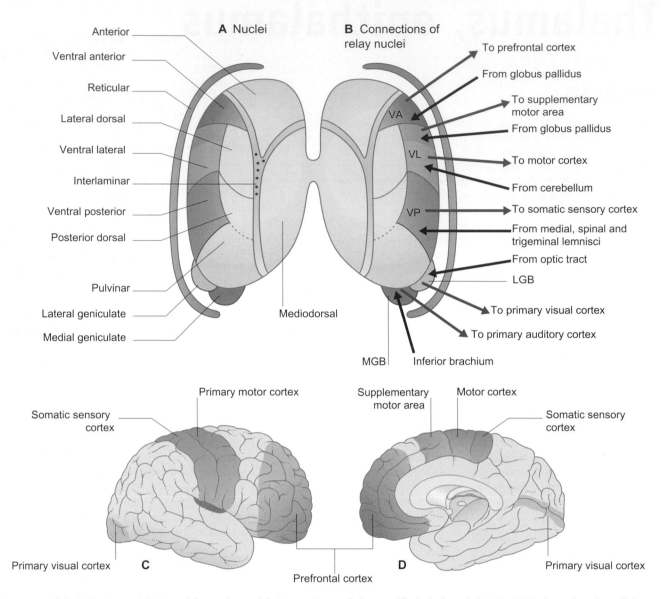

Figure 24.1 (A) Thalamic nuclei viewed from above. **(B)** Connections of the specific (relay) nuclei. LGB, MGB, lateral and medial geniculate bodies; VA, ventral anterior nucleus; VL, ventral lateral nucleus; VP, ventral posterior nucleus. **(C)** Lateral and **(D)** medial surface of hemisphere showing cortical areas receiving projections from the relay nuclei.

the inferior brachium from the inferior colliculus (which carries auditory signals from both ears, Ch. 17), and it projects to the primary auditory cortex in the superior temporal gyrus.

The **lateral geniculate body** (lateral geniculate nucleus) is the principal thalamic nucleus for vision. It receives retinal inputs from both eyes by way of the optic tract, and it projects to the primary visual cortex in the occipital lobe. The visual pathways are described in Chapter 25.

Association nuclei

The association nuclei are reciprocally connected to the association areas of the cerebral cortex.

The **lateral dorsal nucleus** has reciprocal connections with the posterior part of the cingulate cortex,

which is involved in functions related to memory (Ch. 29).

The **mediodorsal nucleus** receives inputs from the olfactory and limbic systems and is reciprocally connected with the entire prefrontal cortex. It has functions in relation to cognition (thinking), judgment, and mood.

The **lateral posterior nucleus** and the **pulvinar** belong to a single nuclear complex. They receive afferents from the superior colliculus and project to the entire visual association cortex and to the entire parietal association cortex. An 'extrageniculate visual pathway' runs from the optic tract to the visual association cortex by way of the superior colliculus and the pulvinar. It has the function of drawing attention to objects of interest in the peripheral field of vision, but it is not itself a source of conscious visual perception.

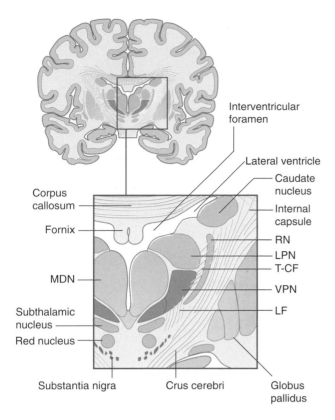

Figure 24.2 Coronal section through the thalamus and related structures. LF, lemniscal fibers; LPN, lateral posterior nucleus; MDN, mediodorsal nucleus; RN, reticular nucleus; TCF, thalamocortical fibers; VPN, ventral posterior nucleus.

Non-specific nuclei

The non-specific nuclei are so called because they are not specific to any one sensory modality. They include the intralaminar and reticular nuclei.

The **intralaminar nuclei** are contained within the internal medullary lamina of white matter. They can be regarded as a rostral continuation of the reticular formation of the midbrain (ascending reticular activating system in Ch. 21). They project widely to the cerebral cortex, as well as to the corpus striatum.

The **reticular nucleus** is shaped like a shield around the front and lateral side of the thalamus. It is separated from the main thalamus by the external medullary lamina. All of the thalamocortical projections pass through the reticular nucleus and give collateral branches to it (*Figure 24.4*). The nucleus reciprocates by sending a matching, inhibitory (GABAergic) supply to the corresponding thalamic nucleus – both to the projection neurons and to a set of GABAergic internuncials within the nucleus.

Afferents belonging to the ascending reticular activating system synapse in the reticular nucleus, the intralaminar nuclei and the nucleus of Meynert in the basal forebrain (Ch. 29).

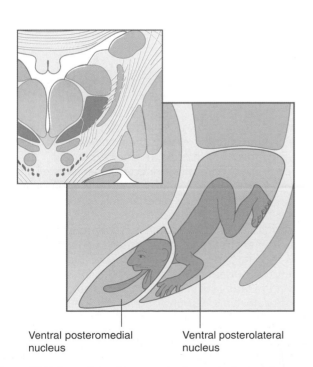

Figure 24.3 Somatic sensory map in the ventral posterior thalamic nucleus. (Redrawn and modified from Ohye (1990) with permission.)

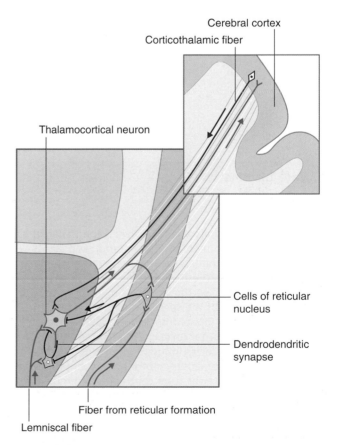

Figure 24.4 Synaptic relationships of a thalamocortical relay neuron in the ventral posterior nucleus of the thalamus. Arrows indicate directions of impulse transmission. Inhibitory neurons are shown in black.

In animal experiments (cat), thalamocortical neurons are subdued by the reticular nucleus during sleep, exhibiting only intermittent short bursts of activity. During wakefulness, thalamocortical neurons fire continuously, apparently because of disinhibition: the reticular nucleus is still active, but its effect seems to be shifted to the inhibitory internuncials.

Not represented in *Table 24.1* are *aminergic afferents* passing to the ventral and intralaminar nuclei, from the midbrain raphe (serotoninergic) and locus ceruleus (noradrenergic). The proven value of tricyclic antidepressants in the therapy of chronic pain may be related to drug-induced prolongation of excitatory aminergic effects on thalamocortical neurons.

Thalamic peduncles

The reciprocal connections between the thalamus and the cerebral cortex travel in four thalamic peduncles, as shown in *Figure 24.5*. The **anterior thalamic peduncle** passes through the anterior limb of the internal capsule to reach the prefrontal cortex and cingulate gyrus. The **superior thalamic peduncle** passes through the posterior limb of the internal capsule to reach the premotor, motor, and somatic sensory cortex. The **posterior thalamic peduncle** passes through the retrolentiform part of the internal capsule to reach the occipital lobe and the posterior parts of the parietal and temporal lobes. The **inferior thalamic peduncle** passes below the lentiform nucleus to reach the anterior temporal and orbital cortex. Each of the four fans becomes incorporated into the corona radiata.

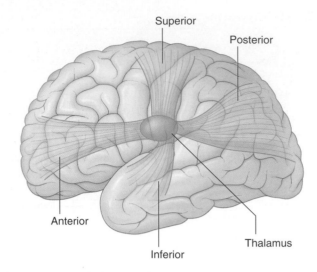

Figure 24.5 The thalamic peduncles (left hemisphere).

EPITHALAMUS

The epithalamus includes the pineal gland (considered in Ch. 23); and the habenula and stria medullaris which are included with the limbic system in Chapter 28.

Core Information

Thalamus

The internal medullary lamina divides the thalamus anatomically into mediodorsal, anterior, and lateral nuclear groups, the lateral being separable into dorsal and ventral tiers. The thalamus may be divided functionally into specific, association, and non-specific nuclear groups. Of the specific nuclei, (1) ventral anterior receives inputs from globus pallidus and projects to prefrontal cortex; (2) the anterior part of ventral lateral receives inputs from globus pallidus and projects to supplementary motor area whereas the posterior part receives from contralateral cerebellum and projects to motor cortex; (3) ventral posterior receives the somatic sensory pathways and projects to the somatic sensory cortex; (4) the medial geniculate nucleus receives the inferior brachium and projects to the primary auditory cortex; and (5) the lateral geniculate nucleus receives from the optic tract and projects to the primary visual cortex. Of the association nuclei, (1) the anterior receives the mammillothalamic tract and projects to the cingulate cortex; (2) the mediodorsal is reciprocally connected to all parts of the prefrontal cortex; and (3) the lateral posterior-pulvinar complex receives from the superior colliculus and projects to the parietal association cortex. Of the non-specific nuclei, (1) the intralaminar nucleus receives inputs from the reticular formation and projects widely to the cerebral cortex, also to the corpus striatum; (2) the reticular nucleus (external to the thalamus proper) receives excitatory collaterals from all thalamocortical and corticothalamic neurons, and returns inhibitory fibers to all nuclei within the thalamus. Reciprocal connections between thalamus and cortex travel in four thalamic peduncles which become incorporated into the corona radiata.

REFERENCES

Guillery, R.W. (1995) Anatomical evidence concerning the role of the thalamus in corticocortical communication: a brief review. *J. Anat.* **187**: 583–592.

Jones, E.G. (1985) *The Thalamus*. New York: Plenum Press.

Kultas-Ilinsky, K. and Ilinsky, I.A. (1986) Neuronal and synaptic organization of the motor nuclei of mammalian thalamus. In *Current Topics in Research on Synapses, Vol. 3*, pp. 77–145. New York: Alan R. Liss.

Lenz, F.A. (1992) Ascending modulation of thalamic function and pain. In *Advances in Pain Research and Therapy* (Sicuteri, F. et al., eds), pp. 177–196. New York: Raven Press.

Mahe, V. and Chevalier, F. (1995) Human circadian clock in disease. *Presse Med.* **24**: 1041–1046.

Ohye, C. (1990) Thalamus. In *The Human Nervous System* (Paxinos, G., ed.), pp. 439–468. San Diego: Academic Press.

Steriade, M. and Llinas, R.R. (1988) The functional states of the thalamus and the associated neuronal interplay. *Physiol. Rev.* **68**: 649–742.

Visual pathways

INTRODUCTION

The visual pathways are of outstanding importance in clinical neurology. They extend from the retinas of the eyes to the occipital lobes of the brain. Their great length makes them especially vulnerable to demyelinating diseases such as multiple sclerosis; to tumors of the brain or pituitary gland; to vascular lesions in the territory of the middle or posterior cerebral artery; and to head injuries.

The visual system comprises the retinas, the visual pathways from the retinas to the brainstem and visual cortex, and the cortical areas devoted to higher visual functions. The retinas and visual pathways are described in this chapter. Higher visual functions are described in Chapters 26 and 27.

RETINA

The retina and the optic nerves are part of the central nervous system. In the embryo, the retina is formed by an outgrowth from the diencephalon called the optic vesicle (Ch. 1). The optic vesicle is invaginated by the lens and becomes the two-layered optic cup.

The outer layer of the optic cup becomes the pigment layer of the mature retina. The inner, nervous layer of the cup gives rise to the retinal neurons.

Figure 25.1 shows the general relationships in the developing retina. The nervous layer contains three principal layers of neurons: **photoreceptors**, which become applied to the pigment layer when the intraretinal space is resorbed;

bipolar neurons; and **ganglion cells** which give rise to the optic nerve and project to the thalamus and midbrain.

Note that the retina is *inverted*: light must pass through the layers of optic nerve fibers, ganglion cells, and bipolar neurons to reach the photoreceptors. However, at the point of most acute vision, the **fovea centralis**, the bipolar and ganglion cell layers lean away all around a central pit (fovea), and light strikes the photoreceptors directly (see Foveal Specialization, later). In the mature eye, the fovea is about 1.5 mm in diameter and occupies the center of the 5 mm wide **macula lutea** ('yellow spot') where many of the photoreceptor cells contain yellow pigment. The fovea is the point of most acute vision and lies in the *visual axis* – a line passing from the center of the visual field of the eye, through the center of the lens, to the fovea (*Figure 25.2*). To *fixate* or *foveate* an object is to gaze directly at it so that light reflected from its center registers on the fovea.

The axons of the ganglion cells enter the optic nerve at the **optic papilla** (*optic nerve head*), which is devoid of retinal neurons and constitutes the physiological 'blind spot'.

The visual fields of the two eyes overlap across two-thirds of the total visual field. Outside this *binocular field* is a *monocular crescent* on each side (*Figure 25.3*). During passage through the lens, the image of the visual field is reversed, with the result that, e.g., objects in the left part of the binocular visual field register on the right half of each retina and objects in the upper part of the visual field register on the lower half. This arrangement is preserved all the way to the visual cortex in the occipital lobe.

From a clinical standpoint, it is essential to appreciate that *vision is a crossed sensation.* The visual field on one side of the visual axis registers on the visual cortex of the opposite side. In effect, the right visual cortex 'sees' the left visual field. Only half of the visual information crosses in the optic chiasma, for the simple reason that the other half has already crossed the midline in space.

Visual defects caused by interruption of the visual pathway are always described *from the patient's point of view*, i.e. in terms of the visual fields, and not in terms of retinal topography.

Structure of the retina

In addition to the serially arranged photoreceptors, bipolar cells and ganglion cells shown in *Figure 25.1*, the retina contains two sets of neurons arranged transversely: **horizontal cells** and **amacrine cells** (*Figure 25.4*). A total of eight layers are described for the retina as a whole. ·

Action potentials are generated by the ganglion cells, providing the requisite speed for conduction to the thalamus and midbrain. For the other cell types, distances are very short and passive electrical change (electrotonus) is sufficient for intercellular communication, whether by gap-junctional contact or transmitter release.

Photoreceptors

The photoreceptor neurons comprise **rods** and **cones**. Rods function only in dim light and are not sensitive to

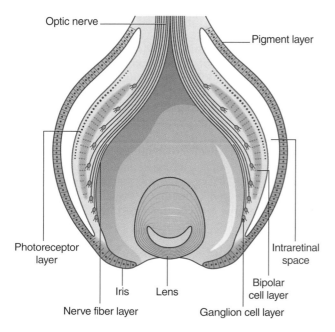

Figure 25.1 Embryonic retina. *Green* and *red* represent rods and cones, respectively.

Optic nerve

Pigment layer

Photoreceptor layer

Intraretinal space

Iris Lens

Bipolar cell layer

Nerve fiber layer

Ganglion cell layer

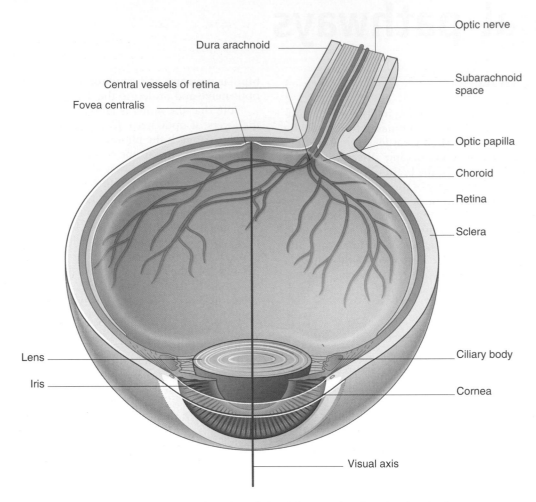

Figure 25.2 Horizontal section of the right eye, showing the visual axis.

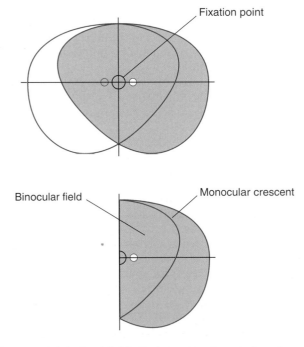

Figure 25.3 (A) Visual fields. Both eyes are targeted on the fixation point. The visual field of the right eye is shaded. **(B)** The right visual field. The white spot (arrow) represents the blind spot of the right eye.

color. They are scarce in the outer part of the fovea and absent from its center. Cones respond to bright light, are sensitive to color (received in the form of electromagnetic wavelength energy) and to shape, and are most numerous in the fovea.

Each photoreceptor has an outer and an inner segment and a synaptic end-foot. In the outer segment, the plasma membrane is folded to form hundreds of membranous discs which incorporate visual pigment (rhodopsin) formed in the inner segment. The synaptic end-foot makes contact with bipolar neurons and horizontal cell processes in the outer plexiform layer.

A surprising feature of the photoreceptors is that they are hyperpolarized by light. During darkness Na$^+$ channels are opened, creating sufficient positive electrotonus to cause leakage of transmitter (glutamate) from the end-feet. Illumination causes the Na$^+$ channels to close.

Cone and rod bipolar neurons

Cone bipolar neurons

Cone bipolar neurons are of two types. ON bipolars are switched on (depolarized) by light, being inhibited by transmitter released in the dark. They converge onto ON ganglion cells. OFF bipolars have the reverse response and converge onto OFF ganglion cells (*Figure 25.5*).

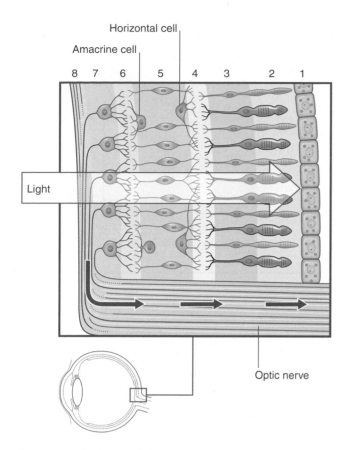

Figure 25.4 The layers of the retina. (1) Pigment layer; (2) photoreceptor layer; (3) outer nuclear layer; (4) outer plexiform layer; (5) inner nuclear layer; (6) inner plexiform layer; (7) ganglion cell layer; (8) nerve fiber layer.

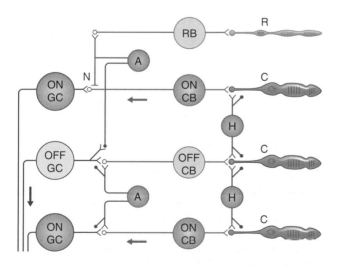

Figure 25.5 Retinal circuit diagram. (Adapted from Massey and Redburn (1987).) A, amacrine cell; C, cone; CB, cone bipolar neuron; GC, ganglion cell; H, horizontal cell; N, nexus (gap junction); R, rod; RB, rod bipolar.

Rod bipolar neurons

Rod bipolar neurons are all hyperpolarized by light. They activate ON and OFF ganglion cells indirectly, by way of amacrine cells (*Figure 25.5*).

Horizontal cells

The dendrites of horizontal cells are in contact with photoreceptors. The peripheral dendritic branches give rise to axon-like processes which make inhibitory contacts with bipolar neurons.

The function of horizontal cells is to inhibit bipolar neurons outside the immediate zone of excitation. The excited bipolars and ganglion cells are said to be on-line; the inhibited ones are off-line.

Amacrine cells

Amacrine cells have no axons. Their appearance is octopus-like, the dendrites all emerging from one side of the cell. Dendritic branches come into contact with bipolar neurons and ganglion cells.

More than a dozen different morphological types of amacrine cells have been identified, as well as several different transmitters including acetylcholine, dopamine, and serotonin. Possible functions include contrast enhancement and movement detection. For the rods, they convert large numbers of rods from OFF to ON with respect to ganglion cells.

Ganglion cells

The ganglion cells receive synaptic contacts from bipolar neurons in the inner plexiform layer. The typical response of ganglion cells to bipolar activity is 'center-surround'. An ON ganglion cell is excited by a spot of light, and inhibited by a surrounding annulus (ring) of light. The inhibition is caused by horizontal cells. OFF ganglion cells give the reverse response.

Coding for color

There are three types of cone with respect to spectral sensitivity. One is sensitive to red, one to green, and one to blue. Groups of each type are connected to ON or OFF ganglion cells.

The characteristic response of ganglion cells is one of *color opponency*:

- Ganglion cells that are on-line for green are off-line for red.
- Ganglion cells that are on-line for red are off-line for green.
- Ganglion cells that are on-line for blue are off-line for yellow, i.e. for green and red cones acting together.

Coding for black and white

White light is a mixture of green, red, and blue. In bright conditions, it is encoded by the three corresponding cones, all of them converging onto common ganglion cells. Both ON and OFF ganglion cells are involved in black-and-white vision, just as in color vision.

In very dim conditions, e.g. starlight, only rod photoreceptors are active, and objects appear in varying shades of gray. The rods are subject to the same rules as cones, showing center-surround antagonism between white and black, and being connected to ON or OFF ganglion cells.

Most rod and cone ganglion cells are small (parvocellular or 'P') having small receptive fields and being responsive to color and shape. A minority are large (magnocellular or

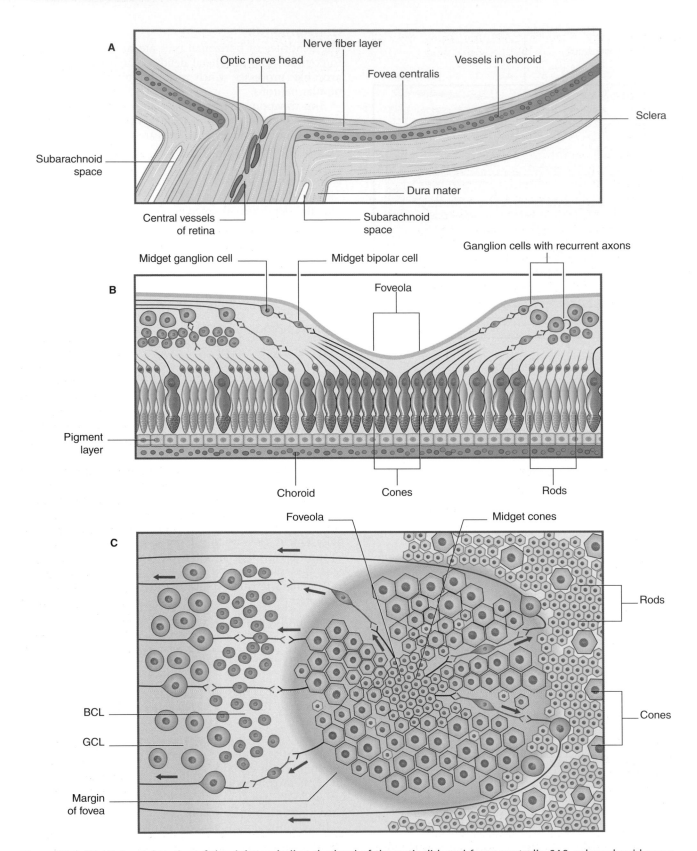

Figure 25.6 (A) Horizontal section of the right eyeball at the level of the optic disk and fovea centralis. SAS, subarachnoid space. **(B)** Enlargement from (A). Recurrent axons sweep around the fovea as shown in C. **(C)** Surface view of fovea centralis and neighbouring retina. Cones have been omitted at intervals to show the 'chain' sequence of neurons. BCL, bipolar cell layer; GCL, ganglionic cell layer.

'M') having large receptive fields and being especially responsive to movements within the visual field.

Foveal specialization

The relative density of cones increases progressively, and their size diminishes progressively, from the edge of the fovea inwards (*Figure 25.6*). The central one-third of the fovea, little more than 100 μm wide and known as the **foveola**, contains only *midget* cones. Two special anatomical features assist the foveal cones in general, and the midget cones in particular, in transducing the maximum amount of information concerning the form and color values of an object under direct scrutiny. First, the more superficial layers of the retina lean outward from the center, and their neurites are exceptionally long, with the result that the outer two-thirds of the foveola are little overlapped by bipolar cell bodies and the inner third is not overlapped at all; light reflected from the object strikes the cones of the foveola without any diffraction. Second, fidelity of central transmission is enhanced by one-to-one synaptic contact between the midget cones and *midget* bipolar neurons, and between these and *midget* ganglion cells. Outside the foveola, the amount of cone-to-bipolar-to-ganglion cell convergence increases progressively.

CENTRAL VISUAL PATHWAYS

Optic nerve, optic tract

The optic nerve is formed by the axons of the retinal ganglion cells. The axons acquire myelin sheaths as they leave the optic disc.

The number of ganglion cells varies remarkably between individuals, from 800 000 to 1.5 million. Since every ganglion cell contributes to the optic nerve, the number of axons in the optic nerve is correspondingly variable.

The retinal ganglion cells are homologous with the sensory projection neurons of the spinal cord. The optic nerve is homologous with spinal cord white matter, and is *not* a peripheral nerve. As explained in Chapter 7, true peripheral nerves, whether cranial or spinal, contain Schwann cells and collagenous sheaths, and are capable of regeneration. The optic nerve contains neuroglial cells of central type (astrocytes and oligodendrocytes) and is not capable of regeneration in mammals. In addition, the nerve is invested with meninges containing an extension of the subarachnoid space – a feature largely responsible for the changed appearance of the fundus oculi when the intracranial pressure is raised (*papilledema*, Ch. 4).

At the optic chiasm, fibers from the nasal hemiretina (medial half-retina) enter the contralateral optic tract whereas those from the temporal (lateral) hemiretina remain uncrossed and enter the ipsilateral tract.

As already noted in Chapter 21, some optic nerve fibers enter the suprachiasmatic nucleus of the hypothalamus. This connection has been invoked to account for the beneficial effect of bright artificial light, for several hours per day, in the treatment of wintertime depression.

Each optic tract winds around the midbrain and divides into a medial and a lateral root.

Medial root of optic tract

The medial root contains 10% of the optic nerve fibers. It enters the side of the midbrain. It contains four distinct sets of fibers:

1 Some fibers, mainly from retinal M cells, enter the superior colliculus and provide for automatic scanning, e.g. reading this page.
2 Some fibers are relayed from the superior colliculus to the pulvinar of the thalamus; they belong to the extrageniculate visual pathway to the visual association cortex (Ch. 26).
3 Some fibers enter the pretectal nucleus and serve the pupillary light reflex (Ch. 20).
4 Some fibers enter the parvocellular reticular formation, where they have an arousal function (Ch. 21).

Lateral root of the optic tract and lateral geniculate body

The lateral root of the optic tract terminates in the lateral geniculate body (LGB) of the thalamus. The LGB shows six cellular laminae, three of which are devoted to crossed fibers and three to uncrossed fibers. The two deepest laminae (one for crossed and one for uncrossed fibers) are magnocellular and receive axons from retinal 'M' ganglion cells concerned with detection of *movement*. The other four are parvocellular and receive the axons of 'P' cells concerned with *particulars*, namely visual detail and color.

The circuitry of the LGB resembles that of other thalamic relay nuclei, and includes inhibitory (GABA) terminals derived from internuncial neurons and from the thalamic reticular nucleus. (The portion of the reticular nucleus serving the LGB is called the **perigeniculate nucleus**.) Corticogeniculate axons arise in the primary visual cortex and synapse upon distal dendrites of relay cells as well as upon inhibitory internuncials. Cortical synapses on relay cells are twice as numerous as those derived from retinal ganglion cells. Cortical stimulation usually enhances the response of relay cells to a given retinal input. A likely, but unproven, function could be that of selective enhancement of particular features of the visual scene, e.g. when searching for an object of known shape or color.

Geniculocalcarine tract and primary visual cortex

The **geniculocalcarine tract**, or **optic radiation**, is of major clinical importance because it is frequently compromised by vascular disorders or tumors in the posterior part of the cerebral hemisphere. It travels from the lateral geniculate body to the primary visual cortex.

The anatomy of the optic radiation is shown in *Figures 25.7–25.10*. Fibers destined for the lower half of the primary visual cortex sweep forward into the temporal lobe, as *Meyer's loop*, before turning back to accompany those traveling to the upper half. The tract enters the retrolentiform part of the internal capsule and continues in the white matter underlying the lateral temporal cortex. It runs alongside the posterior horn of the lateral ventricle before turning medially to enter the occipital cortex.

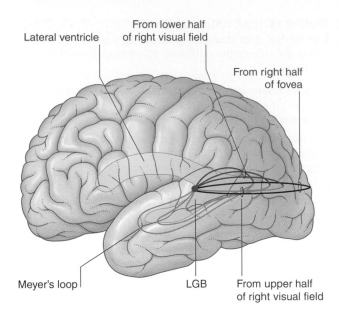

Figure 25.7 Left optic radiation. LGB, Lateral geniculate body.

The **primary visual cortex** occupies the walls of the calcarine sulcus along its entire length (the sulcus is 10 mm deep). It emerges onto the medial surface of the hemisphere for 5 mm both above and below the sulcus, and onto the occipital pole of the brain for 10 mm. Its total area is about 25 cm². In the freshly cut brain, it is easily identified by a thin band of white matter (the *visual stria* of Gennari) within the gray matter – hence an alternative term, *striate* cortex. The left and right eyes are represented in the cortex in alternating stripes called *ocular dominance columns* (*Figure 25.9*).

Retinotopic map

The contralateral visual field is represented upside down. The plane of the calcarine sulcus represents the horizontal meridian. Retinal representation is posteroanterior, with a greatly magnified foveal representation in the posterior half of the calcarine cortex (*Figure 25.10*).

The clinical effects of various lesions of the visual pathway are described in *Clinical Panel 25.1*.

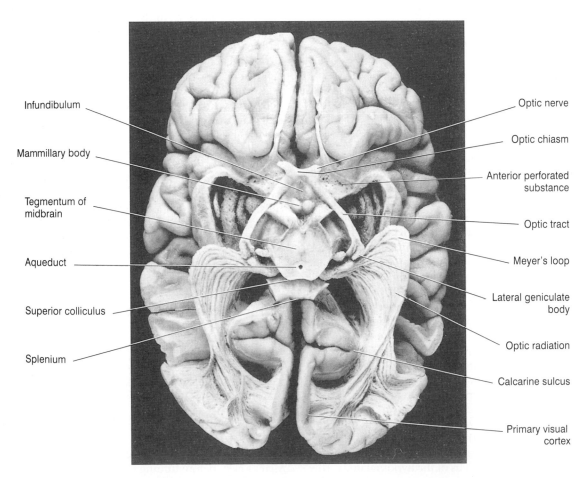

Figure 25.8 A dissection of the visual pathways, viewed from below. (Photograph reproduced from Gluhbegovic, N. and Williams, T. W. (1980) *The Human Brain*, by kind permission of the authors and of J.B. Lippincott, Inc.)

Clinical Panel 25.1   Lesions of the visual pathways

The following points arise in testing the visual pathways:

- The patient may be unaware of quite extensive blindness – sometimes even of a hemianopia.

- Large visual defects can often be detected by simple confrontation, as follows. The patient covers one eye at a time, and focuses on the examiner's nose. The examiner, seated opposite, looks the patient in the eye while bringing one or other hand into view from various directions, with the index finger wiggling.

- In a blind area, the patient does not see blackness; the patient does not see anything.

- Visual defects are described from the patient's viewpoint, in terms of the visual fields.

- Possible sites of injury to the visual pathways are shown in *Figure CP 25.1.1*. The effects produced correspond to the numbers in the following list.

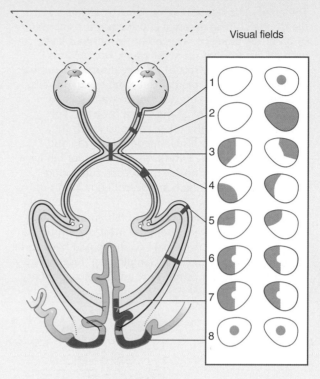

Visual fields

Figure CP 25.1.1 Visual field defects following various lesions of the visual pathways.

	Lesions	Field defects
1	Partial optic nerve	Ipsilateral scotoma[a]
2	Complete optic nerve	Blindness in that eye
3	Optic chiasm	Bitemporal hemianopia
4	Optic tract	Homonymous[b] hemianopia
5	Meyer's loop	Homonymous upper quadrant anopia
6	Optic radiation	Homonymous hemianopia
7	Visual cortex	Homonymous hemianopia
8	Bilateral macular cortex	Bilateral central scotomas

[a] A scotoma is a patch of blindness.
[b] Matching.

Notes on the numbered lesions

1 Eccentric lesions of the optic nerve produce scotomas in the nasal or temporal field of the affected eye. *When a young adult presents with a scotoma, multiple sclerosis must always be suspected.*

2 Total conduction blockage may follow head injury.

3 Compression of the middle of the chiasm is most often caused by an adenoma (benign tumor) of the pituitary gland.

4 Lesions of the optic tract are rare. Although homonymous (matching) visual fields are affected, the outer, exposed half of the tract tends to be more affected than the inner half, and the hemianopia is then described as incongruous.

5 Meyer's loop may be selectively caught by a tumor in the temporal lobe.

6 Lesions involving the optic radiation include tumors arising in the temporal, parietal, or occipital lobe. The visual fields of both eyes tend to be affected to an equal extent (*congruously*). Tumors impinging on the radiation from below produce an upper quadrantic defect at first whereas tumors impinging from above produce a lower quadrantic defect. The stem of the radiation occupies the retrolentiform part of the internal capsule and is often compromised for some days by edema, following hemorrhage from a branch of the middle cerebral artery (classic stroke, Ch. 30).

7 Thrombosis of the posterior cerebral artery produces a homonymous hemianopia. The notches in field chart no. 7 represent macular sparing. Sparing of the macular hemifields is inconstant.

8 Bilateral central scotomas are most often caused by a backward fall with occipital contusion.

Core Information

The embryonic retina is an outgrowth of the diencephalon. The embryonal optic cup is composed of an outer, pigment layer, an inner, nervous layer, with an intraretinal space between. The nervous layer contains three sets of radially disposed neurons, viz. photoreceptors, bipolar cells, and ganglion cells, and two tangential sets, viz. horizontal cells and amacrine cells. Except at the fovea centralis, light must pass through the other layers to reach the photoreceptors. The visual image is inverted and reversed by the lens. Two-thirds of the visual field are binocular, the outer one-sixth on each side being monocular. Visual defects are described in terms of visual fields.

Rod photoreceptors function in dim light and are absent from the fovea. Cones are most numerous in the fovea; they are responsive to shape and have three kinds of sensitivity to color. Ganglion cell responses are concentric, showing center-surround color opponency.

M ganglion cells are relatively large, are movement detectors, and project their axons to the two magnocellular layers of the lateral geniculate body (LGB). P ganglion cells signal particular features of the image as well as color and project to the four parvocellular layers of LGB. LGB is binocular, receiving signals from the contralateral nasal hemiretina (via the optic chiasm) and from the ipsilateral temporal hemiretina. Both sets of axons arrive by the optic tract, which also gives offsets to the midbrain for lower level visual reflexes.

The geniculocalcarine tract (optic radiation) arises from M and P cells of the LGB and swings around the side of the lateral ventricle to reach the primary visual cortex, in the walls of the calcarine sulcus.

Distinctive visual field defects occur following damage at any of the five major components of the visual pathway (optic nerve, optic chiasm, optic tract, optic radiation, visual cortex).

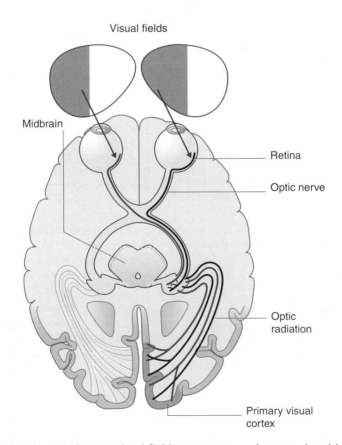

Visual fields

Midbrain

Retina

Optic nerve

Optic radiation

Primary visual cortex

Figure 25.9 Diagram of the visual pathways. The two visual fields are represented separately, without the normal overlap.

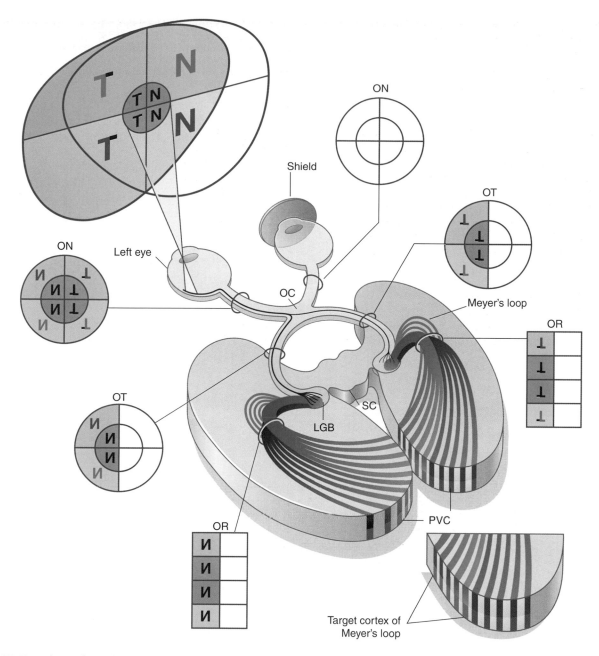

Figure 25.10 Pathway from the visual field of the left eye to the primary visual cortex. T denotes the temporal (outer) half of the left visual field; N denotes the nasal (inner) half of the left visual field.

In the left retina and optic nerve (ON), the neural representation of the image is reversed side to side. It is also inverted top to bottom. The right retina and optic nerve are inactive because this eye is shielded.

At the optic chiasm (OC) the axons forming the nasal half of the left optic nerve cross the midline and form the medial half of the right optic tract (OT). Those forming the lateral half of the nerve form the lateral half of the left optic tract. Each set synapses in the corresponding lateral geniculate body (LGB).

The optic radiations (OR) are fan-like (cf. Figure 25.7) with the axons carrying the foveal input initially in the middle of the fan.

As they approach the occipital pole, the foveal axons (red) in both hemispheres move to the back and enter the posterior part of the primary visual cortex (PVC). Note the striped pattern of delivery to the cortex on both sides. The blank intervals between are the same width and contain the axons and cortex responsible for the visual field of the *right* eye.

SC, superior colliculus.

REFERENCES

Bynke, H. (1984) The visual fields. In *Neuro-ophthalmology, vol. 3* (Lessell, S. and van Dalen, J.T.W., eds), pp. 348–357. Amsterdam: Elsevier.

Celesia, G.G. and DeMarco, P.J. (1994) Anatomy and physiology of the visual system. *J. Clin. Neurophysiol.* **11**: 482–492.

Curcio, C.A. and Kimberly, A.A. (1990) Topography of ganglion cells in human retina. *J. Comp. Neurol.* **300**: 5–25.

Frisen, L. (1980) The neurology of visual acuity. *Brain* **103**: 639–670.

Karten, H.J., Keyser, K.T. and Brecha, N.C. (1990) Biochemical and morphological heterogeneity of retinal ganglion cells. In *Vision and the Brain* (Cohen, B. and Bodis-Wollner, I., eds), pp. 19–33. New York: Raven Press.

Koch, C. (1987) The action of the corticofugal pathway on thalamic nuclei: a hypothesis. *Neuroscience* **23**: 399–406.

Massey, S.C. and Redburn, D.A. (1987) Transmitter circuits in the vertebral retina. *Prog. Neurobiol.* **28**: 55–96.

Vaney, D.I. (1994) Patterns of neuronal coupling in the retina. *Prog. Retl Eye Res.* **13**: 301–355.

Wu, S.M. (1994) Synaptic transmission in the outer retina. *Ann. Rev. Physiol.* **56**: 141–168.

Cerebral cortex

STRUCTURE

The cerebral cortex, or *pallium* (*Gr.* 'shell'), varies in thickness from 2 to 4 mm, being thinnest in the primary sensory areas and thickest in the motor and association areas. More than half of the total cortical surface is hidden from view in the walls of the sulci. The cortex contains about 50 billion neurons; about 500 billion neuroglial cells; and a dense capillary bed.

Microscopy reveals the cortex to have both a laminar and a columnar structure. The general cytoarchitecture varies in detail from one region to another, permitting the cortex to be mapped into dozens of histologically different 'areas'. Although considerable progress has been achieved in relating these to specific functions, the 'areas' are merely nodal points having widespread connections with other parts of the brain.

Laminar organization

A laminar (layered) arrangement of neurons is apparent in sections taken from any part of the cortex. Phylogenetically old elements, including the *paleocortex* of the uncus (concerned with olfaction), and the *archicortex* of the hippocampus in the medial temporal lobe (concerned with memory) are made up of three cellular laminae, whereas six laminae are seen in the **neocortex** (*neopallium*) covering the remaining 90% of the brain.

Cellular laminae of the neocortex   (Figure 26.1)

I   The **molecular layer** contains the tips of the apical dendrites of pyramidal cells (see below), and the most distal branches of axons projecting to the cortex from the intralaminar nuclei of the thalamus.

II   The **outer granular layer** contains small pyramidal and stellate cells.

III   The **outer pyramidal layer** contains medium-sized pyramidal cells and stellate cells.

IV   The **inner granular layer** contains stellate cells receiving afferents from the thalamic relay nuclei. Stellate cells are especially numerous in the primary somatic sensory cortex, primary visual cortex, and primary auditory cortex. The term *granular cortex* is applied to these areas. In contrast, the primary motor cortex contains relatively few stellate cells in lamina IV and is called *agranular cortex*.

V   The **inner pyramidal layer** contains large pyramidal cells projecting to the corpus striatum, brainstem, and spinal cord.

VI   The **fusiform layer** contains modified pyramidal cells projecting to the thalamus.

Columnar organization   (Figure 26.1)

In the somatic sensory cortex, the neurons were discovered (in monkeys) to be arranged functionally in terms of *columns* 50–100 μm in diameter extending radially through all laminae. Within each column, all of the cells are modality-specific. For example, a given column may respond to movement of a particular joint but not to stimulation of the overlying skin. Subsequent research has shown that cell columns comprising several hundred neurons are the functional units or *modules* of the cortex. Some modules are activated by specific thalamocortical inputs, others by corticocortical inputs from the same hemisphere, others again by inputs from the opposite hemisphere. Aggregates of modules create a *cortical mosaic*.

Cell types

The three principal morphological cell types are pyramidal cells, spiny stellate cells, and smooth stellate cells (*Figure 26.2*).

- **Pyramidal cells** have cell bodies ranging in height from 20 to 30 μm in laminae II and III to more than twice that height in lamina V. Tallest of all, at 80–100 μm, are the *giant cells of Betz* in the motor cortex. The single *apical* dendrite of each pyramidal cell reaches out to lamina I. The several *basal* dendrite branches arising from the basal 'corners' of the cell extend radially within their respective laminae. The apical and basal dendrites branch freely and are studded with dendritic spines. The axons of all pyramidal cells give off recurrent branches, capable of exciting neighboring pyramidal cells, before leaving the gray matter. All pyramidal cells are excitatory, and use glutamate (or closely related aspartate) as transmitter.

- **Spiny stellate cells** have spiny dendrites and in general are excitatory. They receive most of the afferent input from the thalamus and from other areas of the cortex, and they form glutamatergic synapses upon pyramidal cells.

- **Smooth stellate cells** have non-spiny dendrites and are inhibitory. They receive recurrent collateral branches from pyramidal cells and they form GABA-ergic synapses upon other pyramidal cells. Inhibitory, GABA-secreting neurons make up about 25% of all neurons in the cerebral cortex. Some synapse upon the bases of dendritic spines of pyramidal cells, some synapse upon their somas, and some synapse upon their initial axonal segments (*Figure 26.3*). The most powerful of the three types is the *chandelier cell*, so named because of the candle-shaped clusters of axoaxonic boutons. As is the case in the cerebellar cortex (Ch. 22), the GABA neurons exert a focusing action in the cerebral cortex by silencing weakly active cell columns.

- **Bipolar cells** are found mainly in the outer laminae. Most contain one or more peptides, such as vasoactive intestinal polypeptide (VIP), cholecystokinin (CCK), or somatostatin. Peptides are also co-liberated with GABA from many smooth stellate cells.

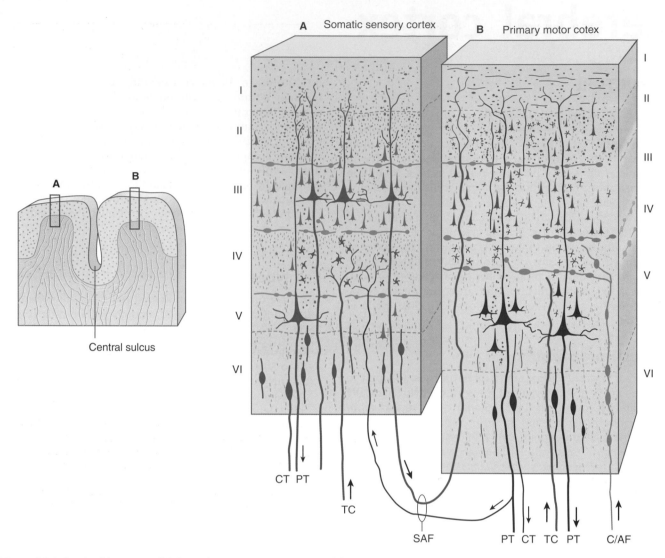

Figure 26.1 Cerebral isocortex. **(A)** Somatic sensory cortex. Cortical laminas I–VI are numbered on the left. Abbreviations, left to right: CT, corticothalamic fiber passing from fusiform neuron to ventral posterior nucleus of thalamus; PT, pyramidal tract fiber running from large pyramidal neuron to a sensory relay nucleus; TC, thalamocortical afferent from ventral posterior nucleus of thalamus; SAF, short association fiber passing to the motor cortex. **(B)** Primary motor cortex. Cortical laminas are numbered on the right. Abbreviations, left to right: SAF, short association fiber collateral passing to somatic sensory cortex; PT, pyramidal tract fiber running to motor nucleus in brain stem or spinal cord; CT, corticothalamic fiber passing to ventral lateral nucleus of thalamus; TC, thalamocortical afferent from ventral lateral nucleus of thalamus; PT as above; C/AF, cholinergic or aminergic fiber.

Human cortical neurons can be captured in fragments of biopsies taken for other purposes. They can be kept alive for several hours and examined for responses to transmitters and transmitter analogs. It appears that a single pyramidal cell may have as many as ten different kinds of receptor scattered over its surface. It also appears that the response of the neuron to a particular transmitter is not completely predictable being modified by concurrent effects of other transmitters.

Afferents

Afferents to a given region of the cortex are derived from five sources:

1 Long and short *association fibers* from small and medium-sized pyramidal cells occupying other parts of the ipsilateral cortex.

2 *Commissural fibers* from medium-sized pyramidal cells projecting through the corpus callosum from matching areas in the opposite hemisphere.

3 *Thalamocortical fibers* from the appropriate specific or association nucleus, e.g. from the ventral posterior thalamic nucleus to the somatic sensory cortex, from the dorsomedial thalamic nucleus to the *prefrontal* cortex (defined below).

4 *Non-specific thalamocortical fibers* from the intralaminar nuclei.

5 *Cholinergic and aminergic fibers* from basal forebrain, hypothalamus, and brainstem. These fibers are represented in *green* in *Figure 26.1*. The relevant nuclei of origin, and the transmitters/modulators involved, are as follows:

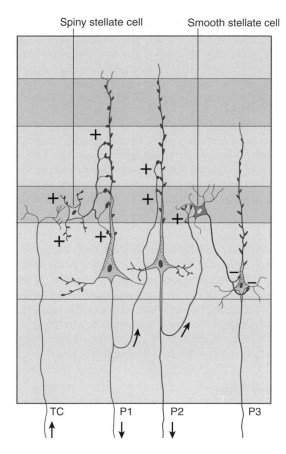

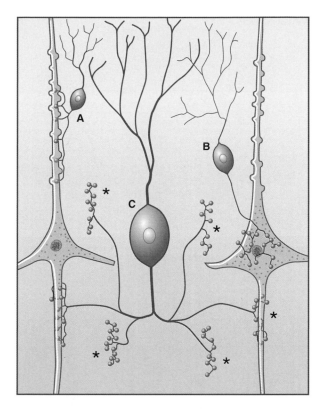

Figure 26.2 Input–output connections. Arrows indicate directions of impulse traffic. +/− Signs denote excitation/inhibition. TC, thalamocortical fiber. Pyramidal cell P1 is excited by the spiny stellate cell; it excites P2 within its own cell column; P3 within a neighboring column is inhibited by the smooth stellate cell.

Figure 26.3 Three morphological types of GABAergic inhibitory neuron. **A**, axodendritic cell, synapsing upon the shaft of the apical dendrite of a pyramidal cell. **B**, basket cell, forming axosomatic synapses on a pyramidal cell; **C**, chandelier cell, forming axoaxonic synapses (*) upon the initial segments of the two pyramidal cell axons shown, and upon four other initial segments not shown. (Based on DeFelipe, 1999.)

- basal forebrain nuclei   acetylcholine
- tuberoinfundibular (hypothalamus)   histamine
- tegmentum (midbrain)   dopamine
- raphe nucleus (midbrain)   serotonin
- cerulean nucleus (pons)   norepinephrine

These five sets of neurons are of particular relevance to psychiatry and are considered in Chapter 30.

Efferents

All efferents from the cerebral cortex are axons of pyramidal cells, and all are excitatory in nature.

Axons of some pyramidal cells contribute to short or long association fibers. Others form commissural or projection fibers.

- Examples of short association fiber projections are those entering the motor cortex from the sensory cortex and vice versa (*Figure 26.1*). Examples of long association fiber projections are the numerous backward projections from the *prefrontal cortex* – the cortex anterior to the motor areas (see below) to sensory association areas.
- The commissural fibers of the brain are *entirely* composed of pyramidal-cell axons running across in the corpus callosum and anterior commissure (and in other, minor commissures) to matching areas in the opposite hemisphere.
- Projection fibers from the primary sensory and motor cortex form the largest input to the basal ganglia (Ch. 28). The thalamus receives projection fibers from all parts of the cortex. Other major projection systems are corticopontine (to the ipsilateral nuclei pontis), corticonuclear (to contralateral motor and somatic sensory cranial nerve nuclei in pons and medulla), and corticospinal (to anterior horn motor neurons).

CORTICAL AREAS

The most widely used reference map is that of Brodmann, who divided the cortex into 47 areas on the basis of cyto-architectural differences. Most of these areas are shown in *Figure 26.4*. Colored in that figure are the three principal primary sensory areas (somatic, visual, auditory) and the single primary motor area, together with the respective *unimodal association areas*. The rest of the neocortex comprises *multimodal (polymodal) association areas* receiving association fibers from more than one unimodal association area (e.g. receiving tactile and visual inputs, or visual and auditory).

Medial surface

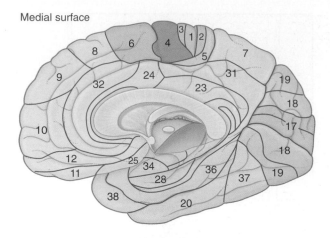

Lateral surface

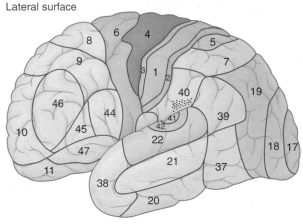

Figure 26.4 Cytoarchitectural areas of Brodmann.

Colored areas
Motor
4 primary motor cortex
6 on medial surface, supplementary motor area
6 on lateral surface, premotor cortex

Sensory
3/1/2 primary somatic sensory cortex, SI
40 secondary somatic sensory cortex, SII (stippled) on deep
surface above insula
17 primary visual cortex
18, 19 visual association cortex
41, 42 primary auditory cortex
22 auditory association cortex
(*Note:* The primary auditory cortex is not in fact visible from
the side, being entirely on the *upper* surface of the superior
temporal gyrus.)

Investigating functional anatomy

Two dominant methods are in use for localization of functions in the human brain. Both techniques depend upon the local increases in blood flow that meet the additional oxygen demand imposed by localized neural activity.

Positron emission tomography

Positron emission tomography (PET) measures oxygen consumption following injection of water labeled with oxygen-15 into a forearm vein. ^{15}O is a positron-emitting isotope of oxygen; the positrons react with nearby electrons in the

blood to create gamma-rays which are counted by gamma-ray detectors. Alternatively, fluorine-18-labeled deoxyglucose may be used to measure glucose consumption. ^{18}F-deoxyglucose is taken up by neurons as readily as glucose.

Image subtraction and *image averaging* are required for meaningful interpretation of PET studies, as explained in the caption to *Figure 26.5*.

For specialized investigations, radiolabeled drugs are used to quantify receptor function, e.g. radiolabeled dopamine in the corpus striatum in relation to Parkinson's disease (Ch. 28); radiolabeled serotonin in brainstem and cortex in relation to depression (Ch. 30), and radiolabeled acetylcholinesterase in relation to Alzheimer's disease (Ch. 30).

Functional magnetic resonance imaging

Functional magnetic resonance imaging (fMRI) does not require introduction of any extraneous material. It depends upon the different magnetic susceptibility of oxygenated versus deoxygenated blood. As it happens, the local increases in blood flow are more than sufficient to meet oxygen demands, and it is the relative excess of oxyhemoglobin that is exploited to generate the MR signal.

Sensory areas

Somatic sensory cortex (areas 3, 1, 2)

Components

The somatic sensory or *somesthetic cortex* occupies the entire postcentral gyrus (*Figure 26.6*). Representation of contralateral body parts is inverted except for the face, and the hand, lips, and tongue have disproportionately large representations. The original of the homunculus diagram shown in *Figure 26.6A* was intended to be only schematic and ignored the extensive overlap of body part representation.

In vertical sections, represented by *Figure 26.7*, the somesthetic cortex is divisible into areas 3, 2, and 1. Area 3 is divided into a smaller area 3a, in receipt of information relayed from muscle spindles, and a larger area 3b, receiving information relayed from cutaneous receptors. Area 3b is highly granular and is regarded as the true primary somatosensory cortex (S1).

Modules in area 1 have peripheral receptive fields confined to a single digit (*Figure 26.7D*). In monkeys, needle electrodes recording from area 1 reveal *feature extraction*, e.g. some modules are rapidly adapting, some are slowly adapting, some respond only to skin stroking in a specific direction, and some respond only to noxious stimulation of the skin. Modules in area 2 (*Figure 26.7E*) have multidigit receptive fields and receive from muscles and joint capsules in addition to skin.

Afferents

In addition to thalamic afferents from the ventral posterior nucleus (*Figure 26.7B*), the somesthetic cortex receives commissural fibers from the opposite somatic sensory cortex through the corpus callosum, and short association fibers from the adjacent primary motor cortex. Many of the fibers from the motor cortex are collaterals of corticospinal fibers traveling to the anterior horn of the spinal cord, and

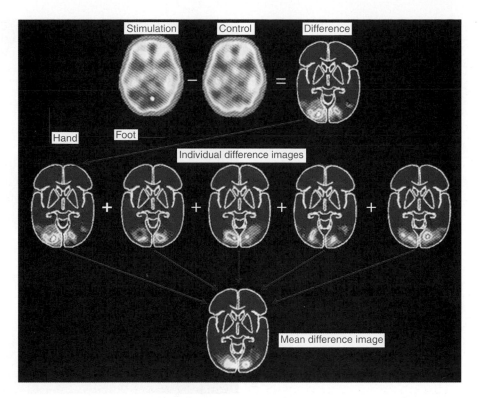

Figure 26.5 Image subtraction and image averaging in PET scans.
Top: The middle image is from a control mode, where the subject lies at rest. Uptake of ^{15}O is active throughout the cortex and subcortical gray matter. The left image is from the same subject staring at dots moving on a screen. The high level of background activity obscures the effect. The right image is produced by subtracting the control value to reveal the additional activity in the visual cortex produced by the staring task.
Middle: Four other subjects have performed the same task. Subtraction of background 'noise' reveals varying differences among the five. Because brains vary in size between individuals, activities in all five brains have been projected onto a common, 'average' brain (hence the identical brain profiles in this row).
Bottom: A mean value for the five brains produces a 'mean difference image' representative of the five as a group.
(Adapted from Posner and Raichle, *Images of Mind*, Sci. Amer. Library, 1994, p. 65, with permission.)

they may contribute to the *sense of weight* when an object is lifted.

It is not unusual for the somesthetic cortex to be compromised by bleeding from a striate branch of the middle cerebral artery supplying the sensory thalamocortical projection, within the upper part of the internal capsule. *Cortical-type sensory loss* in such cases is shown by a reduction in sensory acuity on the opposite side of the body, especially in forearm and hand, evidenced by a raised sensory threshold, poor two-point discrimination, and impaired vibration sense and position sense. The term *stereoanesthesia* is sometimes used with reference to inability to identify an unseen object held in the hand, as a consequence of cortical-type sensory loss.

Efferents

Efferents from the somesthetic cortex comprise association, commissural, and projection fibers. *Association fibers* pass to the ipsilateral motor cortex, to area 5 and to area 40 (the supramarginal gyrus). *Commissural fibers* pass to the contralateral somesthetic cortex. *Projection fibers* descend within the posterior part of the pyramidal tract and terminate upon internuncial neurons in sensory relay nuclei, namely the

ventral posterior nucleus of the thalamus of the same side, and the posterior column and spinal posterior gray horn of the opposite side. As explained in Chapter 13, sensory transmission in the spinothalamic pathway may be suppressed (via inhibitory internuncials, during vigorous activities such as running, whereas in the posterior column–medial lemniscal pathway, transmission may be enhanced (via excitatory internuncials) during exploratory activities such as palpation of textured surfaces.

Somatic sensory association area

This term is sometimes used with respect to area 5, directly behind the somatic sensory cortex. Most area 5 modules are active during reaching movements of the contralateral arm taking place under visual guidance (see under *dorsal visual pathway*, later).

Inferior parietal cortex (area 40)

Clinically, the term *inferior parietal cortex* is commonly used to designate the *supramarginal gyrus* (area 40), although the angular gyrus (area 39) also occupies the inferior parietal *lobule*. Area 40 integrates (brings together) impulse streams

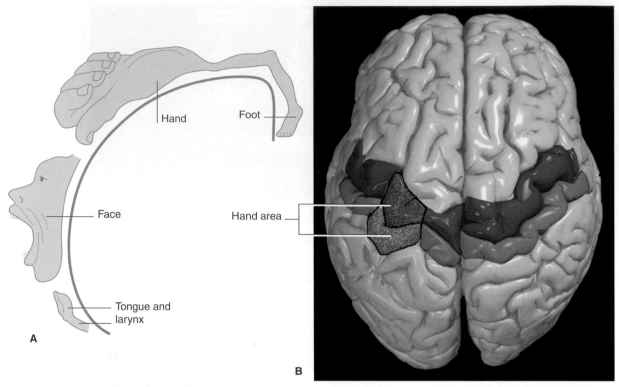

A

Hand

Foot

Face

Hand area

Tongue and larynx

B

Figure 26.6 The primary motor cortex (red) and primary somatosensory cortex (blue) viewed from above. The relatively larger representation of the motor and sensory areas in the left hemisphere is typical of right-handed individuals. On the right hemisphere is shown the extensive overlap of the (left) face and tongue representations. Three-dimensional computerized reconstruction of postmortem brain showing locations of somesthetic cortex (*blue*) and motor cortex (*red*). (Adapted from Kretschmann, H-J. and Weinrich, W. (1998) *Neurofunctional Systems: 3D Reconstructions with Correlated Neuroimaging: Text and CD-ROM*. New York: Thieme.)

The figurine on the left (adapted from Penfield and Rasmussen, 1960) depicts the inverted disposition of the motor homunculus in the left precentral gyrus excepting the face. Overlap among the various body parts is not represented in the figurine.

relayed by tactile, muscular, articular, and kinesthetic afferents in areas 3, 1, and 2, enabling identification of objects by manipulation (manual palpation) alone. This ability is known as *stereognosis*, and it permits (say) a pocketed key to be identified manually (*Figure 26.7*).

Lesions that involve the supramarginal gyrus may be accompanied by *astereognosis*, which is defined as an inability to identify an unseen object held in the hand *despite the presence of normal sensory acuity*.

As will be noted in Chapter 27, area 40 in the right hemisphere is concerned with *physical* (categorical) identification of unseen objects, and in the left hemisphere with *functional* identification. This distinction cannot be made in healthy volunteers because of the normal exchange of information between the two sides through the corpus callosum.

Secondary somatic sensory area

On the medial surface of the parietal operculum of the insula is a small *secondary somatic sensory area* (SII). It receives a nociceptive projection from the thalamus and it is highlighted during PET scans of the brain during peripheral painful stimulation (Ch. 29). SII also appears to collaborate with SI in aspects of tactile discrimination.

Plasticity of the somatic sensory cortex

In monkeys, cortical sensory representations of the individual digits of the hand can be defined very exactly by recording the electrical response of cortical cell columns to tactile stimulation of each digit in turn. These digital maps can be altered by peripheral sensory experience, as the following experiments indicate:

- The median nerve supplies the ventral surface of the outer three digits of the hand whereas the radial nerve supplies their dorsal surfaces. If the median nerve is crushed, the representation of the dorsal surface on the digital map increases at the expense of the ventral representation. The increase begins within hours and progresses slowly over a period of weeks. With regeneration of the median nerve, the cortical map reverts to normal.

- If the middle digit is denervated, the corresponding cortical area is unresponsive for a few hours, then becomes progressively (over weeks) taken over by expansion of the representations of the second and fourth digits.

- If the pad skin of a digit is chronically stimulated, e.g. by having to press a rotating sanded disc in order to

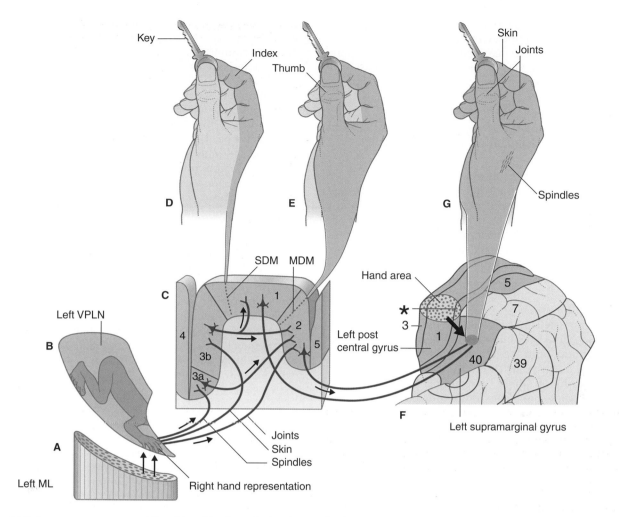

Figure 26.7 Sensory sequence enabling identification of a key by touch alone.

(A) Coded information from the *right* hand is traveling along second-order sensory (crossed) neurons in the medial part of the *left* posterior column–medial lemniscal pathway in the upper brainstem. ML, medial lemniscus.

(B) The hand area of the ventral posterior lateral nucleus (VPLN) of the thalamus contains somas of third-order sensory neurons.

(C) The third-order neurons project to areas 3, 1 (indirectly) and 2 of the somatic sensory cortex.

(D) SDM, single digit module.

(E) MDM, multidigit module.

(F) Surface view of the left parietal lobe.* Indicates the level of section **C** through the hand area. Area 40 receives short association fibers from areas 1, 2 and 5 and integrates information from skin, muscle spindles, and joint capsules.

(G) Connections with tactile memory stores here and in area 5 enable an image of the key to be perceived without the aid of vision.

release pellets of food, representation of the pad may increase to twice its original size over a period of weeks, reverting to normal after the experiment is discontinued.

These experiments show that somatic sensory maps are *plastic*, being modified by peripheral events. A purely anatomical explanation (e.g. sprouting of nerve branches within the CNS, or peripherally) is not appropriate for the earliest changes, which begin within hours. Instead, they can be accounted for on the basis of sensory competition.

Sensory competition

Sensory maps made at the level of the posterior gray horn, posterior column nuclei, thalamus, and somesthetic cortex all show evidence of anatomical overlap. For example, the thalamocortical somesthetic projection for the third digit

overlaps the projections for the second and fourth. Within the zone of overlap, cortical columns are shared by afferents from two adjacent digits. As already explained, smooth stellate cells exert lateral inhibition upon weakly stimulated columns. Under experimental conditions (in cats), the number of columns responding to a particular thalamocortical input can be increased by local infusion of a GABA antagonist drug (bicuculline), which suppresses lateral inhibition. The effect of removal of a peripheral sensory field may be comparable: if one set of thalamocortical neurons falls silent owing to loss of sensory input, it no longer exerts lateral inhibition and cortical columns within its territory are taken over by neighboring, active sets.

In the human somatosensory body map, the digits are represented next to the face. In several well-documented cases of upper limb amputation, patients had later experiences of 'phantom finger' sensations on touching their face on that side with an implement such as a comb held in the other hand. This illusion may occur within 2 weeks of amputation. It can be explained on the basis of the unmasking of pre-existing overlap of thalamocortical neurons.

Visual cortex (areas 17, 18, 19)

The visual cortex comprises the *primary visual cortex* (area 17) and the *visual association cortex* (areas 18 and 19).

Primary visual cortex   (Figure 26.4)

As noted in Chapter 25, the primary visual cortex is the target of the geniculocalcarine tract, which relays information from the ipsilateral halves of both retinas, and therefore from the contralateral visual field. This myelinated tract creates a pale **visual stria** within the primary visual cortex before synapsing upon spiny stellate cells of the highly granular lamina IV. The visual stria (first noted by medical student Francesco Gennari circa 1775) has provided the alternative name, *striate cortex*, for area 17.

The spiny stellate cells belong to *ocular dominance columns*, so named because alternating columns are dominated by inputs from the left and right eyes (Ch. 25). In a surface view of the visual cortex, the columnar arrangement takes the form of whorls, resembling finger prints. The geniculocalcarine projection is so ordered that matching points from the two retinas are registered side by side in contiguous columns. This arrangement is ideal for binocular vision because modules at the edge of a column respond to inputs from both eyes.

Under experimental conditions (monkeys), spiny stellate cells of the primary visual cortex give 'simple' responses to slits of light of a particular orientation. Some of the pyramidal cells give 'complex' responses to bars (broad slits) of a particular orientation; for many cells, the bar must be moving broadside in a specific direction. Other pyramidal cells are 'hypercomplex,' responding to L-shapes. This hierarchy of responses can be explained on the basis of convergence of several simple-cell axons onto complex cells and convergence of complex-cell axons on to hypercomplex cells.

Plasticity of the primary visual cortex

The basic pattern and balance of ocular dominance columns is preserved in animals reared in complete darkness. On the other hand, if one eye is sealed from birth the stripes in area 17 for that eye become abnormally narrow, and those for the open eye abnormally broad. The effect can be explained on the basis of *synaptic competition*. During a critical period (sixth postnatal week in monkeys), the right-eye left-eye projections from the lateral geniculate nucleus overlap extensively. As the cortex matures the redundant axonal arbors (multiple branches) are withdrawn and the column edges become sharply defined. If one eye is deprived of sensory experience from birth, the corresponding geniculocalcarine neurons branch less extensively and those from the 'experienced' eye do not withdraw.

Visual association cortex   (Figure 26.4)

The visual association cortex comprises areas 18 and 19, which are also conjointly called the *peristriate* or *extrastriate*

cortex. Afferents are received mainly from area 17 but they include some direct thalamic projections from the pulvinar. The cell columns are concerned with *feature extraction*. Some columns respond to geometrical shapes, some respond to color, and some are involved in stereopsis (depth perception).

Many of the peristriate columns have large receptive fields. Some of these straddle the physiological 'blind spot' (optic nerve head) and may be responsible for 'covering up' the blind spot during monocular vision.

The projection from the pulvinar to the visual association cortex is considered to be part of the pathway involved in 'blindsight'. This remarkable condition has been observed in patients following thrombosis of the calcarine branch of the posterior cerebral artery. Although blindness in the contralateral field appears complete, these patients are nonetheless able to point to a moving spot of light – without any perception of it, merely a 'feeling' that it is there. The likely pathway concerned is via the medial root of the optic tract, the superior colliculus, and the pulvinar.

The most functionally advanced modules occupy the lateral and medial parts of area 19. The lateral set of modules is colloquially described as belonging to a dorsal, 'where?' visual pathway. The medial set belongs to a ventrally placed, 'what?' pathway.

The 'where?' visual pathway   (Figure 26.8)

Consistent with electrical recordings taken from alert monkeys, PET scans of human volunteers reveal the lateral part of area 19 to be especially responsive to *movement* taking place in the contralateral visual hemifield. The main projection from this area is to area 7, known to clinicians as the *posterior parietal cortex*. In addition to movement perception, area 7 is involved in *stereopsis* (three-dimensional vision) and

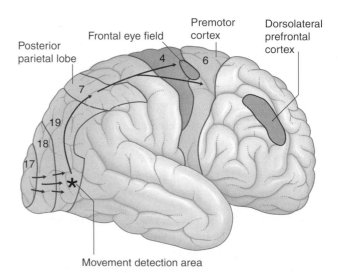

Figure 26.8 Lateral surface of right hemisphere, showing the 'where?' visual pathway from the visual cortex to the parietal and frontal lobes. The asterisk marks the area for detection of movement in the left visual field. Activity of the right frontal eye field facilitates a saccade toward the left visual field.

with *spatial sense*, defined as perception of the position of objects in relation to one another.

Area 7 receives 'blindsight' fibers from the pulvinar, and it projects via the superior longitudinal fasciculus to the ipsilateral frontal eye field and premotor cortex.

In monkeys, cell columns in area 7 are activated when a significant object (e.g. fruit) appears in the contralateral visual hemifield. Through association fibers, the active cell columns increase the resting firing rate of columns in the frontal eye field and premotor cortex, but without producing movement. The effect is called *covert attention*, or *covert orientation*. It becomes *overt* when the animal responds with a saccade with or without a reaching movement directed toward the object. Following a lesion to area 7, the motor responses to significant targets occur late, and reaching movements of the contralateral arm are inaccurate.

In human volunteers, PET scans show increased cortical metabolism in area 7 in response to object movement in the contralateral visual hemifield. During reaching of the opposite arm toward an object, areas 5 and 7 are both active. In humans (as in monkeys), a lesion that includes area 7 is associated with clumsy, inaccurate reaching into the contralateral visual hemifield.

In volunteers, two additional areas of cortex become active when items of special interest appear. Shown in *Figure 26.8*, and mentioned again later, is the *dorsolateral prefrontal cortex* (DLPFC), a significant decision-making area, notably in relation to an *approach* or *withdraw* decision. Shown in *Figure 26.9* is a patch in the cortex of the anterior cingulate gyrus. This area is considered in Chapter 29 but it may be mentioned here that it is activated by the dorsolateral cortex when subjects are *paying attention* to a visual task.

The 'what?' visual pathway (Figure 26.9)

The ventral visual pathway converges onto the anteromedial part of area 19, mainly within the fusiform gyrus (posterior part of the occipitotemporal gyrus). This region is concerned with three kinds of visual identification, indicated in *Figure 26.9B*:

a Relatively lateral are modules activated by the *forms* (shapes) of objects of all kinds, including the shapes of letters. It is regarded as a center for generic (categorical/canonical) object identification (e.g. a dog *as such*, without connotation).

b In the midregion are modules specifically devoted to the generic identification of human faces.

c Relatively medial is the *color recognition area*, essential for recognition of all colors except black and white. A state of *achromatopsia* may occur following a sustained fall in blood pressure within both posterior cerebral arteries, caused, e.g., by an embolus blocking the top of the parent basilar artery. Such patients see everything only in black-and-white (grayscale).

Recognition of individual objects and faces is a function of the anterior part of the 'what?' pathway in the *inferotemporal cortex* (area 20) and in the cortex of the temporal pole (area 38). These two areas are engaged during identification of, for example, *Mary's* face or *my* dog. Failure of facial recognition (*prosopagnosia*) is a frequent and distressing feature of Alzheimer's disease (Ch. 30), where the patient may cease to

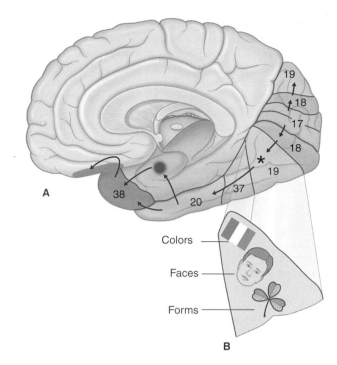

Figure 26.9 (A) Medial view of right hemisphere, showing the 'what?' pathway. The asterisk marks the visual identification area within the fusiform gyrus on the inferior surface. Ventral area 19 is enlarged in **(B)**.

recognize family members despite retaining the sense of familiarity (or otherwise) of common objects.

Threatening sights or faces cause areas 20 and 38 to activate the *amygdala*, especially in the right (emotional) hemisphere; the right amygdala in turn activates the fear-associated *right orbitofrontal cortex* (see Ch. 27).

How are visual association areas activated, e.g. in execution of a decision to look for an apple in a bowl of mixed fruit, or for a particular word in a page of text? In PET studies, the frontal lobe is active whenever attention is being paid to a task at hand. The DLPFC is particularly active during visual tasks involving form and color. During visual searching, the role of the frontal lobe seems to be to activate memory stores within the visual association areas, so that the relevant memories are held on-line during the search. The anterior part of the cingulate cortex is also active.

The V1–V5 nomenclature

Specialists in vision research use the following designations in relation to cortical visual processing:

V1 equates with Brodmann area 17.

V2 and V3 equate with Brodmann areas 18 and 19, respectively.

V4 includes the three sets of identification modules in the fusiform gyrus (anteromedial Brodmann area 19).

V5 equates with the movement detection modules in the lateral occipital cortex (anterolateral Brodmann area 19).

Auditory cortex (areas 41, 42, 22)

The *primary auditory cortex* occupies the anterior transverse temporal gyrus of Heschl, described in Chapter 17. Heschl's gyrus corresponds to areas 41 and 42 on the upper surface of the superior temporal gyrus. Columnar organization in the primary auditory cortex takes the form of *isofrequency stripes*, each stripe responding to a particular tonal frequency. Higher frequencies activate lateral stripes in Heschl's gyrus, lower frequencies activate medial stripes. Because of incomplete crossover of the central auditory pathway in the brainstem (Ch. 17), *each ear is represented bilaterally*. In experimental recordings, the primary cortex responds equally well from both ears in response to monaural stimulation but the contralateral cortex is more responsive during simultaneous binaural stimulation.

The auditory association cortex corresponds to area 22, for speech perception (considered in Ch. 27). Visual and auditory data are brought together in the polymodal cortex bordering the superior temporal sulcus (junction of areas 21 and 22).

Excision of the entire auditory cortex (in the course of removal of a tumor) has no obvious effect on auditory perception. The only significant defect is loss of *stereoacusis*: on testing, the patient has difficulty in appreciating the direction and the distance of a source of sound.

MOTOR AREAS

Primary motor cortex

The primary motor cortex (area 4) is a strip of agranular cortex within the precentral gyrus. It gives rise to 60–80% (estimates vary) of the pyramidal tract (PT). The remaining PT fibers originate in the premotor and supplementary motor areas and in the parietal cortex, as illustrated in Chapter 13.

There is an inverted somatotopic representation of contralateral body parts except the face, with relatively large areas devoted to the hand, circumoral region, and tongue (*Figure 26.6*). The hand area can usually be identified as a backward projecting knob 6–7 cm from the upper margin of the hemisphere.

Ipsilateral body parts are also represented in the somatotopic map, ipsilateral motor neurons being supplied by the 10% of PT fibers that remain uncrossed.

A computerized graphic reconstruction of the motor cortex and corticospinal tracts from a postmortem brain is shown in *Figure 26.10*.

Direct stimulation of the human motor cortex indicates that the cell columns control *movement direction*. Individual PT fibers are known to branch extensively as they approach the anterior gray horn, and to terminate on motor-neuronal dendrites in nuclei serving several different muscles. The pattern of distribution of PT fibers is directed toward *movement synergy*, which in this context means the simultaneous contraction of all of the muscles concerned, with a bias among them suited to the task at hand. The act of picking up a pen, e.g., requires a moderate contraction of opponens pollicis as prime mover, a matching level of contraction of the portion of flexor digitorum profundus providing the tendon to the terminal phalanx of the index finger, and lesser levels of contraction of adductor and flexor brevis pollicis. Steadying the upper limb as a whole during any kind of manipulative activity is a function of the premotor cortex (see later).

Plasticity in the motor cortex

In monkeys and in lower mammals, small lesions of the motor cortex produce an initial paralysis of the corresponding body part, followed within a few days (sometimes within hours) by progressive recovery. The recovery is attributable to a change of allegiance of cell columns close to the lesion, which take on the missing motor function. Instead of inflicting a lesion, it is possible to enlarge the motor territory of a patch of cortex merely by injecting a GABA antagonist drug locally into the cortex. Expansion of motor territories at spinal cord level is already provided for by extensive overlap of projections from area 4 to the motor cell columns in the ventral gray horn.

Sources of afferents to the primary motor cortex

1 *The opposite motor cortex*, through the corpus callosum. The strongest commissural linkages are between matching cell columns that control the vertebral and abdominal musculature. This is to be expected since these muscle groups routinely act bilaterally in maintaining the upright position of the trunk and head. The weakest commissural linkages are between cell columns controlling the distal limb muscles, where the two sides tend to act independently.

2 *Somatosensory cortex.* Cutaneous cell columns in areas 1, 2, and 3 feed forward via short association fibers. Linkages for the hand are especially numerous; the distance is short because the hand areas of the motor and somatic sensory cortex mainly occupy the corresponding walls of the central sulcus. *Proprioceptive* cell columns in area 3a receive afferent relays from the annulospiral endings of muscle spindles; they send short association fibers to the corresponding motor columns for execution of the long-loop stretch reflex (Ch. 22).

3 *Contralateral dentate nucleus.* The cerebellum assists in the selection of appropriate muscles for synergic activities, and in the timing and strength of their contractions.

4 *Supplementary motor area.*

Premotor cortex

The premotor cortex (PMC, area 6 on the lateral surface of the hemisphere) is about six times larger than the primary motor cortex. It receives cognitive inputs from the frontal lobe in the context of motor intentions, and a rich sensory input from the parietal lobe (area 7) incorporating tactile and visuospatial signals. It is especially active when motor routines are run in response to visual or somatic sensory cues, e.g. reaching for an object in full view or identifying an object out of sight by manipulation. The PMC is usually active bilaterally if at all. One explanation is the need for interhemispheric transfer of motor plans through the corpus callosum. It is also the case that the PMC has a major projection to the brain stem nuclei that give origin to the reticulospinal tracts (and a minor one to the pyramidal tract). Lesions confined to the human PMC are rare, but they are characterized by postural instability of the contralateral shoulder and hip. A significant function of the PMC there-

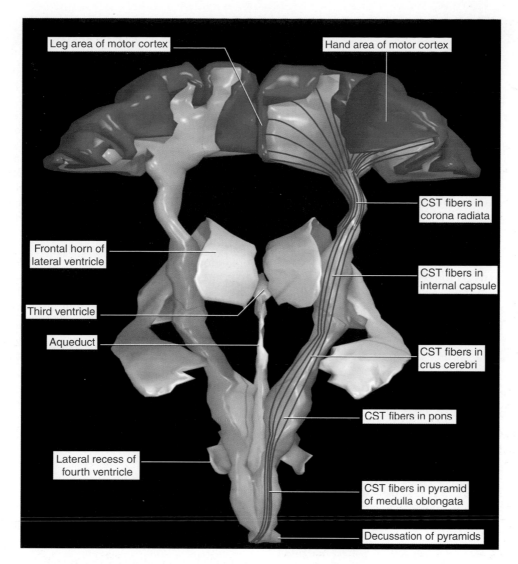

Leg area of motor cortex

Hand area of motor cortex

CST fibers in
corona radiata

Frontal horn of
lateral ventricle

CST fibers in
internal capsule

Third ventricle

Aqueduct

CST fibers in
crus cerebri

CST fibers in pons

Lateral recess of
fourth ventricle

CST fibers in pyramid
of medulla oblongata

Decussation of pyramids

Figure 26.10 Computerized graphic reconstruction of postmortem brain; anterior view showing the precentral gyri, and the relationships of the corticospinal tracts (CST) to the ventricular system. Some corticospinal fibers have been added to the original. (Reproduced from Kretschmann, H-J. and Weinrich, W. (1998) *Neurofunctional Systems: 3D Reconstructions with Correlated Neuroimaging: Text and CD-ROM*. New York: Thieme, with kind permission of the authors and publisher.)

fore seems to be that of bilateral postural fixation, e.g. to fixate the shoulders during bimanual tasks and to stabilize the hips during walking. The PMC may contribute to recovery of function in cases of pure motor hemiplegia (Ch. 30) following a vascular lesion confined to the corticospinal tract within the corona radiata. The PMC shows increased activity on PET scans following such a lesion; the corticoreticulospinal pathway descends anterior to the corticospinal tract.

Supplementary motor area

In contrast to the PMC's responsiveness to external cues, the supplementary motor area (SMA, area 6 on the medial surface of the hemisphere) responds to *internal cues*. In particular, it is involved in *motor planning*, as exemplified by the fact that SMA is activated by the frontal lobe (DLPFC) the moment we *intend* to make a movement, even if the movement is not performed. The principal function of SMA seems to be that of preprogramming movement sequences that

have already been built into motor memory. It functions in collaboration with a motor loop passing through the basal ganglia (Ch. 28) and projects to area 4 as well as contributing directly to the pyramidal tract. Unilateral lesions of SMA are associated with *akinesia* (inability to initiate movement) of the contralateral arm and leg. Bilateral lesions are accompanied by total akinesia, including akinesia for speech initiation.

Cortical eye fields

Figure 26.11 illustrates six *cortical eye fields* involved in scanning movements (saccades). Their connections and functions are summarized in *Table 26.1*.

Dorsolateral prefrontal cortex

This is a higher level cognitive center engaged in assessment of the visual scene, in decisions about making voluntary sac-

Core Information

The cerebral cortex has both a laminar and a columnar organization. The two basic cell types are pyramidal and stellate. Pyramidal cells occupy laminae II, III, V and (as fusiform cells) lamina VI. Lamina IV is rich in spiny stellate cells. Small pyramidal cells link the gyri within the hemisphere; medium-sized pyramidal cells link matching areas of the two hemispheres; the largest ones project to thalamus, brainstem, and spinal cord. Spiny stellate cells are excitatory to pyramidal cells, smooth ones are inhibitory. Columnar organization takes the form of cell columns 50–100 μm wide.

The somatic sensory cortex contains an inverted representation of body parts. Important inputs come from the ventral posterior nucleus of thalamus; important outputs go to the primary motor and inferior parietal cortex. The primary visual cortex receives the geniculocalcarine tract. Cellular responses of differing complexity depend upon convergence of simpler on to more complex cell types. The visual association areas are characterized by feature extraction, e.g. motion, color, shape. Form and color extraction continues into the cortex on the under side of the temporal lobe, motion into the posterior parietal lobe. The primary auditory cortex occupies the upper surface of the superior temporal gyrus and the auditory association cortex is lateral to it.

The primary motor cortex occupies the precentral gyrus. It gives rise to most of the pyramidal tract, the body parts being represented upside down. Its main inputs are from somatosensory cortex, cerebellum (via the ventral posterior nucleus of thalamus), and the premotor and supplementary motor areas. The premotor area operates mainly in response to external cues, the supplementary motor area in response to internally generated cues. Under control of the dorsolateral prefrontal cortex, four distinct cortical areas are involved, in different contexts, in producing contraversive saccades.

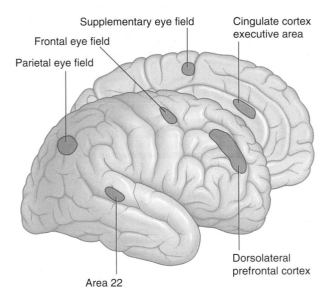

Figure 26.11 Areas of cerebral cortex involved in saccadic movements.

cades and in voluntary repression of reflexive saccades. (*Voluntary* saccades result from internally generated decisions. *Reflexive* saccades are automatic responses to objects appearing in the peripheral visual field. Strictly speaking, reflexive saccades should be called *responsive*; they are not true reflexes, being amenable to voluntary suppression.)

Cingulate cortex

Participates with DLPFC in decision-making, and in assessing the emotional significance, or *valence*, of visual targets.

Supplementary eye field

Occupies the anterior part of the supplementary motor area, and is engaged in motor planning, especially when multiple saccades are required.

Frontal eye field (FEF)

Initiates voluntary saccades in response to one or more of the three inputs listed. Both clinical and experimental (monkey) observations indicate that:

- The FEFs are tonically active, bilaterally.
- Increased activity in the midregion of the FEF on one side causes a horizontal saccade toward the contralateral visual hemispace (a *contraversive saccade*).
- Increased activity in the upper region on one side produces an obliquely downward contraversive saccade; bilateral upper region activation causes both eyes to look straight down.
- Increased lower region activity has corresponding effects with respect to upward gaze.

Parietal eye field (PEF)

Initiates reflexive saccades and prompts FEF to initiate voluntary saccades. PEF is also involved in spatial perception by generating a map of the visual scene.

Area 22

The lower part of the superior temporal cortex is polysensory, some modules responding to both visual and auditory inputs. Inputs from the periphery of the visual scene may initiate reflexive saccades via the superior colliculus.

For prefrontal cortex and frontal lobe dysfunction, see Chapter 27.

Table 26.1 Cortical eye fields

Eye fields	Afferents from	Efferents to	Functions
Dorsolateral prefrontal cortex (DLPFC)	Visual association areas	Ipsilateral FEF, SEF, SC* and CCx	Voluntary saccades
Cingulate cortex (CCx)	DLPFC, FEF, SEF	Ipsilateral FEF and SC	Assessment of emotional significance
Supplementary eye field (SEF)	DLPFC, PEF, area 22	Ipsilateral FEF and SC	Motor planning
Frontal eye field (FEF)	DLPFC, FEF, PEF	Contralateral PPRF**, ipsilateral CCx and SC	Voluntary saccades
Parietal eye field (PEF)	'Where' visual pathway, pulvinar and DLPFC	Ipsilateral FEF and SC	Reflexive saccades
Area 22	Auditory association cortex, PEF	Ipsilateral SC	Saccades to source of sound

*SC, superior colliculus; **PPRF, paramedian pontine reticular formation.
Note: The left PPRF pulls the eyes to the left. The right SC also pulls the eyes to the left, because of a crossed projection from it to the left PPRF.

REFERENCES

Ashe, J. and Ugurbil, K. (1994) Functional imaging of the motor system. *Curr. Opin. Neurobiol.* **4**: 832–839.

Celesia, C.G. (1994) Anatomy and physiology of the visual system. *J. Clin. Neurophysiol.* **11**: 482–492.

Damasio, A.R. (1998) The somatic marker hypothesis and the possible functions of the prefrontal cortex. In *The Prefrontal Cortex: Executive and Cognitive Functions* (Roberts, A.C., Robbins, T.W. and Weiskrantz, L., eds), pp. 36–50. Oxford: Oxford University Press.

DeFelipe, J. (1999) Chandelier cells and epilepsy. *Brain* **122**: 1807–1822.

Desomone, R. and Duncan, J. (1995) Neural mechanisms of selective attention. *Ann. Rev. Neurosci.* **18**: 193–222.

Donoghue, J.P. and Saines, J.N. (1994) Motor areas of the cerebral cortex. *J. Clin. Neurophysiol.* **11**: 382–396.

Edeline, J.-M. (1999) Learning-induced physiological plasticity in the thalamocortical sensory systems. *Progr. Neurobiol.* **57**: 165–224.

Elliott, Lois L. (1994) Functional brain imaging and hearing. *J. Acoust. Soc. Am.* **96**: 1397–1408.

Frith, C.D. and Dolan, R.J. (1997) Higher cognitive processes. In *Human Brain Function* (Frackowiak, R.S.J., Friston, K.J., Frith, C.D. and Dolan, R.J., eds), pp. 329–366. London: Academic Press.

Goel, V., Gold, B., Kapur, S. and Houle, S. (1998) Neuroanatomical correlates of human reasoning. *J. Cog. Neurosci.* **10**: 293–302.

Halsband, U. and Freund, H-J. (1993) Motor learning. *Curr. Opin. Neurobiol.* **3**: 940–949.

Innocenti, G. (1994) Some new trends in the study of the corpus callosum. *Behav. Brain Res.* **64**: 1–8.

Kaas, J.H. (1991) Plasticity of sensory and motor maps in adult mammals. *Ann. Rev. Neurosci.* **14**: 137–167.

Kleinschmidt, A., Nitschke, M.F. and Frahm, J. (1997) Somatotopy in the human motor cortex hand area. *Eur. J. Neurosci.* **9**: 2178–2186.

Klintsova, A.Y. and Greenough, W.T. (1999) Synaptic plasticity in cortical systems. *Curr. Opin. Neurobiol.* **9**: 203–208.

Krimer, L.S., Muly, E.C., Williams, G.V. and Goldman-Rakic, P. (1998) Dopaminergic regulation of cerebral cortical microcirculation. *Nature Neurosci.* **1**: 286–289.

Mesulam, M-M. (1998) From sensation to cognition. *Brain* **121**: 1013–1052.

Mountcastle, V.B. (1997) The columnar organization of the cerebral cortex. *Brain* **120**: 701–722.

Passingham, R. (1977) Functional organization of the motor system. In *Human Brain Function* (Frackowiak, R.S.J., Friston, K.J., Frith, C.D. and Dolan, R.J., eds), pp. 367–404. London: Academic Press.

Paulesu, P. Frackowiak, R.S.J. and Bottini, G. (1997) Maps of somatosensory systems. In *Human Brain Function* (Frackowiak, R.S.J., Friston, K.J., Frith, C.D. and Dolan, R.J., eds), pp. 367–404. London: Academic Press.

Penfield, W. and Rasmussen, T. (1960) *The cerebral cortex of man.* New York: Hafner.

Posner, M.I. (1994) Attention: the mechanisms of consciousness. *Proc. Natl Acad. Sci. USA* **91**: 7398–7403.

Posner, M.I. and Raichle, M.E. (1994) Images of the brain. In *Images of the Mind* (edited by the authors), pp. 57–82. New York: Scientific American Library.

Salin, P-A. and Bullier, J. (1995) Corticocortical connections in the visual system: structure and function. *Physiol. Rev.* **75**: 107–154.

Schwartz, A.B. (1994) Distributed motor processing in cerebral cortex. *Current Opin. Neurobiol.* **4**: 840–846.

Somogyi, P., Tamas, G., Lujan, R. and Buhl, E.H. (1998) Salient features of synaptic organisation in the cerebral cortex. *Brain Res. Rev.* **26**: 111–135.

Tanji, J. (1994) The supplementary motor area in the cerebral cortex. *Neurosci. Res.* **19**: 251–268.

Ungerlieder, L.G. (1995) Functional brain imaging studies of cortical mechanisms for memory. *Science* **270**: 769–775.

Weinberger, N.M. (1995) Dynamic regulation of receptive fields and maps in the adult sensory cortex. *Ann. Rev. Neurosci.* **18**: 129–158.

Yousry, T.A., Schmid, U.D., Alkadhi, H., Schmidt, T., Peraud, A., Buettner, A. and Winkler, P. (1997) Localization of the motor hand area to a knob on the precentral gyrus. *Brain* **120**: 141–157.

Zilles, K. (1990) Cortex. In *The Human Nervous System* (Paxinos, G., ed.), pp. 757–802. San Diego: Academic Press.

Zilles, K. et al (1995) Mapping of human and macaque sensorimotor areas by integrating architectonic, transmitter receptor, MRI and PET data. *J. Anat.* **187**: 515–538.

Hemispheric asymmetries

The two cerebral hemispheres are *asymmetrical* in certain respects. Some of the asymmetries have to do with handedness, language, and complex motor activities; other, more subtle differences come under the general rubric of *cognitive style*. (Limbic asymmetries are described in Ch. 30.)

HANDEDNESS AND LANGUAGE

Handedness indicates the hemisphere that is dominant for motor control. Left hemisphere/right-hand dominance is the rule. The best indicator available for population estimates of handedness is the preferred hand for writing; this criterion indicates a left hemisphere dominance for motor control in about 90% – at any rate for literate communities!

In 90% of subjects, the left hemisphere is dominant for language. In 7.5%, the right hemisphere is dominant in both sexes, and in 2.5%, the two hemispheres have an equal share. Although the left hemisphere is dominant in respect of both motor control and language, the two features are statistically independent; many left-handers have their language areas in the left hemisphere.

Language areas

Although several areas of the cortex, notably in the frontal lobe, are active during speech, two areas are specifically devoted to this function.

Broca's area   (Figure 27.1)
The French pathologist Pierre Broca assigned a motor speech function to the inferior frontal gyrus of the left side in 1861. The principal premotor area for speech occupies the opercular and triangular parts of the inferior frontal gyrus, corresponding to areas 44 and 45 of Brodmann. Both areas are larger on the left side in right-handers. The main output of Broca's area is to cell columns in the face and tongue areas of the adjacent motor cortex. Lesions involving Broca's area are associated with expressive aphasia (see *Clinical Panel 27.1*). Some workers believe that expressive aphasia requires that the lesion should also include the lower end of the precentral gyrus.

Wernicke's area   (Figure 27.1)
The German neurologist Karl Wernicke made extensive contributions to language processing in the late 19th century. He designated the posterior part of area 22 in the superior temporal gyrus of the left hemisphere as a sensory area concerned with understanding the spoken word. The upper surface of Wernicke's area is called the **temporal plane** (*Figure 27.2*). The volume of cerebral cortex in the temporal plane is larger on the left side in 60% of subjects. The horizontal part of the lateral fissure is longer in consequence – a feature readily identified on MRI scans. Lesions involving

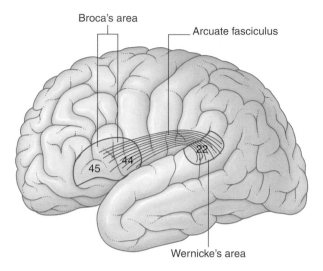

Figure 27.1   Broca's and Wernicke's language areas and the arcuate fasciculus.

Wernicke's area in adults are associated with receptive aphasia (see *Clinical Panel 27.1*).

Wernicke's area is linked to Broca's area by association fibers of the arcuate fasciculus which curve around the posterior end of the lateral fissure within the underlying white matter (*Figure 27.1*). The two areas are also linked through the insula.

It is difficult to assess the significance of the asymmetry of the temporal plane. The 60% incidence of left-sided relative enlargement does not match the 95% left hemisphere dominance for speech. Moreover, the *overall* length of the lateral sulcus is much the same on both sides. The *parietal plane* of the sulcus is longer on the right side because the right supramarginal gyrus is larger than the left one. This feature has been advanced as an explanation for the shorter temporal plane on the right.

Maldevelopment of the left temporal plane is a significant feature in cases of schizophrenia (*Clinical Panel 27.2*).

Right hemisphere contribution
During normal conversation there is some increase in blood flow in areas of the right hemisphere matching those of the left. These areas are believed to be concerned with melodic aspects of speech – the cadences, emphases, and nuances, collectively called *prosody*. Disturbances of the melodic function are called *aprosodias* (*Clinical Panel 27.1*).

Recovery of speech function – when it occurs – depends upon the age of the subject, and in adults upon the extent of the lesion. Occasional cases have been reported of recovery of near-normal speech in right-handed patients, 7 years of age or less, following complete removal of the left hemisphere as a treatment for intractable epilepsy. This can only

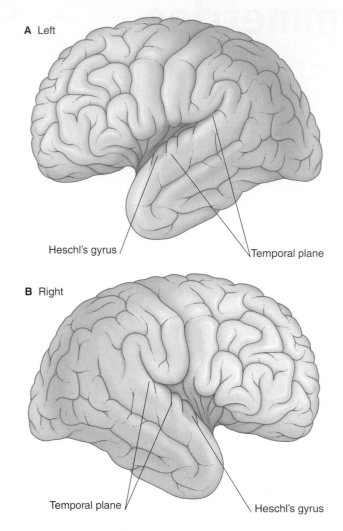

A Left

Heschl's gyrus / Temporal plane

B Right

Temporal plane / Heschl's gyrus

Figure 27.2 Views of the opened lateral sulcus showing the upper surface of the temporal lobes.

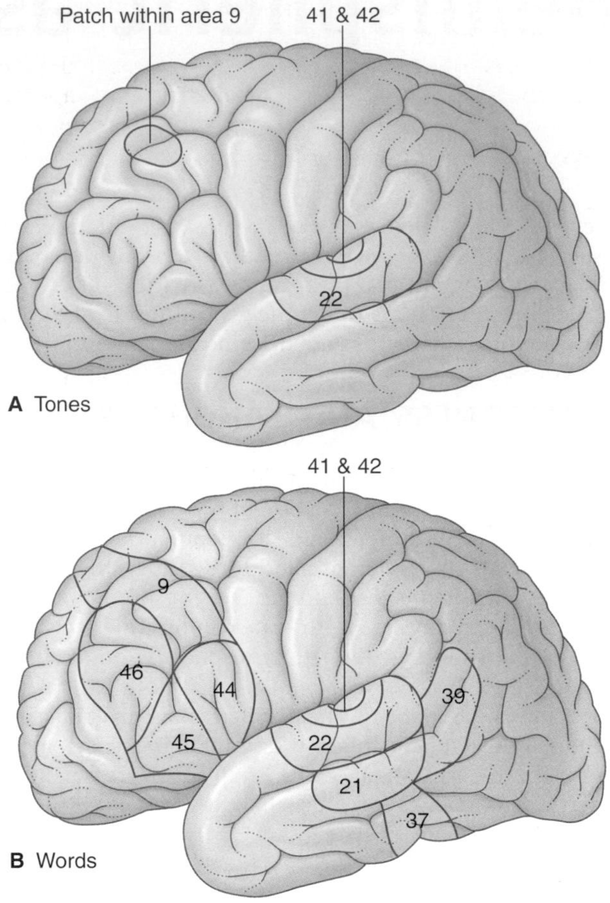

Patch within area 9   41 & 42

22

A Tones

41 & 42

9

46

44

45   22   39

21

37

B Words

Figure 27.3 Regions of increased blood flow during listening **(A)** to tones, and **(B)** to words.

be explained by language processing, including speech, being not fully lateralized at the time of operation. In adults, PET studies have shown increased activity in Broca's and Wernicke's equivalents on the right side following cerebrovascular accidents on the left. However, significant improvement is possible only if the left temporal plane is sufficiently viable to be able to process signals passed to it from the right side through the corpus callosum.

Angular gyrus

The angular gyrus (area 39) belongs descriptively to the inferior parietal lobule. The *left* angular gyrus receives a projection from the inferior part of area 19 (the lingual gyrus, shown in *Figure 2.6*), and itself projects to the temporal plane. It is commonly included as a part of Wernicke's area.

The angular gyrus seems to contain a neural lexicon (dictionary) of words, syllables, and numerical or other symbols, which can be retrieved by visual inputs – or even by visual imagery – and forwarded in the form of impulse trains to Wernicke's area within area 22. During reading, it is engaged in the conversion of written syllables ('graphemes') into the

corresponding sound equivalents ('phonemes'). The angular gyrus is also active during listening to spoken words.

Listening to spoken words

Figure 27.3 contrasts regional increases in blood flow during PET scanning when a volunteer listens to words ('active listening') vs random tone sequences ('passive listening'). As expected, tone sequences activate the primary auditory cortex (bilaterally). Wernicke's area (left side) also becomes active, probably in screening out this non-verbal material from further processing. Area 9 in the frontal lobe is thought to be part of a supervisory, vigilant system.

During active listening to words, areas 21 (middle temporal lobe), 37 (posteroinferior temporal lobe) and 39 (angular gyrus) all participate in auditory word processing. Area 39 identifies phonemes. Areas 21 and 37 identify words in the sound sequence and tap into lexicons stored in memory in a search for meaning – a process called *semantic retrieval*.

Activity in the left dorsolateral prefrontal cortex (DLPFC) expands to include area 46. Engagement of Broca's area is thought to include 'subvocal articulation' of words heard (see Neuroanatomy of Reading, later).

When listening to one's own voice, the areas of the temporal lobe identified above become active. An important function being served here is *metanalysis* (*post hoc* analysis) of speech, whereby 'slips of the tongue' can be identified. Speech metanalysis is singularly lacking in cases of receptive aphasia (*Clinical Panel 27.1*).

Modular organization of language

In alert subjects, electrical studies of the cortex exposed during neurosurgical procedures indicate the presence of a vast cortical mosaic for language. The mosaic of modules extends along the entire length of the frontoparietal operculum above the lateral sulcus and of the temporal operculum below the sulcus. The frontoparietal operculum is predominantly concerned with the motor functions of speaking and writing, and the temporal operculum with the sensory functions of hearing and reading.

It is well known that children have greater facility in acquiring a second language than adults. fMRI and other approaches have shown that the loci of second language acquisition before the age of 7 years overlap extensively with those processing the native language. A second language learned in later years is non-overlapping with the first. One possibility is that in children, the syntactical systems for processing nouns, verbs etc. are able to cope with two languages simultaneously.

It is of interest that following a small vascular lesion in an adult, *either* a late-acquired language *or* the native language may be lost, leaving the other relatively intact.

COGNITIVE STYLE

Hemispheric specializations in relation to information processing have been revealed by various forms of visual, auditory, and tactile tests. Results show that the left hemisphere is superior in processing information that is susceptible to *sequential analysis* of its parts whereas the right is superior in respect of *shapes* and of *spatial relationships*. Accordingly, the left hemisphere is described as being *analytical* and the right as being *holistic*. The right is also 'musical': there is a relative increase in blood flow in the right auditory association area when listening to music, versus a left-sided increase for words.

The analytical character of the left hemisphere is probably due to its unique capacity to perform the 'inner speech' that usually accompanies problem-solving.

Clinical Panel 27.1 The aphasias

Aphasia is a disturbance of language function caused by a lesion of the brain. The usual cause is a stroke produced by vascular occlusion in the anterior cortical territory of the left middle cerebral artery. (Vascular lesions of the forebrain are described in Ch. 30.)

Motor (anterior) aphasia
Patients having a lesion that includes Broca's area suffer from motor aphasia. These patients have difficulty in expressing what they want to say. Speech is slow, labored, and characteristically 'telegraphic' in style. The important nouns and verbs are spoken but prepositions and conjunctions are omitted. The patient comprehends what other people are saying and is well aware of being unable to speak fluently. There is usually an associated agraphia (inability to express thoughts in writing).

If the lesion involves a substantial amount of the cortical territory of the middle cerebral artery, there will be a motor weakness of the right lower face and right arm. Because the lips are affected, the patient will also have *dysarthria* (difficulty in speech articulation) in the form of slurring of certain syllables.

Sensory (posterior) aphasia
A lesion in Wernicke's area is accompanied by a deficit of auditory comprehension. (If the lesion includes the angular gyrus, the ability to read will be compromised

also.) In addition to their difficulty in understanding the speech of others, these patients lose the ability to monitor their own conversation, and usually have difficulty in retrieving correct descriptive names. Speech fluency is normal but two kinds of abnormality occur in the use of nouns:

- Verbal paraphrasia (use of words usually of allied meaning): instead of 'use a knife', 'use a fork'.
- Phonemic paraphrasia (use of made-up but similar-sounding syllables): instead of 'knife and fork', 'bife and dork'.

The most striking feature of Wernicke's aphasia is that, despite garbling to the point of being unintelligible (*jargon aphasia*), the patient may be quite unaware of making mistakes.

Aprosodia
Lesions of the right hemisphere may affect speech in subtle ways. Lesions that include area 44 (corresponding to Broca's area on the left) tend to change the patient's speech to a dull monotone. On the other hand, lesions that involve area 22 (corresponding to Wernicke's area) may lead to listening errors, e.g. being unable to detect inflections of speech; the patient may not know whether a particular remark is intended as a statement or as a question.

Neuroanatomy of reading (Figure 27.4)

Definitions

Orthography (*Gr.* correct writing) Word and sentence construction.

Phoneme (*Gr.* sound) The sound of a syllable. 'Phone' contains one phoneme. 'Phoneme' contains two phonemes!

Phonology The sounds of words. Testing could include: 'How many of these words have two syllables?' or 'How many of these words rhyme with one another?'

Retrieval Matching words, phrases and sentences with those previously entered into memory.

Semantics (*Gr.* meaning) Meaning of words and sentences.

Reading sequence

A *Carry out visual processing*
↓
B *Perform orthographic processing*
↓
C *Perform phonological assembly*
↓
D *Perform semantic retrieval*
↓
E *Execute motor plans*

A *Visual processing* is performed bilaterally in areas 17, 18, and 19. It includes: analysis of letter shapes for their identification; distinguishing between letters in upper *vs* lower case, and between real letters and meaningless shapes ('false fonts'). Processed information in the right extrastriate cortex (areas 18 and 19) is transferred to the left side through the forceps major which traverses the splenium of the corpus callosum – a point of clinical significance (see later).

B *Orthographic processing* means discerning whether or not each letter string in a sentence represents a real or a pseudoword, e.g. 'word' *vs* 'wurd'. Medial area 19 (V4) is especially involved.

C *Phonological processing* means the conversion of graphemes to phonemes. The angular gyrus (area 39) and middle temporal gyrus (area 21) participate.

D *Semantic retrieval* means performance of a memory search, using both orthographical and phonological cues from the text, to extract the meaning of words and sentences. The anterior part of Broca's area (area 45) becomes active at this advanced stage, together with area 37 in the posterior temporal lobe and area 40 (supramarginal gyrus) in the inferior parietal lobule.

E *Execution of motor plans (phonological execution)* is the performance of 'inner speech' ('subvocal articulation'). Both parts of Broca's area become active, as do the adjacent parts of premotor and motor cortex, the supplementary motor area (medial area 6) and the contralateral cerebellar hemisphere. The same four areas become much more active during reading aloud.

The left lateral prefrontal cortex, in and around area 46, is 'switched on' throughout **A–E**. Also active is part of area 32 in the left anterior cingulate cortex, which is involved in all cognitive activities requiring attention.

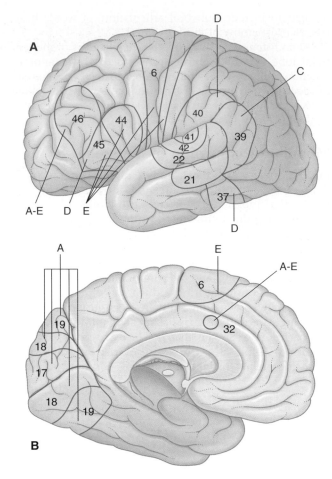

Figure 27.4 Areas of increased cortical blood flow in the left hemisphere observed in PET scans during reading aloud. Arrows at left indicate transfer of coded information from matching areas of the right hemisphere through the splenium of the corpus callosum. For explanation of A–E, see main text.

Schizophrenia (*Clinical Panel 27.3*) is a psychiatric disorder involving the left hemisphere more than the right.

PARIETAL LOBE (Figure 27.5)

The parietal lobe – especially the *right* one – is of prime importance for appreciation of spatial relationships. There is also evidence that the parietal lobe – especially the *left* one – is concerned with initiation of movement.

Inferior parietal lobule and the body schema

Clinically, the term *inferior parietal lobule* refers to area 40, which includes the supramarginal gyrus. Area 40 receives visual information from area 7 and tactile information from area 5; also a limbic input from the posterior cingulate cortex (area 23).

The term *body schema* refers to an awareness of the existence and spatial relationships of body parts, based on previous (stored) and current sensory experience. The reality of body schema has been established by the astonishing condition known as *anosognosia* (*Gr.* 'unawareness of disease')

Clinical Panel 27.2 Developmental dyslexia

It is generally agreed that reading is a more skilled activity than speech, because it requires an exquisite level of integration of visual scanning and auditory (inner speech) comprehension. Reading is thought to activate two pathways in parallel: one passes via the angular gyrus to Wernicke's area and accesses a phonological representation of every syllable in a temporal lobe memory store; the other passes to the left DLPFC and accesses a semantic (meaning) memory store for every word.

Developmental dyslexia affects 3–4% of literate populations. The characteristic feature is a specific and pronounced reading difficulty in children who are the match of their peers in other respects. The performance of dyslexic children can often be improved by special training. Nevertheless, severe dyslexia is known to be associated with significant developmental deficiencies in relevant parts of the brain.

- The magnocells (M cells) of the ganglionic layer of the retina and lateral geniculate nucleus are smaller than normal and their (smaller) axons conduct more slowly. One consequence is that the scanning movements used in reading, controlled by M cell inputs to the superior colliculus (Ch. 25) are so

inefficient that written syllables tend to run together and individual letters may appear to be transposed. The eyes may even be seen to wobble in an unstable manner during reading.

- The magnocellular neurons of the medial geniculate nucleus, which project to the primary auditory cortex (Ch. 17) are also smaller than normal. The effect is one of reduced detection of the frequency and amplitude of sounds, leading to below-normal perception of words that are read aloud.

- A surprising finding is that the *insula* is inactive on PET scans in those with dyslexia on certain language tasks, compared to controls. It has been postulated that the insula may be a station linking the supramarginal and angular gyri to Broca's area, and that a defect in this linkage may be significant in relation to the 'inner speech' that normally takes place during reading.

Explanations for these developmental abnormalities are speculative. An autoimmune response to surface antigens known to be present on the surface of developing ganglion cells of the visual and auditory pathways, with consequent retardation of their growth, has been proposed.

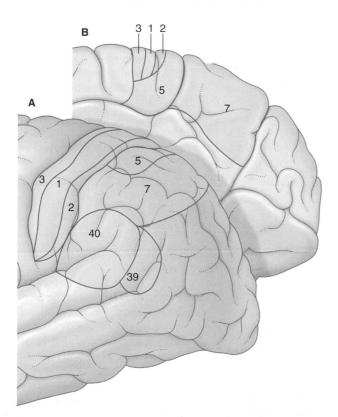

Figure 27.5 Brodmann's areas in the parietal lobe. **(A)** Lateral view; **(B)** medial view. 3/1/2, somesthetic cortex; 5, somesthetic association area; 7, posterior parietal cortex; 39, angular gyrus; 40, supramarginal gyrus.

in which a patient, who has suffered a massive stroke involving the parietal lobe as well as the descending motor pathways, denies ownership of the contralateral, hemiplegic side of the body. A relatively common disorder is that of *hemineglect*, where the contralateral side is ignored but can be used if attention is drawn to it (see *Clinical Panel 27.5*). Hemineglect is much more common following a right parietal lobe lesion than a left one.

Like all of the association areas, each parietal lobe exchanges information with its partner through the corpus callosum. In healthy individuals, the left and right hand are equally adept at distinguishing a key from a coin in a coat pocket without the aid of vision (*stereognosis*, Ch. 26).

Patients with a right hemisphere lesion involving the inferior parietal lobe have difficulty in distinguishing between unseen objects of different shapes with the left hand. They have *astereognosis*. Patients with a comparable lesion in the left hemisphere are able to make this distinction using the right hand but they have difficulty in announcing the *function* of a selected object. The left supramarginal gyrus partici-pates in phonological retrieval, as already noted, and the deficit, although a semantic one, may be related to interference with the 'inner speech' that usually accompanies problem-solving.

Both deficits are forms of *tactile agnosia*. The right hemisphere deficit has become known as *apperceptive* tactile agnosia ('apperception', awareness of perception), and the left one as *associative* tactile agnosia (failure to identify functional associations).

Clinical Panel 27.3 Schizophrenia

Schizophrenia occurs in about 1% of the population in all countries where the incidence has been studied. In about 10% of cases, there is some evidence of a schizophrenic personality in one or more close relatives. MRI brain-imaging studies reveal some degree of atrophy of frontal and temporal parts of the cortex, especially on the left side. There is a reduction or even a reversal of the usual left–right difference in the size of the temporal plane on the upper surface of the temporal lobe. In postmortem studies, a substantial failure of development of the neurons that project from the medial geniculate nucleus to the primary auditory cortex on the left side has also been detected; this may be attributed to failure of the lost cells to establish proper connections with target neurons in the primary auditory cortex. The various anatomical changes can be accounted for, theoretically, on a basis of disordered cell migrations into the developing cortex during the middle trimester of gestation, with consequent failure to establish a full range of connectivities during postnatal growth. The underlying pathology remains relatively stable in adult life, and schizophrenia is described as a psychosis rather than a dementia.

The mode of presentation is quite variable but the behavioral changes permit most patients to be categorized into two classes: those in whom positive symptoms predominate, and those in whom negative symptoms predominate.

- *Positive symptoms* include hallucinations, delusions, and bizarre behavior. Hallucinations are typically auditory (the patient hears voices, and commonly converses with them aloud). Delusions often take a paranoid form, with a belief that one's thoughts and actions are being controlled by some outside agency. Bizarre behavior may include physical aggression in response to the hallucinations or delusions. The positive symptoms are believed to originate in the temporal lobe. Although positive symptoms may cause great alarm, they are much more responsive to treatment than the negative ones.

- *Negative symptoms* are those of withdrawal from society into a private world. The patient has little to say, and in conversation rambles from one inconsequential theme to another. There is a loss of emotional responsiveness ('flattening of affect'). Personal hygiene is a matter of indifference. The negative symptoms are attributed to 'hypofrontality,' i.e. to diminished frontal lobe function. PET scans support this idea, by demonstrating failure of the normal response of the left DLPFC to standard tests of cognitive function.

Treatment of schizophrenia is by means of one of the antipsychotic drugs that block dopamine receptors (e.g. chlorpromazine or haloperidol). These drugs are very effective in terminating bouts of bizarre behavior and in reducing the likelihood of their recurrence. A side effect of these drugs is a tendency to provoke some of the physical symptoms of Parkinson's disease, which is known to be preceded by substantial loss of nigrostriatal dopaminergic neurons (Ch. 28). This is one reason why overactivity of the mesocortical/mesolimbic dopaminergic system (Ch. 21) is considered significant in schizophrenia, although it does not account for the mainly left-sided pathology. Another reason is the fact that symptoms closely resembling the positive ones of schizophrenia may be induced by a 'binge' of amphetamine ('speed'); amphetamine is known to increase the amount of dopamine in the forebrain extracellular space (Ch. 30). In schizophrenia, dopaminergic overactivity seems not to be a matter of overproduction but of greater effectiveness through an increased number of postsynaptic dopamine receptors on the neurons in the cerebral cortex.

Parietal lobe and movement initiation

There are several sites for movement initiation in different behavioral contexts. The present context is the performance of learned movements of some complexity: examples would include turning a door knob, combing one's hair, blowing out a match, and clapping. It is logical to anticipate a starting point within the dominant hemisphere, because they can all be performed in response to verbal command (oral or written). This notion receives support from the observation that, if the corpus callosum has been severed surgically, the patient can perform a learned movement on command using the right hand, but not on attempting it with the left hand.

Failure to perform a learned movement on request is called *ideomotor apraxia*, or *limb apraxia*. It has been repeat- edly observed immediately following vascular lesions at the sites listed and described in *Figure 27.6*.

Ideomotor apraxia can be accounted for if the dominant parietal lobe is considered to contain a repertoire of learned movement programs which, on retrieval, elicit appropriate responses by the premotor cortex on one or both sides under directives from the prefrontal cortex. (The basal ganglia would be involved as well, as described in Ch. 28.)

Ideomotor apraxia is a transient phenomenon. Because parietal blood flow increases almost equally on both sides during reaching movements, the right hemisphere seems to be able to assume a full role for the left arm when no longer overshadowed.

Clinical Panel 27.4   Parietal lobe dysfunction

Anterior parietal cortex

Lesions of the somatic sensory cortex and area 5 tend to occur together, causing cortical-type sensory loss and inaccurate reaching movements into contralateral visual hemispace (e.g. at mealtimes, the patient tends to knock things over).

Supramarginal gyrus

Lesions affecting area 40 are usually vascular (middle cerebral artery) and are usually concomitant with contralateral hemiplegia with or without hemianopia. However, the blood supply to this area is sometimes selectively occluded.

The characteristic result of damage to the supramarginal gyrus is *hemineglect*. The patient ignores the opposite side of the body unless attention is specifically drawn to it. A male patient will shave only the ipsilateral side of the face; a female patient will comb her hair only on the ipsilateral side. The patient will acknowledge a tactile stimulus to the contralateral side when tested alone; simultaneous

testing of both sides will only be acknowledged ipsilaterally (*sensory extinction*).

Aspects of posterior parietal lobe function are affected as well. The patient tends to ignore the contralateral visual hemispace, even if the visual pathways are intact, and there is *visual extinction* (contralaterally) to simultaneous bilateral stimuli, e.g. when the clinician wiggles his/her index fingers in both visual fields simultaneously.

Hemineglect is at least five times more frequent following lesions on the *right* side, irrespective of handedness.

Angular gyrus

An isolated vascular lesion of the left angular gyrus (very rare) produces *alexia* (complete inability to read) and *agraphia* (inability to write); letters on the page are suddenly without any meaning. If the temporal plane has survived, patients can still name words spelt aloud to them. For *ideomotor apraxia*, see main text.

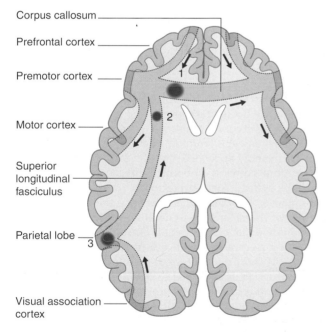

Corpus callosum
Prefrontal cortex
Premotor cortex
Motor cortex
Superior longitudinal fasciculus
Parietal lobe
Visual association cortex

Figure 27.6 Association and commissural pathways serving motor responses to sensory cues. (Adapted from Kertesz, A. and Ferro, J.M. (1984) Lesion size and location in ideomotor apraxia. *Brain* **107**: 921–933.) The premotor cortex is under higher control by the prefrontal cortex.

Lesions at site 1 effectively sever the anterior part of the corpus callosum and produce ipsilateral limb apraxia (left lesion, left limb). Lesions at either site 2 (superior longitudinal fasciculus) or site 3 (angular gyrus) may produce *bilateral* limb apraxia. In practice, a large lesion may render right-limb apraxia impossible to assess because of associated right hemiplegia or receptive aphasia.

PREFRONTAL CORTEX

The prefrontal cortex has two-way connections with all parts of the neocortex except the primary motor and sensory areas, with its fellow through the genu of the corpus callosum, and with the mediodorsal nucleus of the thalamus. It is uniquely large in the human brain and is concerned with the highest brain functions including abstract thinking, decision-making, anticipating the effects of particular courses of action, and social behavior.

The DLPFC, centered in and around area 9, is strongly active in both hemispheres during waking hours. It has been called the *supervisory attentional system*. It participates in all cognitive activities and is essential for conscious learning of all kinds. During conscious learning, it operates *working memory*, whereby memories appropriate to the task ('work') in hand are retrieved and 'held in the mind'. The medial prefrontal cortex has auditory and verbal associations. The orbitofrontal cortex has been described as the *neocortical representative of the limbic system*. It is richly connected to the amygdala, septal area, and the cortex of the temporal pole – three limbic structures described in Chapter 29.

In general terms, the left prefrontal cortex has an 'approach' bias, being engaged in all language-related activities including the 'inner speech' that accompanies investigative activities. The right prefrontal cortex has a 'withdraw' bias, being particularly activated by fearful contexts, whether real or imagined.

Clinical Panel 27.5   Frontal lobe dysfunction

Symptoms of *early* frontal lobe disease typically involve subtle changes in personality and social function rather than diminution of cognitive performance on objective tests. Lack of foresight (failure to anticipate the consequences of a course of action), distractibility (poor concentration), loss of willpower (*abulia*), and difficulty in 'switching cognitive sets' (e.g. inability to switch easily from one subject of conversation to another) are characteristic. These general symptoms are more often associated with bilateral disease with impending dementia, than with a brain tumor. With increasing disease, especially if bilateral, the *gait* is affected. '*Marche à petit pas*' ('Walk with small steps') refers to a characteristic short, shuffling gait often associated with disequilibrium (tendency to fall), and 'freezing' (especially when turning). This syndrome may give rise to a mistaken suspicion of Parkinson's disease.

Large *dorsolateral lesions* are associated with slowing of mental processes of all kinds, leading to hypokinesia, apathy, and indifference to surrounding events. The picture resembles that of the 'withdrawn' type of schizophrenia, and it is of interest that in 'withdrawn' schizophrenic patients cortical blood flow may not show the anticipated increase in the dorsolateral region, in response to appropriate psychological tests.

Large *orbitofrontal* lesions are associated with hyperkinesia, with increased instinctual drives in relation to food and sexual behavior. With disease more pronounced (or only) in the right orbitofrontal cortex, the 'fearful' side of the patient's nature may be lost, leading to puerile jocularity and compulsive laughter. Compulsive crying may be a clue to left-sided disease. A well-known cause of orbitofrontal disturbance is a meningioma arising in the groove occupied by the olfactory nerve; *anosmia* (loss of the sense of smell) may be discovered on testing, and optic atrophy may follow pressure on the optic nerve where it emerges from the optic canal. Hyperkinetic frontal lobe disorders have been treated in the past by means of *lobotomy* – a surgical procedure in which the white matter above the orbital cortex was severed through a supraorbital incision.

Gliomas within the frontal lobe may become large before any cognitive or physical defects appear. Eventually, a left-sided tumor may invade or compress Broca's area and cause motor aphasia. On either side, a progressive hemiparesis may supervene.

Core Information

Hemispheric asymmetries mainly concern handedness, language, and cognitive style. Some 10% of people are left-handers. Language areas are left-sided in 90%, right-sided in 5%, and bilateral in 5%. Broca's motor speech area occupies the inferior frontal gyrus; lesions here give rise to motor aphasia with difficulty in writing. Wernicke's sensory speech area in the planum temporale is required for understanding the spoken word; lesions here result in receptive aphasia, and difficulty in reading if the angular gyrus is involved. The left hemisphere is usually superior in processing information susceptible to sequential analysis; the right hemisphere is superior for analysis of shapes and spatial relationships. The inferior parietal lobule is concerned with the body schema; lesions here may result in neglect of personal and extrapersonal space on the opposite side. Finally, the left parietal lobe may initiate complex motor programs; lesions here may be associated with ideomotor apraxia.

The prefrontal cortex is involved in highest brain functions. The dorsolateral prefrontal cortex (DLPFC) contains a supervisory attentional system especially involved in conscious learning where it operates working memory appropriate to the task at hand. The orbitofrontal cortex is a neocortical representative of the limbic system. The left prefrontal cortex has investigative, 'approach' characteristics, the right has 'withdraw' characteristics. General signs of frontal lobe disease include lack of foresight, distractibility, and difficulty in switching cognitive sets. The gait may take the form of short shuffling steps with instability and 'freezing'. DLPFC lesions lead to slowing of mental process, apathy, and indifference. Orbitofrontal lesions tend to produce a hyperkinetic state with increased instinctual drives and puerile behavior.

REFERENCES

Binder, J.R., Frost, J.A., Hammeke, T.A., Rao, S.M. and Cox, R.W. (1996) Function of the left planum temporale in auditory and linguistic processing. *Brain* **119**: 1239–1247.

Bottini, G., Cappa, S.F., Sterzi, R. and Vignolo, L.A. (1995) Intramodal somaesthetic recognition disorders following right and left hemisphere damage. *Brain* **118**: 395–399.

Eden G.F. and Zeffiro, T.A. (1998) Neural systems affected in developmental dyslexia revealed by functional neuroimaging. *Neuron* **21**: 279–282.

Galaburda, A.M., Menard, M.T. and Rosen, T.D. (1994) Evidence for aberrant auditory anatomy in developmental dyslexia. *Proc. Natl Acad. Sci. USA* **91**: 8010–8013.

Heiss, W.D., Kessler, J., Thiel, A., Ghaemi, M. and Karbe, H. (1999) Differential capacity of left and right hemispheric areas for compensation of poststroke aphasia. *Ann. Neurol.* **45**: 430–438.

Hynd, G.W., Marshall, R., Hall, J. and Edmonds, J.E. (1995) Learning disabilities: neuroanatomic asymmetries. In *Brain Asymmetry* (Davidson, R.J. and Hugdahl, K., eds), pp. 617–636. Cambridge, Mass: MIT Press.

Jancke, L., Schlaug, G., Huang, Y. and Steinmetz, H. (1994) Asymmetry of the planum parietale. *Neuroreport* **5**: 1161–1163.

Kertesz, A., Polk, M., Black, S.E. and Howell, J. (1992) Anatomical asymmetries and functional laterality. *Brain* **115**: 589–605.

Knecht, S., Deppe, M., Drager, B., Bobe, L., Ringelstein, E-B. and Henningsen, H. (2000) Language lateralization in healthy right-handers. *Brain* **123**: 74–81.

Liotti, M., Gay, C.T. and Fox, P.T. (1994) Functional imaging and language. *J. Clin. Neurophysiol.* **11**: 175–190.

Marsden, C.D. and Thompson, P.D. (1996) Frontal gait disorders. In *Brain Asymmetry* (Davidson, R.J. and Hugdahl, K., eds), pp. 188–193. Cambridge, Mass: MIT Press.

Naas, R. (1994) Advances in reading difficulties. *Current Opin. Neurol.* **7**: 179–186.

Passingham, R.E. (1998) Attention to action. In *The Prefrontal Cortex: Executive and Cognitive Functions* (Roberts, A.C., Robbins, T.W. and Weiskranz, L., eds), pp. 131–143. Oxford: Oxford University Press.

Paulesu, P., Frith, U., Snowling, M., Gallagher, A., Morton, J., Frackowiak, R.S.J. and Frith, D. (1996) Is developmental dyslexia a disconnection syndrome? Evidence from PET scanning. *Brain* **119**: 143–157.

Perelle, I.B. and Ehrman, N.D. (1994) An international study of human handedness: the data. *Behav. Genet.* **24**: 217–225.

Posner, M.J. and Abdullaev, Y.G. (1999) Neuroanatomy, circuitry and plasticity of word reading. *Neuro. Report* **10**: R12–R23.

Powers, R.E. (1999) The neuropathology of schizophrenia. *J. Neuropath. Exp. Neurol.* **58**: 679–690.

Price, C.J. (2000) The anatomy of language: contributions from functional imaging. *J. Anat.* **197**: 335–339.

Pugh, K.R., Shaywitz, B.A., Shaywitz, S.E., Constable, R.T., Skudlarski, P., Fulbright, R.K., Bronen, R.A., Shankweiler, D.P., Katz, L., Fletcher, J.M. and Gore, J.C. (1996) Cerebral organization of the functional processes in reading. *Brain* **119**: 1221–1238.

Reed, C.L., Caselli, R.J. and Farah, M.J. (1996) Tactile agnosia. *Brain* **119**: 875–888.

Rumsey, J.M., Donohue, B.C., Brady, D.R., Nace, K., Giedd, J.N. and Andreason, P. (1997) An MRI study of planum temporale asymmetry in males with developmental dyslexia. *Arch Neurol.* **54**: 1481–1489.

Sakata, H. and Taira, M. (1994) Parietal control of hand action. *Current Opin. Neurobiol.* **4**: 847–856.

Silbersweig, D.A. et al. (1995) A functional neuroanatomy of hallucinations in schizophrenia. *Nature* **378**: 176–179.

Stein, J.F. (1994) Developmental dyslexia, neural timing, and hemispheric lateralization. *Intl J. Neurophysiol.* **18**: 241–249.

Tzourio, N., Crivello, F., Mellet, E., Nkanga-Ngila, B. and Mazoyer, B. (1998) Functional anatomy of dominance for speech comprehension in left handers vs right handers. *Neuroimage* **8**: 1–16.

Basal ganglia

INTRODUCTION

The term *basal ganglia* is used to designate the areas of basal forebrain and midbrain known to be involved in the control of movement (*Figure 28.1*). It includes:

- The **striatum** (caudate nucleus, putamen of lentiform nucleus, nucleus accumbens).
- The **pallidum** (globus pallidus of lentiform nucleus), which comprises a **lateral segment** and a **medial segment**. The medial segment has a midbrain extension known as the **reticular part (pars reticulata)** of the **substantia nigra**.

- The **subthalamic nucleus**.
- The pigmented, **compact part (pars compacta)** of **substantia nigra**.

BASIC CIRCUITS

It is possible to demonstrate at least four circuits which commence in the cerebral cortex, traverse the basal ganglia, and return to the cortex. They comprise:

1 A *motor loop*, concerned with learned movements;

2 A *cognitive loop*, concerned with motor intentions;

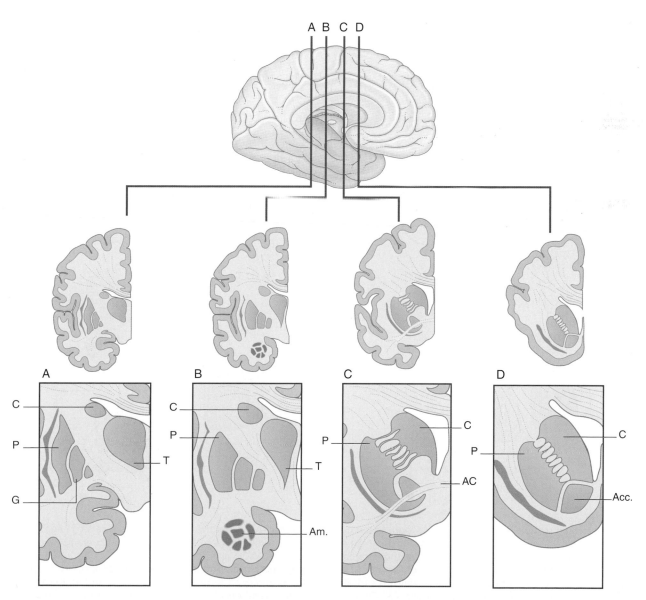

Figure 28.1 Four coronal sections of the brain, viewed from behind. Ventral parts are enlarged below. Acc., nucleus accumbens; AC, anterior commissure; Am., amygdala; C, caudate nucleus; G, globus pallidus; P, putamen; T, thalamus.

3 A *limbic loop*, concerned with emotional aspects of movement;

4 An *oculomotor loop*, concerned with voluntary saccades.

Motor loop

The motor loop commences in the sensorimotor cortex and returns there via striatum, thalamus and SMA (supplementary motor area).

Figure 28.2 is derived from *Figure 28.1A*. It is a schematic coronal section including the posterior part of the striatum, depicting component parts of the motor loop. Two pathways are known. The 'direct' pathway traverses the corpus striatum and thalamus and involves five consecutive sets of neurons (*Figure 28.2A*). The 'indirect' pathway engages the subthalamic nucleus in addition and involves seven sets of neurons (*Figure 28.2B*). The anatomy of the two thalamic projections from the medial pallidum (**ansa lenticularis** and **lenticular fasciculus**) is shown in *Figure 28.3*.

All projections from the cerebral cortex arise from pyramidal cells and are excitatory (glutaminergic). So, too, is the projection from thalamus to SMA. Those from striatum and from both segments of pallidum arise from medium-sized spiny neurons and are inhibitory. They are GABAergic, and also contain neuropeptides of uncertain function.

The *nigrostrial pathway* projects from the compact part of the substantia nigra to the striatum, where it makes two kinds of synapses upon the projection neurons there (*Figure 28.4*). Those upon 'direct' pathway neurons are facilitatory, by way of dopaminergic Type 1 (D_1) receptors on the dendritic spines; those upon 'indirect' pathway neurons are inhibitory, by way of Type 2 (D_2) receptors. Cholinergic internuncial neurons within the striatum are excitatory to projection neurons, and they are inhibited by dopamine.

A healthy substantia nigra is tonically active, favoring activity in the 'direct' pathway. Facilitation of this pathway is necessary for the SMA to become active before and during movement. SMA activity immediately prior to movement can be detected by means of recording electrodes attached to the

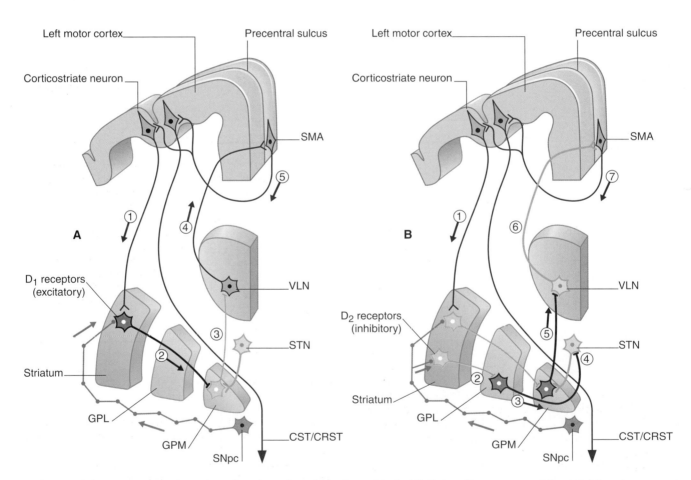

Figure 28.2 Coronal section through the motor loop, based on *Figure 28.1A*. **(A)** Shows the sequence of five sets of neurons involved in the 'direct' pathway from sensorimotor cortex to thalamus with final return to sensorimotor cortex via SMA. **(B)** shows the sequence of seven sets of neurons involved in the 'indirect' pathway.

The *red/pink* neurons are excitatory utilizing glutamate. The *black/gray* neurons are inhibitory utilizing γ-aminobutyric acid. The *brown*, nigrostriatal neuron utilizes dopamine which is excitatory via D_1 receptors on target pallidal neurons and inhibitory via D_2 receptors on the same and other pallidal neurons. CST/CRST, corticospinal, corticoreticular fibers; GPL, GPM, lateral and medial segments of globus pallidus; SMA, supplementary motor area; SNpc, compact part of substantia nigra; STN, subthalamic nucleus; VLN, ventral lateral nucleus of thalamus.

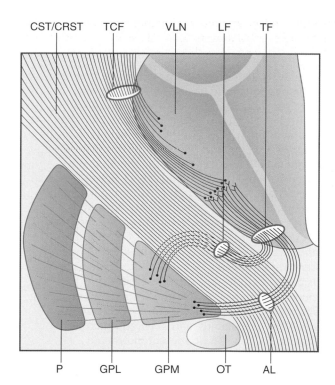

Figure 28.3 Part of the projection from the medial segment of globus pallidus (GPM) to the ventral lateral nucleus (VLN) of the thalamus sweeps around the base of the internal capsule as the **ansa lenticularis** (AL); the remainder traverses this region as the **lenticular fasciculus** (LF). The two parts come together as the **thalamic fasciculus** (TF) before entering the thalamus. CST/CRST, corticospinal and corticoreticular fibers. GPL, lateral segment of globus pallidus; OT, optic tract; P, putamen; TCF, thalamocortical fibers.

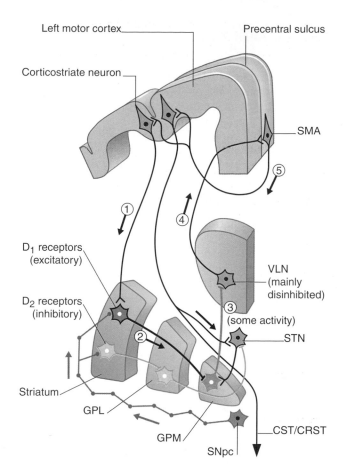

Figure 28.4 Activities in the striatal motor loops, prior to movement.

The SMA (supplementary motor area) is activated through the 'direct pathway' as follows: (1) Corticostriate fibers from the sensorimotor cortex activate those GABAergic spiny neurons in striatum having D_1 receptors tonically facilitated by nigrostriatal inputs. (2) The activated striatal neurons inhibit medial pallidal (GPM) neurons (3) with consequent *disinhibition* of ventral lateral nucleus (VLN) thalamocortical neurons (4) and activation of SMA (5), which both modifies ongoing corticostriate activity and initiates impulse trains along corticospinal (CST) and corticoreticular (CRST) fibers.

Activity along the 'indirect pathway' is relatively slight because of tonic dopaminergic inhibition of the relevant striatal neurons via D_2 receptors. However, the subthalamic nucleus (STN) is tonically activated by corticosubthalamic fibers, curtailing the inhibition of GPM. GPL, lateral segment of globus pallidus; SNpc, compact part of substantia nigra. (Cerebello-thalamocortical projection is not shown.)

scalp. This activity is known as the (electrical) *readiness potential,* and its manner of production is described in the caption to *Figure 28.4.* Impulses pass from SMA to the motor cortex, where a cerebello-thalamocortical projection selectively enhances pyramidal and corticoreticular neurons within milliseconds prior to discharge.

The putamen and globus pallidus are somatotopic, permitting selective facilitation of neurons relevant to (say) arm movements via the direct route, with simultaneous disfacilitation of unwanted (say) leg movements via the indirect route. For suppression of unwanted movements, the subthalamic nucleus (STN), acting upon the body map in the medial pallidal segment, is especially important, since we know that destruction of STN results in uncontrollable spontaneous movements of one or more body parts on the opposite side (see later).

Progressive failure of dopamine production by the compact part of substantia nigra is the precipitating cause of *Parkinson's disease (Clinical Panel 28.1).*

Misdiagnosis

PD has two principal kinds of presentation. In one, *tremor* is the predominant feature. In the other, *akinesia and rigidity* predominate. It is now known that more than one in five people initially diagnosed and treated as suffering from PD either do not have PD at all, or have a 'Parkinson plus' syndrome.

Benign essential tremor is more than twice as prevalent as PD and is often mistaken for it. It is characterized initially by a faint trembling at 8–10 Hz, most noticeable when the arms are fully outstretched. Later, head-bobbing – *not* a feature of PD – and orthostatic (when upright) trunk tremor may appear, and a tremulous diaphragm may impart a vocal tremor. Benign essential tremor is sometimes called *familial tremor* because of autosomal dominant inheritance, and *senile tremor* when observed in the elderly.

Clinical Panel 28.1 Hypokinesia: Parkinson's disease

Parkinson's disease (PD) affects about 1% of people over 50 years of age in all countries. The primary underlying pathology is degeneration of nigrostriatal neurons, resulting in diminished dopamine content within the striatum. [^{18}f]Fluorodopa is a mildly radioactive compound which, when injected intravenously, binds with dopamine receptors in the striatum. In symptomatic PD, a significant reduction of FDOPA binding (and therefore of receptors) is revealed by means of PET scanning (*Figure CP 28.1.1*). One consequence is *increased* striatal activity, with a shift from the direct to the indirect motor pathway (*Figure CP 28.1.2*).

Nigrostriatal degeneration seems to take the form of a *dying back neuropathy*, because dopamine is lost from the striatum earlier than in the midbrain. One possibility is that a toxic metabolite of dopamine is retrieved from the extracellular fluid during dopamine retrieval. This could account for the fact that the cerebrospinal fluid of PD patients is toxic to dopaminergic neurons in cell culture dishes.

Some 60% of nigral neurons have been lost before the first symptoms appear. This delay is accounted for by (a) increased dopamine production by surviving neurons, and (b) increased production ('upregulation') of dopamine receptors in the target striatal neurons.

The following symptoms/signs are characteristic: tremor, bradykinesia, rigidity, and impairment of postural reflexes. Not all are expressed in every patient:

Tremor
Tremor, at 3–6 Hz (*Hertz*, times per second) in one limb is the initial feature in two-thirds of cases. The commonest sequence of limb involvement is from one upper limb to ipsilateral lower limb within 1 year, followed by contralateral limb involvement within 3 years. Rhythmic tremor of lips and tongue, pronation–supination of the forearm, and flexion–extension of the fingers may be obvious. A 'pill-rolling' movement of index and middle fingers against the thumb pad is characteristic Typically, the tremor only involves muscle groups that are 'at rest' and vanishes during voluntary movement. A tremulous patient has no difficulty in raising and draining a tumblerful of water, hence the term *resting tremor* used to distinguish it from the *intention tremor* of cerebellar disease. Intention tremor is absent at rest (unless cerebellar dysfunction is severe) and is brought on by voluntary movement.

Tremor is associated with rhythmic bursting activity of cells in the striatum, pallidum and ventral lateral nucleus (VLN) of thalamus, and in anterior horn cells of the spinal cord. The contribution of disordered autogenic inhibition to both tremor and rigidity is described below.

Rigidity
Rigidity affects all of the somatic musculature simultaneously, but a predilection for flexors imposes a stooped posture. Passive flexion and extension of the major joints evince resistance through the full range of movement. The term 'lead pipe rigidity' is used to distinguish this type of resistance from the 'claspknife rigidity' of the spastic state that accompanies upper motor neuron lesions. The clinician may detect a subtle underlying tremor in the form of ratchety, 'cogwheel' sensation.

Head of caudate nucleus   Putamen

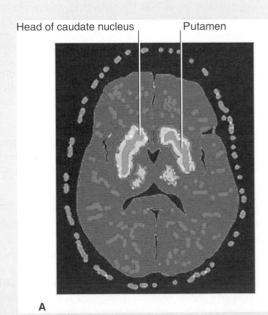 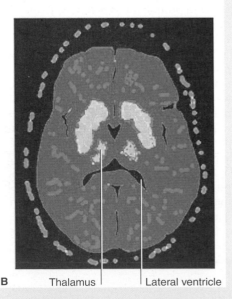

A   B   Thalamus | Lateral ventricle

Figure CP 28.1.1 Diagram showing typical results of brain scans following intravenous injection of [^{18}f]Fluorodopa. Intensity of uptake is indicated as red (greatest), yellow, green, blue (least). **(A)** Control; **(B)** Parkinson's disease.

Clinical Panel 28.1 *Continued*

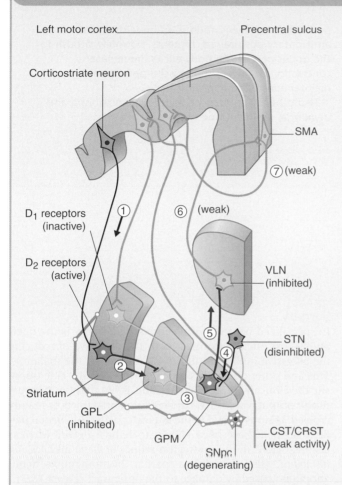

Left motor cortex

Precentral sulcus

Corticostriate neuron

SMA

⑦ (weak)

① ⑥ (weak)

D₁ receptors
(inactive)

D₂ receptors
(active)

VLN
(inhibited)

⑤ STN
(disinhibited)
④

②

Striatum

③

GPL
(inhibited)

CST/CRST
(weak activity)

GPM

SNpc
(degenerating)

Figure CP 28.1.2 Consequences of degeneration of the pathway from the compact part of the substantia nigra (SNpc) to the striatum (S) in Parkinson's disease. The effects arise from loss of tonic facilitation of spiny striatal neurons bearing D₁ receptors, together with loss of tonic inhibition of those bearing D₂ receptors. The 'direct pathway' is disengaged, the 'indirect pathway' is activated by default. (1) Corticostriate neurons from the sensorimotor cortex now strongly activate those GABAergic neurons (2) in the striatum that synapse upon others (3) in the lateral pallidal segment (GPL). The double effect is *disinhibition* of the subthalamic nucleus (STN). STN discharges strongly (4) onto the GABAergic neurons of the medial pallidal segment (GPM); these in turn discharge strongly (5) into the ventral lateral nucleus (VLN) of thalamus, resulting in reduced output along thalamocortical fibers (6) traveling to the supplementary motor area (SMA). Inputs (7) from SMA to corticospinal and corticoreticular fibers (CST/CRST) become progressively weaker, with pathetic consequences for initiation and execution of movements.

Historically, rigidity has been abolished by section of dorsal nerve roots, thus proving its peripheral sensory origin. It can also be alleviated by a surgical lesion of the pallidum or of the VL nucleus of the thalamus. Because muscle spindle stretch reflexes are not

exaggerated in PD, attention has focused on the Golgi tendon organ afferents responsible for autogenetic inhibition. As illustrated in Chapter 8, these afferents synapse upon inhibitory, 1b internuncials which, when activated by muscle contraction, dampen activity of motor neurons supplying the same muscle and any homonymous contributors to the same movement (e.g. impulses generated in biceps brachii tendon organs will depress both brachialis and biceps motor neurons). In PD patients, autogenetic inhibition is reduced, and it is also delayed to the extent that it becomes entrained with the pulses descending from the brain, with the effect of contributing to the tremor. It may also contribute to the rigidity because in PD there is some degree of co-contraction of prime movers and antagonists.

Given that muscular contraction is required to activate tendon organs, why do patients display 'resting tremor', with supposedly inactive muscles? It transpires that, when the forearms (say) are resting on the lap or on the arms of a chair, the forearm/hand muscles are *not* fully at rest. If the limb is properly supported at elbow and wrist, the tremor disappears. The tremor also disappears during sleep.

Normally, both corticospinal and reticulospinal fibers are tonically facilitatory to 1b inhibitory internuncials. In PD, activation of the primary motor cortex by SMA is known to be both reduced and oscillatory, thus accounting for the pronounced effects in the forearm and hand. Impaired reticulospinal activity is more likely to be significant with respect to the lower limbs.

In addition to its massive projections into the pallidum, the putamen projects to another group of GABAergic neurons, namely the reticular part of the substantia nigra. The compact part of the substantia nigra also projects to the reticular part. The reticular part projects in turn to the brainstem locomotor center (Ch. 21). In PD, the overactive putamen would be expected to have the knock-on effect of inhibiting impulse traffic in the projections from the locomotor area to the pontine and medullary reticular reticulospinal tracts.

Difficulty in writing is a common early feature. The individual written letters become small and irregular. Loss of writing skill is attributable to co-contraction of wrist flexors and extensors, owing to marked reduction of supraspinal activation of 1a internuncials synapsing on antagonist motor neurons.

Bradykinesia

Bradykinesia means slowness of movement. Patients report that routine activities, such as opening a door, require deliberate planning and consciously guided execution. Electromyographic studies of the limb musculature show a reduction of the 'initial agonist burst' of electrical charge accompanying the first contraction of relevant prime movers. Normally, the basal ganglionic contribution to movement comes on stream some milliseconds after the premotor cortex and cerebellum have raised the firing rate of motor-cortex neurons to threshold at spinal lower motor neuron level. In PD, the boost to lower motor neuron activation is weak, because of the weakened contribution from SMA.

Impairment of postural reflexes
Patients go off balance easily, and tend to fall stiffly ('like a telegraph pole') in response to a mild accidental

push. The underlying fault is an impairment of anticipatory postural adjustments: normally, a push to the upper part of the body elicits immediate contraction of lower limb muscles appropriate for the maintenance of equilibrium.

Two other symptoms, *oculomotor hypokinesia* and *dementia*, are mentioned in the main text.

The cause is unknown, and levodopa (L-dopa) (see below) is ineffective.

Multisystem atrophy is a 'Parkinson plus' degenerative disorder of brainstem, basal ganglia, and central autonomic neurons. Patients present with one or more of the following:

- akinesia/rigidity with little or no tremor
- one or more signs of autonomic failure: postural hypotension, bladder/bowel dysfunction, impotence, dry eyes and mouth, pupillary abnormalities, impaired sweating
- bilateral pyramidal tract degeneration leading to pseudobulbar palsy (Ch. 15) and 'upper motor neuron signs' (Ch. 13) in the limbs
- poor ocular convergence.

L-dopa is of little value.

Clinical neurology texts describe other relevant disorders, e.g. *progressive supranuclear palsy* and *corticobasal degeneration*.

Treatment of Parkinson's disease

Drugs

The first line of treatment of PD is administration of L-dopa, which can cross the blood–brain barrier and is metabolized to dopamine by surviving nigral neurons. Some 75% of patients benefit, with a reduction of symptoms by 50% or more. After several months of L-dopa therapy, many patients develop spontaneous choreiform movements (described in *Clinical Panel 2*) owing to excessive striatal response. After a year or more, the effectiveness of L-dopa declines with the progressive loss of nigral neurons, and dopamine agonist drugs are often used instead, to stimulate striatal post-synaptic dopamine receptors.

Anticholinergic drugs reduce activity of the cholinergic internuncials in the striatum. They ameliorate tremor in particular, but the required dosage is liable to produce the autonomic side effects listed in *Clinical Panel 10.3*, (Ch. 10)

Surgery

In specialized neurosurgical centers, *pallidotomy* is the operation most often performed, with the objective of reducing the excessive inhibition of the VL nucleus of the thalamus. This and other operations are performed on the side opposite the clinically more disabled side, given that the eventual motor output, via cortico- and reticulospinal tracts, is mainly crossed. Lesions placed in the anterior part of the medial pallidal segment have been shown to reduce *rigidity* whereas lesions placed in the midregion reduce *akinesia* and *postural instability*. (Occasionally, a partial homonymous hemianopia is caused by damage to the optic tract (*Figure 28.3*).) *Tremor* may be abolished by a lesion placed in the VL nucleus of thalamus, where thalamocortical neurons are known to fire in synchrony with tremor.

An alternative to lesioning is to paralyze neurons by high-frequency (130 Hz) stimulation through implanted electrodes. The paralysis is caused by *depolarization block*, whereby target neurons are forbidden the time required for repolarization. This approach is being used in the STN to dramatic effect in patients with full-blown tremor, bradykinesia, and rigidity. All three are greatly ameliorated in most cases. Unilateral stimulation may be sufficient for bilateral relief, of rigidity in particular. The bilateral effect of depolarization block has been accounted for (in monkey experiments) by paralysis of an excitatory projection from STN to the GABAergic reticular part of the substantia nigra which, as already mentioned, gives an inhibitory supply to the cross-connected right and left locomotor center. In other words, STN blockage *disinhibits* the locomotor center.

Fetal nigral transplantation is being carried out in several specialized centers. Briefly, the procedure involves implantation of fetal substantia nigral cells into the putamen while patients are under immune suppression. Long-term clinical benefit has been observed, but some patients have developed uncontrollable athetoid muscle spasms.

What are the normal functions of the motor loop?

Although movements can be produced on the opposite side of the body by direct electrical stimulation of the healthy putamen, the basal ganglia do not normally initiate movements. Nevertheless, they are active during movements of all kinds, whether fast or slow. They seem to be involved in *scaling the strength* of muscle contractions and, in collaboration with SMA, in *organizing the requisite sequences* of excitation of cell columns in the motor cortex. They come into action after the corticospinal tract has already been activated by 'premotor' areas including the cerebellum. Because patients with PD have so much difficulty in performing internally generated movement sequences, it is believed that the putamen provides a reservoir of learned motor programs which it is able to assemble in appropriate sequence for the movements decided upon, and to transmit the coded information to SMA.

Cognitive loop

The head of the caudate nucleus receives a large projection from the prefrontal cortex, and it participates in *motor learning*. PET scan studies have demonstrated increased contralateral blood flow through the head of the caudate when novel motor actions are performed with one hand. There is also increased activity in the anterior part of the contralateral putamen, globus pallidus and ventral anterior (VA) nucleus of the thalamus. The VA nucleus completes an 'open' cognitive loop through its projection to the premotor cortex, and a 'closed' loop through a return projection to the prefrontal cortex. The cortical connections of the caudate suggest that it participates in *planning ahead*, particularly with respect to complex motor intentions. When the novel motor task has been practiced to the level of automatic execution, the motor loop becomes active instead.

Limbic loop

Figure 28.5 depicts the *limbic* basal ganglia loop. This loop passes from the inferior prefrontal cortex through the **nucleus accumbens** (anterior end of the striatum, *Figure 28.1D*) and ventral pallidum, with return via the mediodorsal nucleus of the thalamus to the inferior prefrontal cortex.

The limbic loop is likely to be involved in giving motor expression to emotions, e.g. through smiling or gesturing, or adoption of aggressive or submissive postures. The loop is rich in dopaminergic nerve endings, and their decline may account for the mask-like facies and absence of spontaneous gesturing characteristic of Parkinson's disease, and for the *dementia* which may set in after several years.

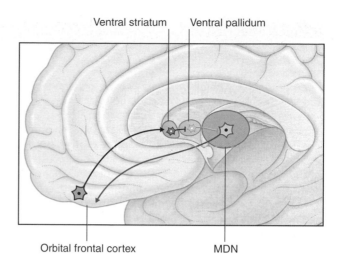

Ventral striatum   Ventral pallidum

Orbital frontal cortex   MDN

Figure 28.5 The limbic basal ganglia loop, right hemisphere. The medial dorsal nucleus of thalamus (MDN) is being released by means of disinhibition.

Oculomotor loop

The oculomotor loop commences in the *frontal eye field* and *posterior parietal cortex* (area 7). It passes through the caudate nucleus and through the reticular part of the substantia nigra (SNpr). It returns via the ventral anterior nucleus of the thalamus to the frontal eye field and prefrontal cortex. SNpr sends an inhibitory GABAergic projection to the superior colliculus, where it synapses upon cells controlling automatic saccades (Ch. 20). These cells are also supplied directly from the frontal eye field.

While the eyes are fixated, SNpr is tonically active. Whenever a deliberate saccade is about to be made toward another object, the oculomotor loop is activated and the superior colliculus is *disinhibited*. The superior colliculus then discharges to reinforce the activity of the direct pathway. Maximum speed (80 km/h) is achieved instantly, the eyeballs are flicked to the target, and SNpr resumes its vigilance.

In PD, *oculomotor hypokinesia* can be revealed by special tests. Saccades toward targets in the peripheral visual field tend to be slow, and sometimes inadequate. This hypokinesia can be explained on the basis of faulty disinhibition of the superior colliculus following associated neuronal degeneration within SNpr.

Other disorders involving the basic ganglia include several *hyperkinetic states* briefly described in *Clinical Panel 28.2*.

Clinical Panel 28.2   Other extrapyramidal disorders

Cerebral palsy

Cerebral palsy is an umbrella term covering a variety of motor disorders arising from damage to the brain during fetal life or in the perinatal period. The incidence is about 2 per 1000 live births in all countries.

The most frequent type of congenital motor disorder is *spastic diplegia*. During the early postnatal months affected children are usually 'floppy' (atonic), changing to a spastic state (of the lower limbs in particular) by the end of the first year. Remarkably, many children who are spastic at the age of 2 will be completely normal by the age of 5. Most of the remainder 'grow into their disability' and become more severely affected.

The ventricular system in spastic diplegia is dilated, owing to maldevelopment of periventricular oligodendrocytes in the 6th to 8th month of gestation, notably those myelinating corticospinal fibers destined for lumbosacral segments of the spinal cord. Intrauterine infection (*Figure CP 28.2.1*), ischemia, and metabolic disorders are etiological suspects.

Extrapyramidal or *dyskinetic* cerebral palsy is statistically correlated with perinatal asphyxia. In this condition, the striatum is particularly affected, perhaps because it is normally highly active metabolically in establishing synaptic connections with the pallidum.

Choreoathetosis is characteristic. *Chorea* refers to momentary spontaneous twitching of muscle groups in a more or less random manner, interfering with voluntary movements. *Athetosis* refers to writhing movements which are continuous except during sleep and may be so severe as to prevent sitting or standing. Waxing and waning of muscle tone commonly cause the head to roll about. Both movements are regarded as escape phenomena resulting from damage to the striatum.

Huntington's chorea

Huntington's chorea is an autosomal (chromosome 4) dominant, inherited disease which occurs in 50% of the offspring of affected families. Onset of symptoms is usually delayed until the 40s. The clinical history is one of chronic, progressive chorea, often with athetoid movements superimposed. Sooner or later, a progressive dementia sets in.

Hemiballism

Hemiballism (or hemiballismus) tends to occur in the elderly. It is known to result from thrombosis of a small branch of the posterior cerebral artery supplying the STN. The condition is perhaps the most remarkable one in the whole of clinical neurology. It is marked by the abrupt onset of wild, flailing movements of the contralateral arm, sometimes of the leg as well. The appearances suggest that the thalamocortical pathway from VLN to SMA has become intensely overactive.

This question may well be asked: if vascular destruction of STN results in hemiballism, why does STN paralysis by high-frequency stimulation not have the same effect? Occasionally it does, requiring immediate withdrawal of the electrode. But, in general, the VLN–SMA pathway remains sufficiently inhibited by underactivity in the 'direct' pathway.

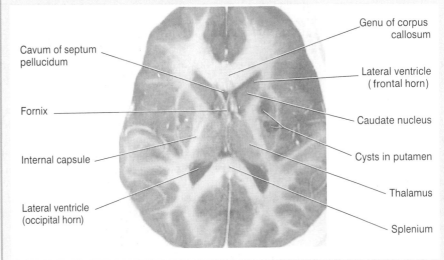

Cavum of septum pellucidum

Genu of corpus callosum

Fornix

Lateral ventricle (frontal horn)

Internal capsule

Caudate nucleus

Cysts in putamen

Lateral ventricle (occipital horn)

Thalamus

Splenium

Figure CP 28.2.1 Horizontal MRI slice at the level of the corpus striatum from a 2-year-old girl suffering from severe choreoathetosis as a result of intrauterine damage to her basal ganglia by toxoplasmosis. The putamen on both sides has been partly replaced by cysts. (MRI kindly provided by Professor J. Paul Finn, Director MRI Facility, Northwestern University School of Medicine, Chicago.)

Core Information

The basal ganglia are nuclear groups involved in movement control. They comprise the striatum (including nucleus accumbens), pallidum, subthalamic nucleus (STN), substantia nigra, and thalamic motor nuclei: VLN, VA, and MD. The pallidum has a lateral and a medial segment (GPL, GPM), the latter tapering into the midbrain as the reticular part of substantia nigra (SNpr). Four circuits commence in the cerebral cortex, pass through the basal ganglia, and return to the cortex. The compact part of substantia nigra (SNpc) stands aside of the circuits but influences them by way of the nigrostriatal pathway.

Cortical inputs to striatum and STN are excitatory. Striatal outputs are inhibitory to the pallidum; so, too are the pallidal outputs to STN and thalamus. STN is excitatory to GPM.

The 'direct' pathway, striatum → GPM, is facilitated by the normal tonic activity of nigrostriatal dopaminergic neurons. The 'indirect' pathway, striatum → GPL → STN → GPM is inhibited. In the *motor loop*, facilitation of the direct pathway is necessary for the SMA to become active before and during movement. SMA activity immediately prior to movement is detectable as the readiness potential, and is produced by silencing of GPM neurons with consequent liberation (disinhibition) of thalamocortical neurons to SMA, with follow-through to the motor cortex for initiation of movement.

Striatum and pallidum are somatotopically organized, permitting selective activation of body parts; STN is especially important for inhibition of unwanted movements.

The main function of the motor loop seems to be the appropriate sequencing of serial order actions for the execution of learned motor programs. In PD, the loss of nigrostriatal dopaminergic neurons causes the 'indirect pathway' to become dominant, with follow-through suppression of VL and reduced SMA activity, thus accounting for the characteristic bradykinesia. PD symptomatology also includes rigidity, tremor, and impairment of postural reflexes. Benign essential tremor and multisystem atrophy are too often misdiagnosed as PD.

The *cognitive loop* begins in the association cortex, and returns via VA nucleus of thalamus to the premotor and prefrontal cortex. It is actively engaged during motor learning, and also seems concerned with planning ahead for later movements.

The *limbic loop* begins in cingulate cortex and amygdala, passes through nucleus accumbens, and returns to SMA; it is probably involved in giving physical expression to the current emotional state.

The *oculomotor loop* disinhibits SNpr, thereby liberating the superior colliculus to execute a saccade.

Hyperkinetic states include many cases of cerebral palsy; also Huntington's chorea and hemiballism.

REFERENCES

Alheid, G.F., Heimer, L. and Switzer, R.C. (1990) Basal ganglia. In *The Human Nervous System* (Paxinos, G., ed.), pp. 483–582. San Diego: Academic Press.

Berger, W., Discher, M., Trippel, M., Ibrahim, I.K. and Dietz, V. (1992) Developmental aspects of stance regulation, compensation and adaptation. *Exp. Brain Res.* 90: 610–619.

Brooks, D.J. (1995) The role of the basal ganglia in motor control: contributions from PET. *J. Neurol. Sci.* 128: 1–13.

Brown, P. and Steiger, M.J. Basal ganglia disorders. In *Clinical Disorders of Balance Posture and Gait* (Bronstein, A.M., Brandt, T. and Woollacott, M., eds), pp. 156–166. London: Arnold.

Burne, J.A. and Lippold, O.C.J. (1996) Loss of tendon organ inhibition in Parkinson's disease. *Brain* 119: 1115–1121.

Ceballos-Baumann, A.O., Boecker, H., Bartenstein, P., von Halkenhayn, H.R., Riescher, H., Conrad, B., Moringlane, J.R. and Alesch, F. (1999) A PET study of subthalamic nucleus stimulation in Parkinson's disease. *Arch. Neurol.* 56: 997–1003.

Chase, T.N., Oh, J.D. and Blanchet, P.J. (1998) Neostriatal mechanisms in Parkinson's disease. *Neurology* 51 (Suppl 2): S30–S35.

Crossman, A.R. (2000) Functional anatomy of movement disorders. *J. Anat.* 196: 519–525.

Henderson, J.M. and Dunnett, S.B. (1998) Targeting the subthalamic nucleus in the treatment of Parkinson's disease. *Brain Res. Bull.* 46: 467–474.

Hornykiewicz, O. (1998) Biochemical aspects of Parkinson's disease. *Neurology* 51 (Suppl 2): S2–S9.

Kuban, K.C.K. and Leviton, A. (1994) Cerebral palsy. *New Engl. J. Med.* 330: 188–195.

Le, W-D., Rowe, D.B., Jankovic, J., Xie, W. and Appel, S.H. (1999) Effects of cerebrospinal fluid from patients with Parkinson's disease on dopaminergic cells. *Arch. Neurol.* 56: 194–202.

Leonard, B.E. (1997) Drug treatment of Parkinson's disease. In *Fundamentals of Psychopharmacology* (same author), pp. 233–248. Chichester: Wiley.

Lozano, A.M., Lang, A.E., Hutchison, W.D. and Dostrovsky, J.O. (1998) New developments in understanding the etiology of Parkinson's disease and its treatment. *Curr. Opin. Neurobiol.* 8: 783–790.

Menon, G. and Menon, V. (1995) *Parkinson's Disease and Related Disorders*. Published by G. Kamath for Menon Foundation.

Meunier, S., Pol, S., Houeto, J.L. and Vidailhet, M. (2000) Abnormal reciprocal inhibition between antagonist muscles in Parkinson's disease. *Brain* 123: 1017–1026.

Pfann, K.D., Penn, R.D., Shannon, K.M. and Corcos, D.M. (1998) Pallidotomy and bradykinesia. *Neurology* 51: 796–803.

Poewe, W.H. and Wenning, G.K. (1998) The natural history of Parkinson's disease. *Ann. Neurol.* 44 (Suppl 1): S1–S9.

Stanley, F.J. (1994) The aetiology of cerebral palsy. *Early Hum. Dev.* 36: 81–88.

Summers, J.J. (1994) The pathogenesis of gait hypokinesia in Parkinson's disease. *Brain* 117: 1169–1181.

Weiss, P., Stelmach, G.E. and Hefter, H. (1997) Programming a movement sequence in Parkinson's disease. *Brain* 120: 91–102.

Wichmann T. and DeLong, M.R. (1996) Functional and pathophysiological models of the basal ganglia. *Curr. Opin. Neurobiol.* 6: 751–758.

Olfactory and limbic systems

OLFACTORY SYSTEM

The olfactory system is remarkable in four respects:

1 The somas of the primary afferent neurons occupy a surface epithelium.

2 The axons of the primary afferents enter the cerebral cortex directly; second-order afferents are not interposed.

3 The primary afferent neurons undergo continuous turnover, being replaced from basal stem cells.

4 The pathway to the highest cortical centers (in the frontal lobe) is entirely ipsilateral.

The olfactory system comprises the olfactory epithelium and olfactory nerves; the olfactory bulb and tract; and several areas of olfactory cortex.

Olfactory epithelium

The olfactory epithelium occupies the upper one-fifth of the lateral and septal walls of the nasal cavity. The epithelium contains three cell types (*Figure 29.1*):

1 **Olfactory neurons**. These are bipolar neurons, each with a dendrite extending to the epithelial surface and an unmyelinated axon contributing to the olfactory

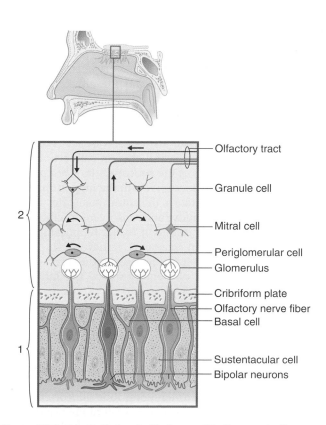

Figure 29.1 Connections of olfactory epithelium and olfactory bulb. The second glomerulus from the left is 'on line' (see text).

nerve. The dendrites are capped by immotile cilia containing molecular receptor sites. The axons run upward through the cribriform ('sieve-like') plate of the ethmoid bone and enter the olfactory bulb. The axons (some 3 million on each side) are grouped into fila (bundles) by investing Schwann cells. The collective fila constitute the **olfactory nerve**.

2 **Sustentacular cells** are interspersed among the bipolar neurons.

3 **Basal stem cells** lie between the other two cell types. Olfactory bipolar neurons are unique among mammalian neurons in that they undergo a continuous cycle of growth, degeneration, and replacement. The basal cells transform into fresh bipolar neurons, which survive for about a month. Replacement declines over time, accounting for the general reduction in olfactory sensitivity with age.

Olfactory bulb   (Figure 29.1)

The olfactory bulb consists of three-layered allocortex surrounding the commencement of the olfactory tract. The chief cortical neurons are some 50 000 **mitral cells**, which receive the olfactory nerve fibers and give rise to the olfactory tract.

Contact between olfactory fibers and mitral cell dendrites takes place in some 2000 **glomeruli**, which are sites of innumerable synapses and have a glial investment. Glomeruli which are 'on-line' (active) inhibit neighboring, 'off-line' glomeruli through the mediation of GABAergic **periglomerular cells** (cf. the horizontal cells of the retina). Mitral cell activity is also sharpened at a deeper level by **granule cells**, which are devoid of axons (cf. the amacrine cells of the retina). The granule cells receive excitatory dendrodendritic contacts from active mitral cells and they suppress neighboring mitral cells through inhibitory (GABA) dendrodendritic contacts.

Central connections

Mitral cell axons run centrally in the **olfactory tract** (*Figure 29.2*). The tract divides in front of the anterior perforated substance into **medial** and **lateral olfactory striae**.

The medial stria contains axons from the **anterior olfactory nucleus**, which consists of multipolar neurons scattered within the olfactory tract. Some of these axons travel to the septal area via the diagonal band (see later, under Limbic System). Others cross the midline in the anterior commissure and inhibit mitral cell activity in the contralateral bulb (by exciting granule cells there). The result is a relative enhancement of the more active bulb, providing a directional cue to the source of olfactory stimulation.

The lateral olfactory stria terminates in the **piriform lobe** of the anterior temporal cortex. The human piriform lobe includes the cortical part of the amygdala, the uncus, and the anterior end of the parahippocampal gyrus. The highest center for olfactory discrimination is the posterior part of the orbitofrontal cortex, which receives connections from the piriform lobe via the mediodorsal nucleus of the thalamus.

A routine test of olfactory function is to ask the patient to identify strong-smelling substances such as coffee and chocolate through each nostril in turn. Loss of smell, or **anosmia**, may not be detected by the patient without testing if it is unilateral. If it is bilateral, the complaint may be one of loss of taste because the flavor of foodstuffs depends on the olfactory qualities of volatile elements; in such cases, the four primary taste sensations (sweet, sour, salty, bitter) are preserved. Unilateral anosmia may be caused by a *meningioma* compressing the olfactory bulb or tract, or by a head injury with fracture of the anterior cranial fossa. Anosmia may be a clue to a fracture, and should prompt tests for leakage of cerebrospinal fluid into the nasal cavity.

Olfactory auras are a typical prodromal feature of *uncinate epilepsy* (see *Clinical Panel 29.2*).

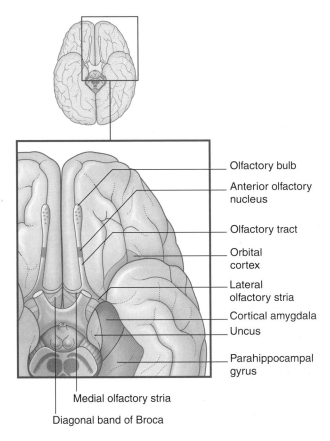

Olfactory bulb

Anterior olfactory nucleus

Olfactory tract

Orbital cortex

Lateral olfactory stria

Cortical amygdala

Uncus

Parahippocampal gyrus

Medial olfactory stria

Diagonal band of Broca

Figure 29.2 Brain viewed from below, showing cortical olfactory areas.

The medial forebrain bundle links the olfactory cortical areas with the hypothalamus and brainstem. These linkages trigger autonomic responses such as salivation and gastric contraction, and arousal responses through the reticular formation.

Points of clinical interest are mentioned in *Clinical Panel 29.1*.

LIMBIC SYSTEM

The limbic system comprises the limbic cortex (so-called *limbic lobe*) and related subcortical nuclei. The term 'limbic'

(Broca, 1878) originally referred to a *limbus* or rim of cortex immediately adjacent to the corpus callosum and diencephalon. The limbic cortex is now taken to include the three-layered *allocortex* of the hippocampal formation and septal area together with transitional *mesocortex* in the parahippocampal gyrus, cingulate gyrus, and insula. The principal subcortical component of the limbic system is the amygdala, which merges with the cortex on the medial side of the temporal pole. Closely related subcortical areas are the hypothalamus and reticular formation, and the nucleus accumbens. Cortical areas closely related to the limbic system are the orbitofrontal cortex and the temporal pole (*Figure 29.3*).

Figure 29.4 is a graphic reconstruction of mainly subcortical limbic areas.

Parahippocampal gyrus

The parahippocampal gyrus is a major junctional region between the cerebral neocortex and the allocortex of the hippocampal formation. Its anterior part is the **entorhinal cortex** (area 28 of Brodmann), which is six-layered but has certain peculiar features. The entorhinal cortex can be said to face in two directions. Its *neocortical face* exchanges massive numbers of afferent and efferent connections with all four association areas of the neocortex. Its *allocortical face* exchanges abundant connections with the hippocampal formation. In the broadest terms, the entorhinal cortex receives a constant stream of cognitive and sensory information from the association areas, transmits it to the hippocampal formation for consolidation (see later), retrieves it in consolidated form, and returns it to the association areas where it is encoded in the form of memory traces. The fornix and its connections form a second, circuitous pathway from hippocampus to neocortex.

Hippocampal formation

The hippocampal formation comprises the **subiculum**, the **hippocampus proper**, and the **dentate gyrus** (*Figure 29.5*). All three are composed of temporal lobe allocortex which has tucked itself into an S-shaped scroll along the floor of the lateral ventricle. The band-like origin of the fornix from the subiculum and hippocampus is the **fimbria**. The hippocampus is also known as *Ammon's horn* (after an Egyptian

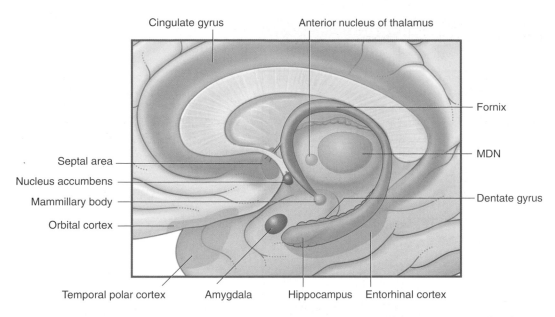

Cingulate gyrus

Anterior nucleus of thalamus

Fornix

MDN

Septal area

Nucleus accumbens

Mammillary body

Orbital cortex

Dentate gyrus

Temporal polar cortex   Amygdala   Hippocampus   Entorhinal cortex

Figure 29.3 Medial view of cortical and subcortical limbic areas. MDN, mediodorsal nucleus of thalamus.

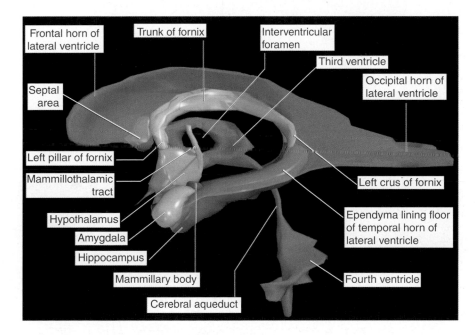

Frontal horn of
lateral ventricle

Trunk of fornix

Interventricular
foramen

Third ventricle

Occipital horn of
lateral ventricle

Septal
area

Left pillar of fornix

Mammillothalamic
tract

Left crus of fornix

Ependyma lining floor
of temporal horn of
lateral ventricle

Hypothalamus

Amygdala

Hippocampus

Mammillary body

Fourth ventricle

Cerebral aqueduct

Figure 29.4 Three-dimensional computerized reconstruction of postmortem brain showing components of the limbic system in relation to the ventricular system. (Excerpt of figure, from Kretschmann, H-J. and Weinrich, W. (1998) *Neurofunctional Systems: 3D Reconstructions with Correlated Neuroimaging: Text and CD-ROM*. New York: Thieme, with kind permission of the authors and the publisher.)

deity with a ram's head). For research purposes, it is divided into four *cornu ammonis* (CA) zones (*Fig. 29.6A*).

The principal cells of the subiculum and hippocampus are **pyramidal cells**; those of the dentate gyrus are **granule cells**. The dendrites of both granule and pyramidal cells are studded with dendritic spines. The hippocampal formation is also rich in inhibitory (GABA) internuncial neurons.

It should be mentioned that in general discussions related to memory, it is customary to use the term 'hippocampus' as synonymous with 'hippocampal formation'.

Connections

Afferents

The largest afferent connection of the hippocampal formation is the **perforant path**, which projects from the entorhinal cortex onto the dendrites of dentate granule cells (*Figure 29.6B*). The subiculum gives rise to a second, *alvear* path which contributes to a sheet of fibers on the ventricular surface of the hippocampus, the **alveus**.

The axons of the granule cells are called **mossy fibers**;

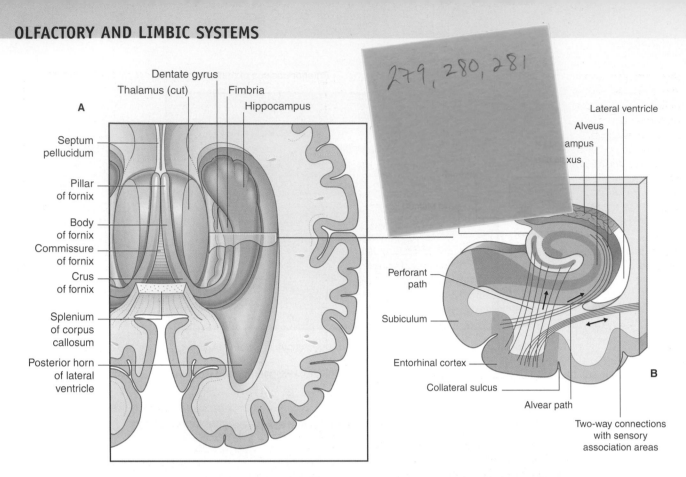

279, 280, 281

Figure 29.5 Hippocampal formation. **(A)** View from above. **(B)** Enlargement from **A** showing the entorhinal cortex and the three component parts of the hippocampal formation.

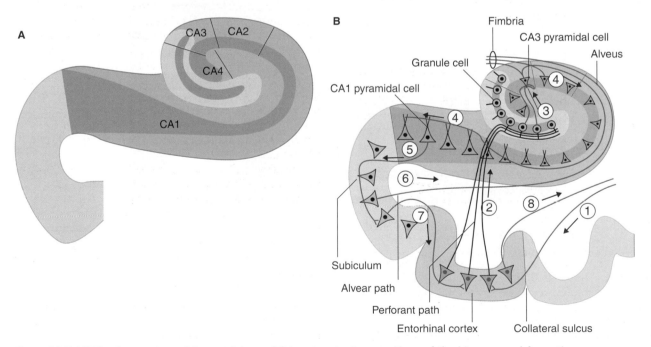

Figure 29.6 (A) The four sectors of Ammon's horn. **(B)** Input–output connections of the hippocampal formation.

1 Afferent from sensory association cortex.
2 Entorhinal cortex projecting perforant path fiber to dentate gyrus.
3 Dentate granule cell projecting to CA3.
4 CA3 principal neuron projecting into fimbria and CA1.
5 CA1 principal cell projecting to subiculum.
6 Subicular principal cell projecting into fimbria.
7 Subicular principal cell projecting into entorhinal cortex.
8 Entorhinal pyramidal cell projecting to sensory association cortex.

they synapse upon pyramidal cells in the CA3 sector. The axons of the CA3 pyramidal cells project into the fimbria; before doing so they give off *Schaffer collaterals* which run a recurrent course from CA3 to CA1. CA1 projects into the entorhinal cortex.

Auditory information enters the hippocampus from the association cortex of the superior and middle temporal gyri. The supramarginal gyrus (area 40) transmits coded information about personal space (the *body schema* described in Ch. 27) and extrapersonal (visual) space. From the occipito-temporal region on the inferior surface, information concerning object shape and color, and facial recognition, is projected to cortex called *perirhinal*, or *transrhinal*, immediately lateral to the entorhinal cortex. From here, it enters the hippocampus. A return projection from entorhinal to perirhinal cortex is linked to the temporal polar and prefrontal cortex.

In addition to the discrete afferent connections mentioned above, the hippocampus is diffusely innervated from several sources, mainly by way of the fornix:

- A dense *cholinergic* innervation, of particular significance in relation to memory, is received from the septal nucleus.

- A *noradrenergic* innervation is received from the cerulean nucleus.

- A *serotoninergic* innervation enters from the raphe nuclei of the midbrain. The linkage between serotonin depletion and major depression is mentioned in Chapter 23.

- A *dopaminergic* innervation enters from the ventral tegmental area of the midbrain. The linkage between dopamine and schizophrenia is mentioned in Chapter 27.

Efferents

The largest efferent connection is a massive projection via the entorhinal cortex to the association areas of the neocortex. A second, forward projection is the **fornix** (*Figure 29.5A*). The fornix is a direct continuation of the **fimbria**, which receives axons from the subiculum and hippocampus proper. The **crus** of the fornix arches up beneath the corpus callosum, where it joins its fellow to form the **trunk** and links with its opposite number through a small **hippocampal commissure**. Anteriorly, the trunk divides into two **pillars**. Each pillar splits around the anterior commissure, sending *precommissural* fibers to the septal area and *postcommissural* fibers to the anterior hypothalamus, mammillary body, and medial forebrain bundle. The mammillary body projects into the anterior nucleus of thalamus, which projects in turn to the cingulate cortex, completing the *Papez circuit* from cingulate cortex to hippocampus, with return to cingulate cortex via fornix, mammillary body and anterior thalamic nucleus (*Figure 29.7*).

The term *medial temporal lobe* is clinically inclusive of the hippocampal formation, parahippocampal gyrus, and amygdala. The term is most often used in relation to seizures (*Clinical Panel 29.2*).

Memory function of the hippocampal formation

The evidence for a *mnemonic* (memory) function in the hippocampal formation is discussed at considerable length in psychology texts. Some insights are listed below.

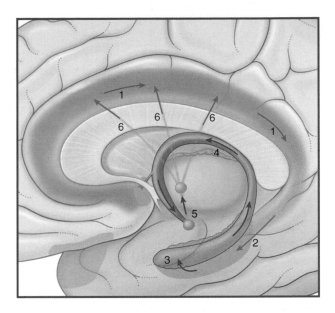

Figure 29.7 The Papez circuit.

1 Backward-projecting neurons in the cingulate gyrus;
2 Projection into the entorhinal cortex;
3 Projection into hippocampus;
4 Fornix;
5 Mammillothalamic tract;
6 Projections from anterior nucleus of thalamus to cingulate cortex.

- Bilateral damage or removal of the anterior part of the hippocampal formation is followed by *anterograde amnesia*, a term used to denote absence of conscious recall of newly acquired information for more than a few minutes. When asked to name a commonplace object, the subject will have no difficulty because access to long-term memories does not require the anterior hippocampus. However, when the same object is shown a few minutes later, the subject will not remember having seen it. This is known as a loss of *declarative* (data-based) memory.

  Procedural (how-to-do) memory is preserved. If asked to assemble a jigsaw puzzle, the subject will do it in the normal way. When asked to repeat the exercise the next day, the subject will do it faster although there will be no recollection of having seen the puzzle previously. *The hippocampus is not required for procedural memory*. The cerebellum appears to be the primary store for procedural memory, perhaps linked to the motor teaching function of the inferior olivary nucleus (Ch. 22).

- *Long-term potentiation* (LTP) is uniquely powerful in dentate gyrus and hippocampus. It is regarded as vital for preservation (consolidation) of memory traces. Under experimental conditions, LTP is most easily demonstrated in the perforant path–dentate granule cell connections and in the Schaffer collateral–CA1 connections. A strong, brief (milliseconds) stimulus to the perforant path or Schaffer collaterals induces the target cells to show long-lasting (hours) sensitivity to a fresh stimulus. LTP is associated with a cascade of biochemical events in the target neurons, following

Clinical Panel 29.2 Temporal lobe epilepsy

Next to vascular disorders, seizures (epileptic attacks) are the commonest group of problems encountered in clinical neurology. Some 3% of the population suffer two or more attacks during their lifetime.

The term 'seizure' refers to a transient alteration of behavior brought about by abnormal burst-firing of neurons in the cerebral cortex. Seizures are divided into two main categories:

- *Primary generalized tonic–clonic seizures* are characterized by sudden onset of unconsciousness with falling. The body stiffens for up to a minute (tonic stage) and then exhibits jerky movements of all four limbs and chewing movements of the mouth for a second minute (clonic stage). A third minute is spent in more relaxed unconsciousness. Electroencephalographic (EEG) recordings taken at the onset of this kind of *ictus* (attack) show simultaneous bilateral burst-firing all over the cortex.

- *Primary partial seizures* are more common. They nearly always originate in a focus of run-away neural activity within the temporal lobe and spread over the general cortex within seconds to trigger a *secondary* tonic–clonic seizure. Premonitory 'auras' at the beginning of temporal lobe seizures include well-formed visual or auditory hallucinations (scenes, sound sequences), a sense of familiarity with the surrounding scene ('*déjà vu*'), a sense of strangeness ('*jamais vu*') or a sense of fear. Attacks originating in the uncus are ushered in by unpleasant olfactory or gustatory auras.

Drug treatment of seizures (see below) is not always successful, and surgery is frequently undertaken in intractable cases. Following accurate localization of the ictal (seizure) focus by means of recording electrodes inserted into the exposed temporal lobe, a tissue block including the focus may be removed, with abolition of seizures in four out of five cases. Histological examination of the surgical biopsy typically reveals *hippocampal sclerosis*: the picture is one of glial scarring, with extensive neuronal loss in CA2 and CA3 sectors. The granule cells of the dentate gyrus are relatively well preserved. Loss of inhibitory, GABA internuncials has been blamed in the past but these cells have recently been shown to persist. Instead, the granule cells appear to be *disinhibited*, because of loss of minute, excitatory, **basket cells** from among their dendrites.

Because 30% of sufferers from temporal lobe epilepsy have first-degree relatives similarly afflicted, often from childhood, a genetic influence must be significant. One possibility could be 'faulty wiring' of the hippocampus during mid-fetal life. Histological preparations show areas of congenital misplacement of hippocampal pyramidal cells, some lying on their sides or even in the subjacent white matter.

The sclerosis is regarded as a typical CNS healing process following extensive loss of neurons. The neuronal loss in turn seems to be inflicted by *glutamate toxicity* – a known effect of excessively high rates of discharge of pyramidal cells in any part of the cerebral cortex. Dentate granule cells are the main source of burst-firing, which is no surprise in view of their natural role in long-term potentiation and kindling (see main text).

Anticonvulsant drugs are of a broadly predictable nature. Most of them enhance GABA-mediated inhibitory processes. Some are used in order to stabilize the membranes of excitatory nerve terminals, making their ion channels less permeable to sodium and/or calcium.

---

activation of appropriate glutamate receptors. It is accompanied by the rapid (within minutes), transient appearance of new synaptic contacts and the expansion of old ones.

LTP is described as an *associative* phenomenon, because it requires that the powerful, depolarizing stimulus must be coupled with a weak stimulus to the depolarized neuron from another source. LTP is promoted by *opioid peptides*, which are co-released from perforant path neurons, and by *norepinephrine* and *dopamine*. The two amines may have a bearing on the attentional or motivational state at the time of learning.

- In both human and animal experiments, *cholinergic activity in the hippocampus* seems to be significant for learning. In human volunteers, central ACh blockade (by administration of scopolamine) severely impairs memory for lists of names or numbers whereas a cholinesterase inhibitor (physostigmine) gives above-normal results. Clinically, hippocampal cholinergic activity is severely reduced in Alzheimer's disease (AD), which is particularly associated with amnesia (see *Clinical Panel 29.3*).

- *Kindling* ('lighting a fire') is a property unique to the hippocampal formation and amygdala, although its relationship to learning is not obvious. Kindling is the progressively increasing group response of neurons to a repetitive stimulus of uniform strength. In both humans and experimental animals, it can spread from mesocortex to neocortex and cause generalized convulsive seizures.

- The contribution of the fornix projection to memory is uncertain. Indirect evidence has been adduced from *diencephalic amnesia*, a state of anterograde amnesia which may follow bilateral damage to the diencephalon. Such damage may interrupt the *Papez circuit* linking the fornix to the cingulate gyrus by way of the mammillary

Clinical Panel 29.3   Alzheimer's disease

Dementia is defined as a severe loss of cognitive function without impairment of consciousness. AD is the commonest cause of dementia, afflicting 5% of people in their seventh decade and 20% of people in their ninth. AD patients fill 20% of all beds in psychiatric institutions.

MRI brain scans usually reveal severe atrophy of the cerebral cortex, with widening of the sulci and enlargement of the ventricular system. The primary sensory and motor areas, and the upper regions of the prefrontal cortex, are relatively well preserved.

Postmortem histological studies of the cerebral cortex reveal:

- Extensive loss of pyramidal neurons throughout the brain.
- *Amyloid plaques* and *neurofibrillary tangles*, notably in the hippocampus and amygdala. The plaques begin in the walls of small blood vessels and have been explained in terms of an enzyme defect resulting in abnormal, *beta-amyloid* protein production. The tangles are made up of clumps of microtubules associated with an abnormal variant of a microtubule-associated *tau* protein. The tangles are progressively replaced by amyloid.
- Loss of up to 50% of the cholinergic neurons from the basal nucleus of Meynert and from the septal area, together with their extensive projections through the cerebral isocortex and mesocortex. Indeed, degenerating ACh terminals seem to contribute to the neurofibrillary tangles in the temporal lobe.

Hypometabolism can be shown on PET scans arranged to detect glucose utilization. This is attributable in part to loss of pyramidal cells, and in part to loss of cholinergic innervation of the pyramidal cells remaining. Healthy pyramidal neurons have excitatory ACh receptors in their cell membranes.

Although the pattern of degeneration varies from case to case, its general trend is to commence in the medial temporal lobe and to travel upward and forward. The following clinical features are explained in that sequence:

Dwindling hippocampal function. Anterograde amnesia leads to *forgetfulness*, e.g. recounting a personal event within minutes of telling it (loss of present-time episodic memory); difficulty in finding one's way around familiar streets, or alarming misjudgments while driving an automobile (hippocampal activity is required to sustain parietal lobe *spatial sense*); *attentional deficit*, whose earliest manifestation is an inability to switch attention from one thing to another.

Dwindling occipitotemporal function. Damage to area 37 leads to an inability to read and write. Damage to the temporal polar region leads to distressing failure to recognize the faces of family and friends. Involvement of the supramarginal and angular gyri leads to an inability to write.

Dwindling frontal lobe function. Usually within 3 years of onset, the patient is 'spaced out', staring at walls and seemingly unaware of what is going on in the room. This 'vacant' state lasts for up to 5 or 6 years antemortem.

An unusual variant, known as *early-onset AD*, shows clear evidence of an autosomal dominant trait. The illness appears during the fourth or fifth decade. Chromosomal analyses have revealed a specific mutation in the gene coding for amyloid precursor protein on the long arm of chromosome 21. This mutation is also found in Down's syndrome, where sufferers surviving into middle age usually develop AD.

---

body and the anterior nucleus of the thalamus. Complete transection of the fornix may have the same effect, although amnesia is not an invariable result.

Left vs right hippocampal functions

In keeping with known hemispheric asymmetries, the left anterior hippocampus and dorsolateral prefrontal cortex (DLPFC) are engaged in encoding novel material involving language function. Also consistent is the finding that the right hippocampus and right inferior parietal lobe are engaged in spatial tasks such as driving a car (*Figure 29.8*). Blood flow in the DLPFC increases more on the left side during driving, presumably because of the 'inner speech' that occurs when exploring novel territory.

Anterior vs posterior hippocampal functions

The hippocampus is about 8 cm in length, and there is evidence for anteroposterior functional specialization with respect to novelty vs familiarity, e.g. when novel material is being read on a screen the left anterior hippocampus is especially active, but with development of familiarity with repeated exposure, activity shifts to the posterior part, suggesting that this region is involved in encoding material into long-term memory. Consistent with this observation is the clinical observation that development of retrograde amnesia requires posterior damage. This retrograde amnesia most often follows head injury and is episodic rather than declarative, e.g. the patient may have no recollection of his or her past life but retains the ability to retrieve the identity of common objects from long-term memory stores; these are believed to reside in the relevant association areas of the neocortex.

Insula

The anterior insula is a cortical center for pain (*Box 29.1*). The central region is continuous with the frontoparietal and

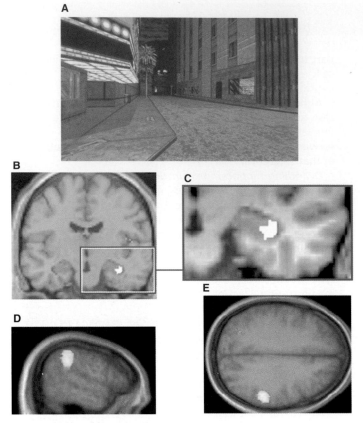

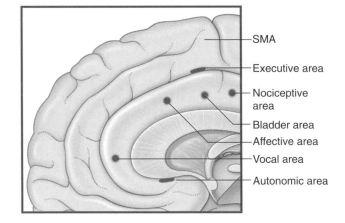

Figure 29.8 Navigation in a virtual environment. **(A)** Scene from a virtual town. Subjects navigated through the town using a keypad to stay clear of obstacles. PET scans taken during the virtual journey showed increased activation, **(B)** and **(C)**, within the right hippocampus and **(D)** and **(E)** within the right supramarginal gyrus. (Kindly provided by Dr Eleanor Maguire, Wellcome Department of Cognitive Neurology, Institute of Neurology, University College, London, UK, and with permission from the Editor of *Current Opinion in Neurobiology*.)

temporal opercular cortex, and it seems to have a *language* rather than a limbic function. During language tasks, PET scans show activity there as well as in the opercular speech receptive and motor areas – but not in people with congenital dyslexia, where it remains silent (Ch. 27). The posterior insula is interconnected with the entorhinal cortex and the amygdala, and is therefore presumed to participate in emotional responses – perhaps in the context of pain evaluation.

Cingulate cortex and posterior parahippocampal gyrus

The cingulate cortex is part of the Papez circuit, receiving a projection from the anterior nucleus of the thalamus and becoming continuous with the parahippocampal gyrus behind the splenium of the corpus callosum.

The *anterior* cingulate cortex belongs to the *rostral limbic system* which includes the amygdala, ventral striatum, orbitofrontal cortex, and anterior insular cortex.

Six functional areas can be discerned in the anterior cingulate cortex (*Figure 29.9*).

1 An *executive area* is connected directly with the DLPFC and with the supplementary motor area (SMA). The executive area becomes active prior to execution of willed movements, including voluntary saccades (Ch. 26) – and even prior to the SMA itself. The executive area is thought to have special significance, together with the DLPFC, in generating *appropriate motor plan selection* by the SMA.

Figure 29.9 Functional areas in the anterior cingulate cortex. SMA, supplementary motor area.

2 A *pain perception area* receives afferents from the medial dorsal nucleus of the thalamus (*Box 29.1*).

3 An *emotional area* lies close to the pain perception area. When volunteers 'think happy' while undergoing PET scans, the anterior cingulate cortex 'lights up' and the amygdala 'switches off'. A reverse result occurs when volunteers 'think sad'. Anterior cingulectomy has often been performed in the past, yielding successful control of aggressive psychiatric disorders.

Box 29.1 Pain and the brain

The International Association for the Study of Pain has given the following definition:
Pain is an unpleasant sensory and emotional experience associated with actual or potential tissue damage or described in terms of such damage.
This definition emphasizes the *affective* (emotional) component of pain. Its other component is *sensory-discriminative* ('where and how much?').

The current consensus is that there exists a *lateral*, sensory-discriminative pathway and a *medial* affective pathway in relation to pain (*Figure Box 29.1.1*).

Lateral pain pathway

For the trunk and limbs, the lateral pathway arises in the posterior gray horn of the spinal cord and projects as the lateral spinothalamic tract to the posterior part of the contralateral ventral posterior lateral nucleus of thalamus. For the head and neck, it commences in the spinal nucleus of the trigeminal nerve and occupies the trigeminothalamic projection to the contralateral posterior medial thalamic nucleus. The onward projection is mainly to the primary somatic sensory cortex (SI), partly to the upper bank of the lateral sulcus (SII). The arrangement is somatotopic, as can be seen on PET scanning when a noxious heat stimulus is applied to different parts of the body. Animal investigations demonstrate intensity responsive, nociceptive-specific neurons in SI, having appropriately small peripheral receptive fields, ideal candidates for encoding the 'where and how much' aspects of pain.

Nociceptive neurons in SII are less numerous, and many receive visual inputs as well. They may be concerned with facilitating visual attention to the source of the stimulus.

Medial pain pathway

The medial pathway is polysynaptic, via spinoreticular and trigeminoreticular tracts to the contralateral medial dorsal thalamic nucleus (among others), with onward projection to the anterior cingulate cortex (ACCx). That the ACCx is concerned with the affective component of pain experience is strongly supported by the effect of surgical undercutting (cingulotomy) or removal (cingulectomy) as a treatment for chronic pain. Patients report that the intensity of their pain is unchanged but that it lost its aggressive nature. Precisely the same result follows morphine injection – presumably because the anterior cingulate has the greatest number of opiate receptors in the cerebral cortex.

Following cingulotomy, edema of the bladder control area frequently causes temporary urinary incontinence. More importantly, more than half of all patients show permanent 'flatness of affect', i.e. low experience of either elation or depression.

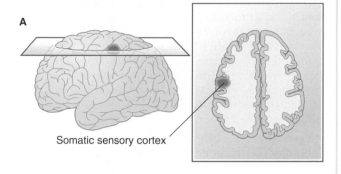

A

Somatic sensory cortex

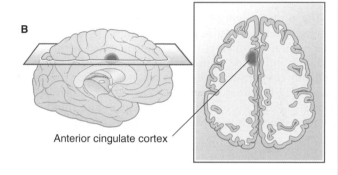

B

Anterior cingulate cortex

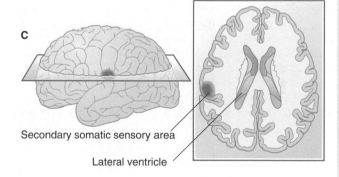

C

Secondary somatic sensory area

Lateral ventricle

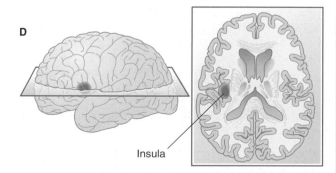

D

Insula

Figure Box 29.1.1 Areas showing increased metabolic activity following application of noxious heat to the right forearm.

4 A *bladder control area* becomes increasingly active during bladder filling (Ch. 21).

5 A *vocalization area* becomes active, together with the DLPFC, during *decision-making* about appropriate sentence construction for speech activity. Electrical stimulation of this area causes jumbling of speech. *Stammering* in children is associated with *reduced* blood flow in the left anterior cingulate gyrus during speech. Blood flow there is also reduced in people suffering from *Tourette's syndrome*, which is characterized by brief, loud utterances of a single syllable or phrase, often offensive to the ear.

6 An *autonomic area*, below the rostrum of the corpus callosum, elicits autonomic and respiratory responses when stimulated electrically. This area is thought to participate in eliciting the visceral responses typical of emotional states.

The posterior cingulate gyrus (area 23 of Brodmann) merges with the posterior parahippocampal gyrus (area 36). This cortical complex is richly interconnected with visual, auditory, and tactile/spatial association areas. The complex evidently contains memory stores related to these functions because PET studies reveal increased activity there when scenes or experiences are conjured up in the mind. The complex is also engaged during reading (Ch. 27).

Amygdala

The **amygdala** (*Gr.* almond; also called the *amygdaloid body* or *amygdaloid complex*) is a large group of nuclei above and in front of the temporal horn of the lateral ventricle and anterior to the tail of the caudate nucleus. *The amygdala is primarily associated with the emotion of fear*, as illustrated by the effect of looking at an angry or fearful face (*Figure 29.10*). Current clinical and basic science ambition is to gain diagnostic and therapeutic insights into the role of the amygdala with regard to various *phobias* and *anxiety states* prevalent in both the young and the adult population. The connections of the amygdala (inasmuch as these are understood) are consistent with the present perception of a 'bottleneck' position in the perception and expression of fear.

Afferent pathways

Within the amygdala, nuclear groups receiving afferents are predominantly laterally placed and are usually referred to collectively as the **lateral nucleus**. In *Table 29.1* and related Figures, the afferents are segregated into subcortical and cortical.

Subcortical access, depicted in *Figure 29.11*, is thought to be especially important in infancy and childhood, at a time when the amygdala is developing faster than the hippocampus and is capable of acquiring fearful memory traces

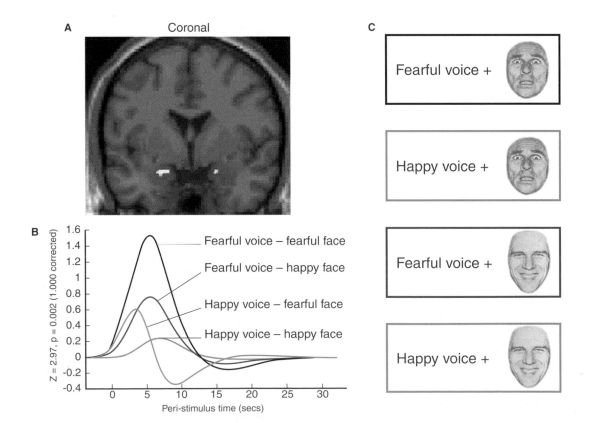

Figure 29.10 Cross-modal emotional responses. **(A)** Coronal structural MRI image showing a superimposed fMRI map of bilateral activation of the amygdala in a volunteer observing a fearful face accompanied by a fearful voice (see **C**). At the opposite end of the spectrum, amygdalar activity was below normal level in the presence of a happy face and voice. **(B)** The associated graph shows experimental condition-specific fMRI responses in the amygdala. (Kindly provided by Professor R.J. Dolan, Wellcome Department of Cognitive Neurology, Institute of Neurology, University College, London, UK.)

Table 29.1 Afferents to lateral nucleus of amygdala

Nature	Subcortical source	Cortical source
Tactile	Ventral posterior nucleus of thalamus	Parietal lobe
Auditory	Medial geniculate body	Superior temporal gyrus
Visual	*Lateral geniculate body	Occipital cortex
Olfactory		Piriform lobe
Mnemonic (memory)		Hippocampus/ entorhinal cortex
Cardiac	Hypothalamus	
Nociceptive		Insula
Cognitive		Orbital cortex
Attention-related	Cerulean nucleus	Basal nucleus of Meynert

*Afferents from LGB to amygdala have yet to be clearly identified.

Table 29.2 Efferents from central nucleus of amygdala

Target nucleus/pathway	Function/effect
Peri-aqueductal gray matter (to medulla/raphespinal tract)	Antinociception
Peri-aqueductal gray matter (to medullary reticulospinal tract)	Freezing
Cerulean nucleus	Arousal
Norepinephrine medullary neurons (projection to lateral gray horn)	Tachycardia/ hypertension
Hypothalamus/dorsal nucleus of vagus (to heart)	Bradycardia/fainting
Hypothalamus (liberation of corticotropin-releasing hormone)	Stress hormone secretion
Parabrachial nucleus (to medullary respiratory nuclei)	Hyperventilation

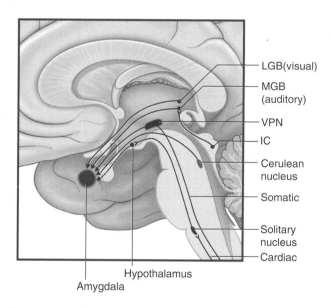

Figure 29.11 Subcortical afferents to lateral nucleus of amygdala. IC, inferior colliculus; LGB, MGB, lateral, medial geniculate body; VPN, ventral posterior nucleus of thalamus.

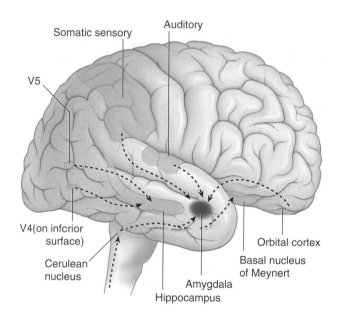

Figure 29.12 Cortical afferents to lateral nucleus of amygdala. V4, object/face recognition area; V5, motion detection area.

without hippocampal participation. Such memories cannot be *consciously* recalled at any later time despite generating physical responses of an 'escape' nature. The general-sense and special-sense pathways listed and depicted are sufficiently comprehensive to account for the acquisition of almost any specific 'unexplained' phobia (e.g. enclosed spaces, smoke, heights, dogs, faces).

As indicated in *Table 29.2* and *Figure 29.12*, all sensory association areas of the cortex have direct access to the lateral nucleus of the amygdala. These areas are also linked to the prefrontal cortex through long association fiber bundles, rendering all conscious sensations subject to cognitive evaluation.

Activity of the visual association cortex is especially important in connection with phobias and anxiety states. Area V4 at the inferior surface of anterior area 19 is a link in the object/face recognition pathway. V5, at the lateral surface of anterior area 19, is a link in the movement detection pathway. Both are connected to the amygdala via the hippocampus, where fearful visual memories may be recalled by the current visual scene. The visual association cortex is also important in that fearful visual images conjured in the mind independently of current sensation, may activate the amygdala. This capability has resonance in relation to *post-traumatic stress disorder*, where a seemingly innocent scene may cause the afflicted individual to 'relive' a horrific visual experience, up to 20 years or more after the event. In the multimodal anterior region of the superior temporal gyrus, where sound and vision coalesce, a door banged shut may induce a 'virtual reality' re-enactment of a horrific encounter, e.g. of a haunting war experience.

The orbital prefrontal cortex of the right side, with its bias toward 'withdrawal' rather than 'approach' (Ch. 27), is commonly active (in PET scans) along with the right amygdala in fearful situations, e.g. when a specific phobia is presented to a susceptible subject. On the one hand, this offers the 'downside' potential to 'feed on one's fear'. On the other hand, expert social/psychological conditioning may eventually suffice to reduce the 'negative drive' of the orbital cortex. When conditioning is combined with use of anxiolytic drugs, specific phobias may be abolished completely.

The insula is omitted from Figure 29.12 but, as noted earlier, its posterior part also has direct access to the amygdala, probably related to the emotional evaluation of pain.

Finally, the basal nucleus of Meynert is listed. The cholinergic projection from this nucleus is thought to be of significance in facilitating cortical cell columns in the context of situations having negative emotional valence. Meynert activity appears to be heightened in association with *anxiety*, generating a raised level of autonomic activity involving the amygdala (and/or the adjacent bed nucleus of the stria terminalis, mentioned below).

Efferent pathways   (Table 29.2)

Easily identified in the postmortem brain is the **stria terminalis** (*Figure 29.13*). which, upon emerging from the central nucleus of the amygdala, follows the curve of the caudate nucleus and accompanies the thalamostriate vein along the upper surface of the thalamus. The stria sends fibers to the septal area and hypothalamus before entering the medial forebrain bundle and (downstream) the central tegmental tract. Some fibers of the stria terminate in a *bed nucleus*, above the anterior commissure. The bed nucleus is regarded

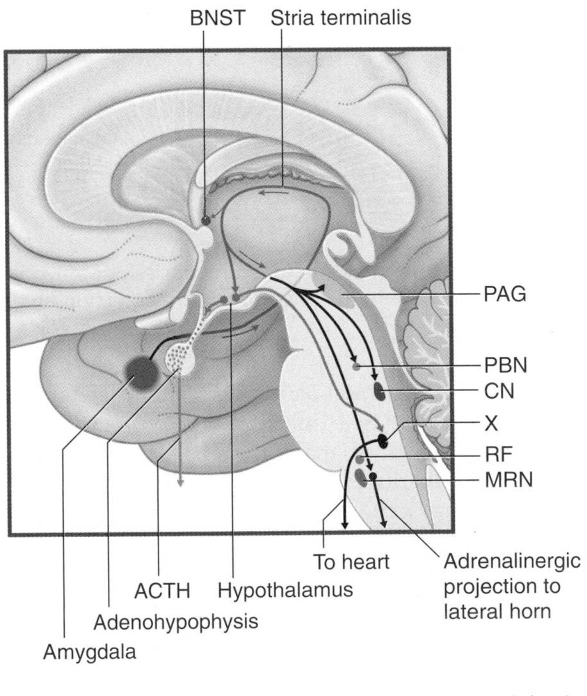

by some workers as part of the 'extended amygdala'; it may be more active than the amygdala proper, on PET scans, in anxiety states.

A second efferent projection, the **ventral amygdalofugal pathway** (see later), passes medially to synapse within the nucleus accumbens.

Notes on the efferent target connections

Peri-aqueductal gray matter (PAG). A source of *supraspinal antinociception* was described in Chapter 21, namely the opioid-containing axons from the hypothalamus which disinhibit the excitatory projection from the PAG to the serotoninergic cells of origin of the raphespinal tract. The excitatory cells of the *dorsal* PAG are directly stimulated by axon terminals entering from the amygdala via the medial forebrain bundle.

In laboratory animals, stimulation of the *ventral* PAG causes *freezing*, where a fixed, flexed posture is adopted. The ventral PAG contains neurons projecting to the cells of origin of the medullary reticulospinal tract. This tract activates flexor motor neurons during the walking cycle, and intense activation may cause a frightened person to 'go weak at the knees' and perhaps fall down.

Cerulean nucleus. Facilitation of excitatory cortical neurons by the noradrenergic projection from this pontine nucleus is to be expected.

Medullary adrenalinergic neurons. As noted in Chapter 21, these neurons are a component of the baroreflex pathway sustaining the blood pressure against gravitational force. Sudden stimulation by the direct projection from the amygdala may send the heart dullthudding and cause a major elevation of systemic blood pressure.

Hypothalamus. Fibers of the stria terminalis synapse upon two sets of hypothalamic neurons. The first, located in the anterolateral region, sends axons into the dorsal longitudinal fasciculus to synapse in cells of origin of the vagal supply to the heart. The well-known condition, referred to by psychiatrists as *blood trauma phobia* (fainting at the sight of blood at the scene of an accident), is characterized by initial sympathetic excitation followed by vagus-induced bradycardia causing the individual to collapse (faint).

The second set of neurons secrete corticotropin-releasing hormone (CRH) into the adenohypophysis via the hypophysial portal system, with consequent release of adrenocorticotropin (ACTH). Curiously, these CRH neurons send collateral branches into the central nucleus of the amygdala, with positive feedback enhancement of its activity.

Parabrachial nucleus. In individuals subject to *panic attacks*, hyperventilation, together with a sense of fear, may be triggered by what may appear to be relatively trivial environmental challenges. Normally, the respiratory alkalosis produced by washout of carbon dioxide reduces the respiratory rate causing the blood pH to return to normal, whereas susceptible individuals continue to hyperventilate. Because specific serotonin reuptake inhibitors (SSRIs) are highly successful in treatment, the prevailing view is that the normal inhibitory role of serotoninergic terminals within the nucleus accumbens (see below) has become deficient. However, overactivity of the cerulean nucleus has also been implicated because the drug yohimbine can induce a panic attack, apparently through norepinephrine release.

Figure 29.13 Efferents from central nucleus of amygdala via stria terminalis. The only postsynaptic pathways shown are autonomic. The peri-aqueductal gray matter (PAG) projects to the magnocellular reticular formation (RF) giving rise to the medullary reticulospinal tract; PAG also projects to magnus raphe neurons (MRN) giving rise to the raphespinal tract. ACTH, adrenocorticotrophic hormone; BNST, bed nucleus of stria terminalis. CN, nucleus ceruleus; MCN, magnus raphe nucleus; PBN, parabrachial nucleus; X, dorsal nucleus of vagus.

Limbic striatal loop. This circuit is depicted in Chapter 28, passing from the prefrontal cortex through the nucleus accumbens and medial dorsal nucleus of thalamus, with return to the prefrontal cortex. However, the central nucleus of the amygdala participates in this circuit through an excitatory projection to the nucleus accumbens. In the right hemisphere, this projection is likely to facilitate a withdrawal response; in the left, it may facilitate an approach response.

Bilateral ablation of the amygdala has been carried out in humans for treatment of *rage attacks*, characterized by irritability, building up over several hours or days to a state of dangerous aggressiveness. This controversial operation has been successful in eliminating such attacks. In monkeys, bilateral ablation leads to placidity, together with a tendency to explore objects orally and to exhibit hypersexuality (*Kluver–Bucy syndrome*). A comparable syndrome has occasionally been observed in humans.

At the other end of the spectrum, PET studies of incarcerated murderers have revealed that the amygdala of the majority remains 'silent' even when gruesome scenes are presented on screen.

The nucleus accumbens is considered again below, in the context of drug dependency.

Nucleus accumbens

The full name is *nucleus accumbens septi pellucidi*, 'the nucleus leaning against the septum pellucidum'. More accurately, the nucleus abuts against septal nuclei located in the base of the septum. *Figures 29.14 and 29.17C* show this relationship. The nucleus accumbens is one of many deep-seated brain

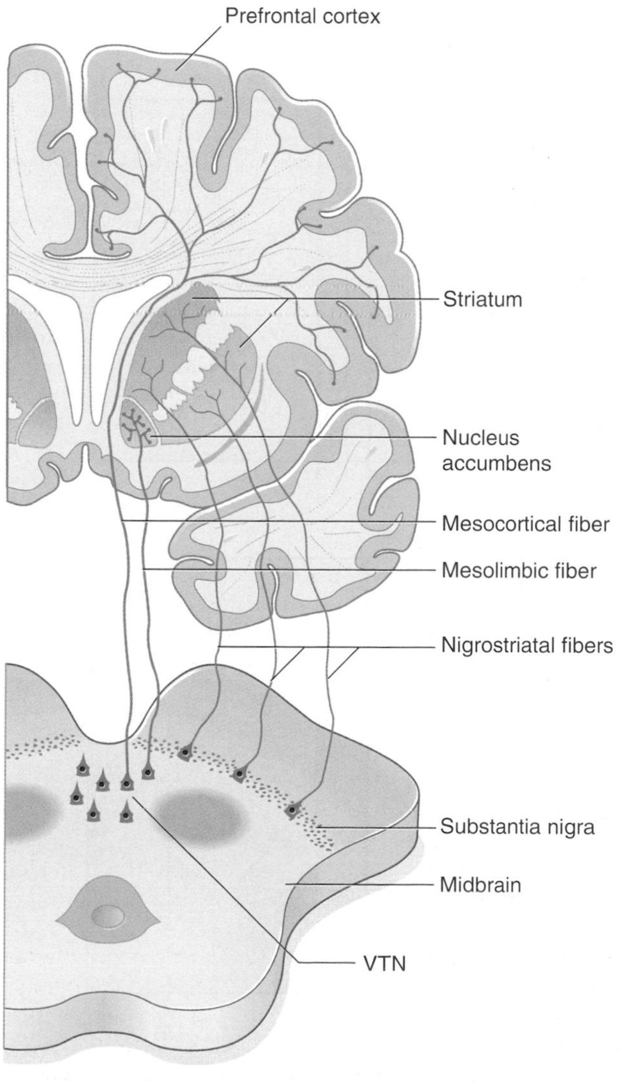

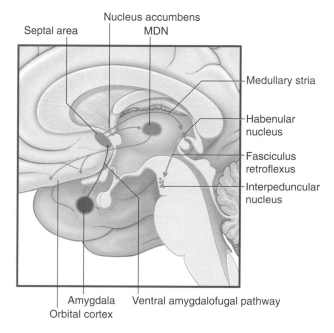

Figure 29.15 Connections of the septal area. MDN, mediodorsal nucleus of thalamus.

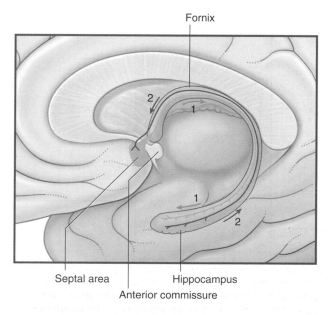

Figure 29.16 Septohippocampal pathway (1) with return projection from hippocampus (2).

Figure 29.14 Coronal section at the level of the nucleus accumbens highlighting distribution of dopaminergic fibers arising in the ventral tegmental nuclei (VTN) of the midbrain.

areas where electrodes have been inserted on a therapeutic trial basis (notably in the hope of providing pain relief). Stimulation here induces an intense sense of well-being, comparable to that experienced by intake of drugs of addiction such as heroin (*Clinical Panel 29.4*). This 'high' feeling is attributed to flooding of the nucleus, and of the medial prefrontal cortex, by synaptic and volume release of dopamine. Normally, dopamine is released in small amounts and quickly retrieved from the extracellular space by a specific dopamine reuptake transporter.

Septal area

The septal area comprises the **septal nuclei**, merging with the cortex directly in front of the anterior commissure, together with a small extension into the septum pellucidum. (*Figure 29.15*).

Afferents to the septal nuclei are received from:

- the amygdala, via the *diagonal band* (of Broca), a slender connection passing alongside the anterior perforated substance;
- the olfactory tract, via the medial olfactory stria;
- the hippocampus, via the fornix; and
- brainstem monoaminergic neurons, via the medial forebrain bundle.

The two chief *efferent* projections are the:

- **stria medullaris**, a glutamatergic strand running along the junction of side wall and roof of the third ventricle to synapse upon cholinergic neurons in the **habenular nucleus**. The habenular nuclei of the two sides are connected through the **habenular commissure** located close to the root of the pineal gland, as shown earlier, in *Figure 14.19*. The habenular nucleus sends the cholinergic **habenulo-interpeduncular tract (fasciculus**

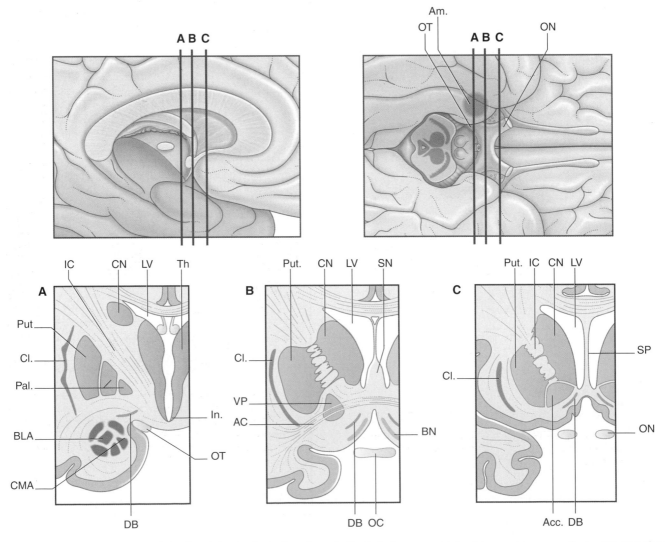

Figure 29.17 Coronal sections of the basal forebrain in the planes indicated. Am., amygdala; Acc., nucleus accumbens; AC, anterior commissure; BLA, basolateral amygdala; BN, basal nucleus of Meynert; Cl., claustrum; CMA, corticomedial amygdala; CN, caudate nucleus; DB, diagonal band of Broca; IC, internal capsule; In., infundibulum; LV, lateral ventricle; OC, optic chiasm; ON, optic nerve; OT, optic tract; Pal., pallidum; Put., putamen; SN, septal nucleus; SP, septum pellucidum; Th., thalamus; VP, ventral pallidum.

Clinical Panel 29.4   Drugs of dependency

Experimental evidence from the injection of drugs of abuse has yielded the following results (*Figures CP 29.4.1 and 29.4.2*):

- Cocaine binds with the dopamine reuptake transporter, blocking reuptake of the normal secretion with consequent dopamine accumulation in the extracellular space.

- Amphetamine and methamphetamine are potent dopamine-releasing agents and also tend to block the re-incorporation of dopamine into synaptic vesicles. These two drugs are also significantly active within the terminal dopaminergic network in the prefrontal cortex.

- Cannabinoids activate specific, excitatory, cannabinoid receptors on dopamine nerve endings.

- Nicotine attaches to specific excitatory receptors in the plasma membrane of parent somas in the midbrain.

- Opioids such as morphine and dihydromorphine (heroin) activate specific *inhibitory* receptors located in the plasma membrane of GABAergic internuncial neurons within the nucleus. These neurons normally exert a tonic braking action on the projection cells of the ventral tegmental nuclei. Opioid-induced hyperpolarization of the internuncials leads to functional disinhibition of the projection cells, with consequent increased activity of both mesolimbic and mesocortical neurons.

- Ethanol also interferes with normal GABAergic activity. It binds to postsynaptic GABA membrane receptors throughout the brain without activating them; again, the target neurons become more excitable.

Serotoninergic and noradrenergic neurons projecting to limbic system and hypothalamus have also been implicated in connection with drug dependency, notably in expressing some of the effects of abrupt drug withdrawal.

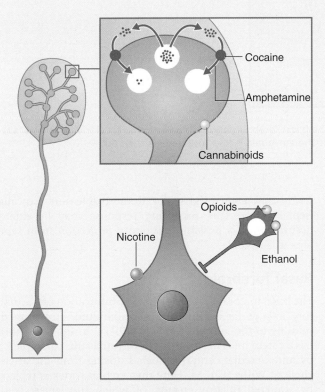

Figure CP 29.4.1 Mesolimbic neuron supplying nucleus accumbens, showing sites of action of some drugs of dependency.

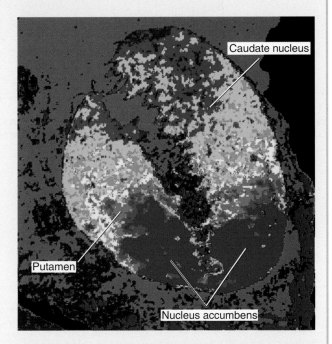

Figure CP 29.4.2 Intense activation (red) of D_3 receptors (D_2 variants) in the nucleus accumbens of a cocaine addict. (From Staley, J.K. and Mash, D.C. (1996) Adaptive increase in D_3 dopamine receptors in the brain reward circuits of human cocaine fatalities. J. Neurosci **16**: 6100–6106 with permission.)

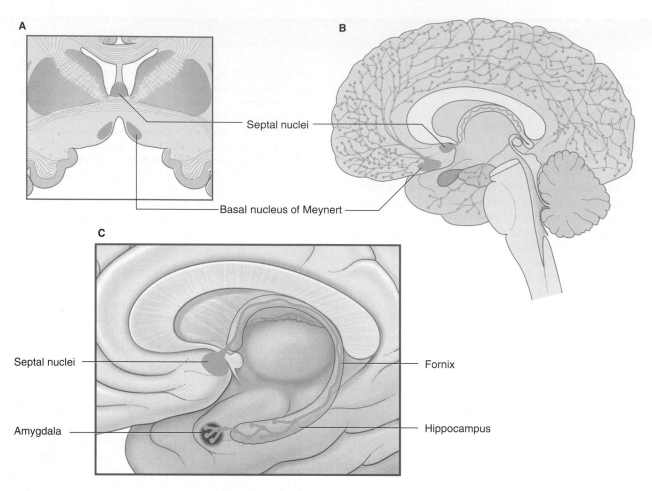

Figure 29.18 Cholinergic innervation of the cerebral cortex from the basal forebrain nuclei. **(A)** Section at level indicated in **B**. **(B)** Cortical innervation. **(C)** Septohippocampal pathway via the fornix. The amygdala is also supplied via this route.

retroflexus) to synapse in the **interpeduncular nucleus** of the reticular formation in the midbrain (*Figure 14.19*). The interpeduncular nucleus is believed to participate in the sleep–wake cycle together with the cholinergic neurons beside the cerulean nucleus, identified earlier (*Figure 21.3*).

- **septohippocampal pathway** running to the hippocampus by way of the fornix. (*Figure 29.16*). It is responsible for generating the slow-wave *hippocampal theta rhythm* detectable in EEG recordings from the temporal lobe. Glutamatergic neurons in this pathway are pacemakers determining the *rate* of theta rhythm; cholinergic neurons determine the *size* of the theta waves. Theta rhythm is produced by synchronous discharge of groups of hippocampal pyramidal cells, and is significant in the development of biochemical alterations within pyramidal glutamate receptors during the long-term potentiation involved in laying down episodic memory traces. The strength of theta rhythm is greatly reduced in AD, reflecting the substantial loss of both cholinergic neurons and episodic memory formation and retrieval in this disease.

Electrical stimulation of the human septal area produces sexual sensations akin to orgasm. In animals, an electrolytic lesion may evince signs of extreme displeasure (so-called 'septal rage'). This surprising response may be due to destruction of a possible inhibitory projection from septal area to amygdala.

Basal forebrain

The basal forebrain extends from the bifurcation of the olfactory tract as far back as the infundibulum, and from the midline to the amygdala (*Figure 29.17*). In the floor of the basal forebrain is the **anterior perforated substance**, pierced by anteromedial central branches arising from the arterial circle of Willis (Ch. 5). Here the cerebral cortex is replaced by scattered nuclear groups, of which the largest is the **magnocellular basal nucleus** of Meynert.

The *cholinergic neurons of the basal forebrain* have their somas mainly in the septal nuclei and basal nucleus of Meynert (*Figure 29.18*). The basal nucleus projects to all parts of the cerebral neocortex, which also contains scattered intrinsic cholinergic neurons.

The septal and basal nuclei, and small numbers contained in the diagonal band of Broca, are often referred to as the *basal forebrain nuclei*.

In the neocortex, the cholinergic supply from Meynert's nucleus is tonically active in the waking state, contributing to

Core Information

Olfactory system

The olfactory system comprises the olfactory epithelium in the nose, the olfactory nerves, olfactory bulb and olfactory tract, and several patches of olfactory cortex. The epithelium comprises bipolar olfactory neurons, supporting cells, and basal cells which renew the bipolar neurons at a diminishing rate throughout life. Central processes of the bipolar neurons form the olfactory nerves, which penetrate the cribriform plate of the ethmoid bone and synapse upon mitral cells in the bulb. Mitral cell axons form the olfactory tract, which has several low-level terminations in the anterior temporal lobe. Olfactory discrimination is a function of the orbitofrontal cortex, which is reached by way of the mediodorsal nucleus of the thalamus.

Limbic system

The limbic system comprises the limbic cortex and related subcortical nuclei. The limbic cortex includes the hippocampal formation, septal area, parahippocampal gyrus, and cingulate gyrus. The principal subcortical nucleus is the amygdala. Closely related are the orbitofrontal cortex, temporal pole, hypothalamus and reticular formation, and the nucleus accumbens.

The anterior part of the parahippocampal gyrus is the *entorhinal cortex*, which receives cognitive and sensory information from the cortical association areas, transmits it to the hippocampal formation for consolidation, and returns it to the association areas where it is encoded in the form of memory traces.

The hippocampal formation comprises the subiculum, hippocampus proper, and dentate gyrus. Sectors of the hippocampus are called cornu ammonis (CA) 1–4.

The perforant path projects from the entorhinal cortex on to the dendrites of dentate granule cells. Granule cell axons synapse on CA3 pyramidal cells which give Schaffer collaterals to CA1. CA1 back-projects to the entorhinal cortex which is heavily linked to the association areas.

The fornix is a direct continuation of the fimbria, which receives axons from the subiculum and hippocampus. The crus of the fornix joins its fellow to form the trunk. Anteriorly the pillar of the fornix divides into precommissural fibers entering the septal area and postcommissural fibers entering anterior hypothalamus, mammillary bodies, and medial forebrain bundle.

Bilateral damage to or removal of the hippocampal formation is followed by anterograde amnesia, with loss of declarative memory. Procedural memory is preserved. Long-term potentiation of granule and pyramidal cells is regarded as a key factor in the consolidation of memories.

The insula has functions in relation to pain and to language. The anterior cingulate cortex has functions in relation to motor response selection, emotional tone, bladder control, vocalization, and autonomic control. The posterior cingulate responds to the emotional tone of what is seen or felt.

The amygdala, above and in front of the temporal horn of the lateral ventricle, is the principal brain nucleus associated with the perception of fear. Its afferent, lateral nucleus receives inputs from olfactory, visual, auditory, tactile, visceral, cognitive, and mnemonic sources. The central, efferent nucleus sends fibers via the stria terminalis to the hypothalamus, activating corticotropin release and vagus-mediated bradycardia, and to the brainstem activating dorsal and ventral peri-aqueductal gray matter and influencing respiratory rate and autonomic activity. The amygdalofugal pathway from the central nucleus facilitates defensive/evasive activity via the limbic striatal loop.

The nucleus accumbens is a clinically important component of the mesolimbic system in the context of drug dependency, based upon its abundance of dopaminergic nerve terminals derived from ventral tegmental nuclei. Dopamine levels in the extracellular space in nucleus accumbens and medial prefrontal cortex are raised by cocaine and amphetamines which interfere with local dopamine recycling, and by cannabinoids which activate specific terminal receptors. Nicotine activates specific receptors in the parent tegmental neurons. Opioids and ethanol interfere with the normal braking action of GABA tegmental internuncials.

The septal area comprises two main nuclear groups. One sends a set of glutamatergic fibers in the stria medullaris thalami to the habenular nucleus, which in turn sends the cholinergic fasciculus retroflexus to the interpeduncular nucleus which participates in the sleep–wake cycle. The other forms the septohippocampal pathway to synapse upon hippocampal pyramidal cells. Glutamatergic and cholinergic elements govern the rate and strength, respectively, of hippocampal theta rhythm which facilitates formation of episodic memories.

The basal forebrain is the gray matter in and around the anterior perforated substance. It includes the cholinergic, nucleus basalis of Meynert which projects to all parts of the neocortex, and the cholinergic, septal nucleus projecting to the hippocampus. Both lose about half of their neurons in AD, and the neocortical distribution is vulnerable to stroke.

the 'awake' pattern on EEG recordings. All areas of the neo-cortex are richly supplied. Tonic liberation of ACh tonically activates muscarinic receptors on cortical neurons, causing a reduction of potassium conductance making them more responsive to other excitatory inputs. The cholinergic supply promotes long-term potentiation and training-induced synaptic strengthening of neocortical pyramidal cells.

The general psychic slow-down often observed in patients following a stroke may be accounted for by interruption of cholinergic fiber bundles in the subcortical white matter caused by arterial occlusion within the territory of the anterior or middle cerebral artery. The result may be virtual cholinergic denervation of the cortex both at and posterior to the site of the lesion.

REFERENCES

Baxendale, S.A. (1995) The hippocampus – functional and structural correlations. *Seizure* 4: 105–117.

Braak, H. and Braak, E. (1998) Evolution of neuronal changes in the course of Alzheimer's disease. *J. Neural Transm.* (Suppl) 53: 127–140.

Coplan, J.D. and Lydiard, R.B. (1998) Brain circuits in panic disorder. *Biol. Psychiatry* 44: 1264–1266.

Cummings, J.L., Vinters, H.V., Cole, G.M. and Khacthaturian, Z.S. (1998) Alzheimer's disease: etiologies, pathophysiology, cognitive reserve, and treatment opportunities. *Neurology* 51(Suppl): S2–S17.

Dekker, A.J.A.M., Connor, D.J. and Thal, L.J. (1991) The role of cholinergic projections from the nucleus basalis in memory. *Neurosci. Behav. Rev.* 15: 299–317.

De Lacalle, S., Lim, C., Sobreviela, T., Mufson, E.J., Hersh, L.B. and Saper, C.B. (1994) Cholinergic innervation of the human hippocampal formation including the entorhinal cortex. *J. Comp. Neurol.* 345: 321–344.

Devinsky, O., Morrell, M.J. and Vogt, B.A. (1995) Contributions of anterior cingulate cortex to behavior. *Brain* 118: 279–306.

Dolan, R.J., Paulesu, E. and Fletcher, P. (1997) Human memory systems. In *Human Brain Function* (Frackowiak, R.S.J., Friston, K.J., Frith, C.D. and Dolan, R.J. eds), pp. 367–404. London: Academic Press.

Duvernoy, H.M. (1998) *The Human Hippocampus*, 2nd edn, with drawings by J.L. Vannson. Berlin: Springer.

Eseri, M.M. and Morris, J.H. (1997) *The Neuropathology of Dementia*. Cambridge: Cambridge University Press.

Francis, P.T., Palmer, A.M., Snape, M. and Wilcock, G.K. (1999) The cholinergic hypothesis of Alzheimer's disease: a review of progress. *J. Neurol. Neurosurg. Psychiat.* 66: 137–147.

Frith, C.D. et al. (1996) Is developmental dyslexia a disconnection syndrome? Studies with PET. *Brain* 119: 143–158.

Garza-Trevino, E.S. (1994) Neurobiological factors in aggressive behavior. *Hosp. Commun. Psychiat.* 45: 690–699.

Hyman, S.E. (1998) Brain neurocircuitry of anxiety and fear. *Biol. Psychiatry* 44: 1401–1403.

Jay, V. and Becker, L.E. (1994) Surgical pathology of epilepsy. *Pediat. Pathol.* 14: 731–750.

Jellinger, K.A. (1998) The neuropathological diagnosis of Alzheimer disease. *J. Neural Transm.* (Suppl) 53: 97–118.

Kuhl, D.E., Koeppe, R.A., Minoshima, S., Synder, S.E., Ficaro, E.P., Foster, N.L., Frey, K.A. and Kilbourn, M.R. (1999) In vivo mapping of cerebral acetylcholinesterase activity in aging and Alzheimer's disease. *Neurology* 52: 691–699.

LeDoux, J.E. (1995) Emotion: clues from the brain. *Ann. Rev. Psychol.* 46: 209–235.

Leonard, B.E. (1997) *Fundamentals of Psychopharmacology*, 2nd edn. Chichester: Wiley.

Maguire, E.A., Burgess, N. and O'Keefe, J. (1999) Human spatial navigation: cognitive maps, sexual dimorphism, and neural substrates. *Curr. Opin. Neurobiol.* 9: 171–177.

Malenka, R.C. (1994) Synaptic plasticity in the hippocampus. *Cell* 78: 835–838.

Meldrum, B.S. (1994) The role of glutamate in epilepsy and other CNS disorders. *Neurology.* 44(Suppl 8): S14–S22.

Merskey, H. (1986) Classification of chronic pain. Descriptions of chronic pain syndromes and definitions of pain terms. *Pain* 3(Suppl 1): S1–S225.

Mishkin, M., Varghka-Khadem, F. and Gadian, D.G. (1998) Amnesia and the organization of the hippocampal system. *Hippocampus* 8: 212–216.

Perry, R.J. and Hodges, J.R. (1999) Attention and executive deficits in Alzheimer's disease. *Brain* 122: 383–404.

Selden, N.R., Gitleman, D.R., Salammon-Murayama, N., Parrish, T. and Mesulam, M-M. (1998) Trajectories of cholinergic pathways within the cerebral hemispheres of the human brain. *Brain* 121: 2249–2257.

Shin, C. (1994) Mechanism of epilepsy. *Ann. Rev. Med.* 45: 379–389.

Treede, R.D., Kenshalo, D.R., Gracely, R.H. and Jones, A.K.P. (1999) The cortical representation of pain. *Pain* 79: 105–111.

Villanueva, L. and Nathan, P.W. (2000) Multiple pain pathways. In *Progress in Pain Research and Management, vol. 16*, pp. 371–386. Seattle: IASP Press.

Willis, W.D. (1995) From nociception to cortical activity. In *Advances in Pain Research and Therapy, vol. 22* (Brom, B., ed.), pp. 1–19. Philadelphia: Lippincott–Raven.

Cerebrovascular disease

INTRODUCTION

Cerebrovascular disease is the third leading cause of death in adults, being superseded only by heart disease and cancer. The most frequent expression of cerebrovascular disease is that of a *stroke*, which is defined as a focal neurological deficit of vascular origin which lasts for more than 24 hours if the patient survives. The most frequent example is a hemiplegia caused by a vascular lesion of the internal capsule. However, it will be seen that many varieties of stroke symptomatologies are recognized, based upon place and size.

The three chief underlying disorders are atherosclerosis within the large arteries supplying the brain, heart disease, and hypertension.

- Atherosclerosis signifies fatty deposits in the intimal lining of the internal carotid and vertebrobasilar system – most notably in the internal carotid trunk or in one of the vertebral arteries. The deposits pose a dual threat: in situ enlargement may cause progressive occlusion of a main artery; and breakaway deposits may form emboli (plugs) blocking distal branches within the brain. However, gradual occlusion is often redeemed by routing of blood through alternative channels. For example, an internal carotid artery (ICA) may be progressively occluded over a period of 10 years or more without apparent brain damage; the contralateral ICA utilizes the circle of Willis to perfuse both pairs of anterior and middle cerebral arteries; and it is not unusual in such cases for external carotid blood to assist, by retrograde flow from the facial artery through the ophthalmic artery on the affected side. Similarly, occlusion of the stem of one of the three cerebral arteries may be compensated for through small (< 0.5 mm) anastomotic arteries in the depths of cortical sulci, perfused by the other two cerebrals. The number of such small arteries varies greatly between individuals. The crescent-shaped anastomotic region is known as the *border zone (Figure 30.1)*. On the other hand, all of the arteries penetrating the brain substance are end arteries, i.e. their communication with neighboring penetrating arteries are too fine to save brain tissue in the event of blockage.

- Many cerebral emboli originate as blood clots in the left side of the heart, in association with coronary or valvular disease.

- Hypertension is obviously associated with cerebral hemorrhage, which may be so massive as to rupture into the ventricular system and cause death within minutes or hours. Less obvious are lacunae ('small pools') up to 2 cm in diameter, derived from necrotic (dead) brain tissue around small arteries that have become occluded by mural thickening in response to the hypertension.

An area of brain destruction produced by vascular occlusion or hemorrhage is an *infarct*. Cerebral infarcts become swollen after a few days, and some become large enough to produce distance effects by causing subfalcal or tentorial herniation of the brain in the manner of a tumor (Ch. 4).

It is usually easy to distinguish the symptoms/signs of vascular disease from those of a tumor. A vascular stroke takes up to 24 hours to evolve whereas the time frame for tumors is usually weeks or months. However, hemorrhage into a tumor may cause it to expand suddenly and to mimic the effects of a stroke. Very often the hemorrhage is into a metastatic tumor, notably from lung, breast, or prostate; in fact, a stroke may be the first manifestation of a cancer in one of these organs.

Some 10% of vascular strokes are caused by rupture of a berry aneurysm into the brain. As explained later, berry aneurysms usually bleed directly into the subarachnoid space because they originate in or near the circle of Willis, but they may arise at an arterial bifurcation point within the brain. A ruptured aneurysm is always a prime suspect when a stroke comes 'out of the blue' in someone less than 40 years old.

ANTERIOR CIRCULATION OF THE BRAIN

Clinicians refer to the ICA and its branches as the *anterior circulation* of the brain, and the vertebrobasilar system (including the posterior cerebral arteries) as the *posterior circulation*. The anterior and posterior circulations are connected by the posterior communicating arteries (*Figure 30.2*).

About 75% of cerebrovascular accidents (CVAs) originate in the anterior circulation.

Internal capsule

The following details supplement the account of the arterial supply of the internal capsule in Chapter 5.

The blood supply is shown in *Figure 30.3*. The three sources of supply are the **anterior choroidal**, a direct branch of the internal carotid; the **medial striate**, a branch of the anterior cerebral, and **lateral striate (lenticulostriate)** branches of the middle cerebral artery.

The contents of the internal capsule are shown in *Figure 30.4*. The anterior choroidal branch of the internal carotid artery supplies the lower part of the posterior limb and the retrolentiform part of the internal capsule, and the inferolateral part of the lateral geniculate body. Some of its branches (not shown) supply a variable amount of the temporal lobe of the brain and the choroid plexus of the inferior horn of the lateral ventricle.

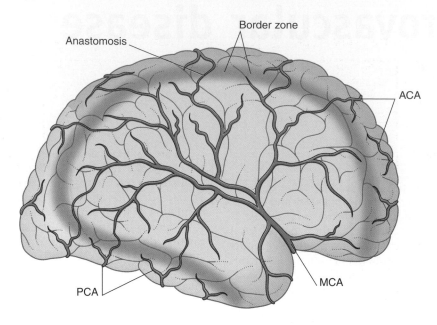

Figure 30.1 Border zone of anastomotic overlap between the middle cerebral artery (MCA) and the anterior and posterior cerebral arteries (ACA, PCA).

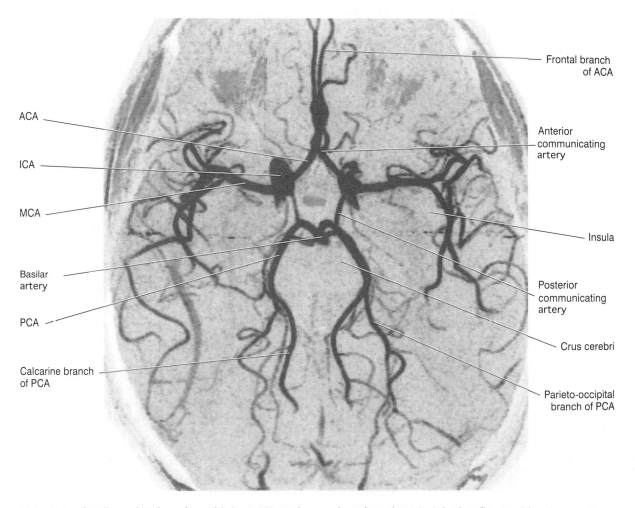

Figure 30.2 Circle of Willis and its branches. This is an MR angiogram based on the principle that flowing blood generates a different signal to that of stationary tissue, without injection of a contrast agent. Conventional angiograms, e.g. those in Chapter 5, require arterial perfusion with a contrast agent. The vessels shown here are contained within a single thick MR 'slice'. Some, e.g. the calcarine branch of the posterior cerebral artery could be followed further in adjacent slices. ACA, anterior cerebral artery; ICA, internal carotid artery; MCA, middle cerebral artery; PCA, posterior cerebral artery. (From a series kindly provided by Professor J. Paul Finn, Director, MRI Facility, Northwestern University School of Medicine, Chicago.)

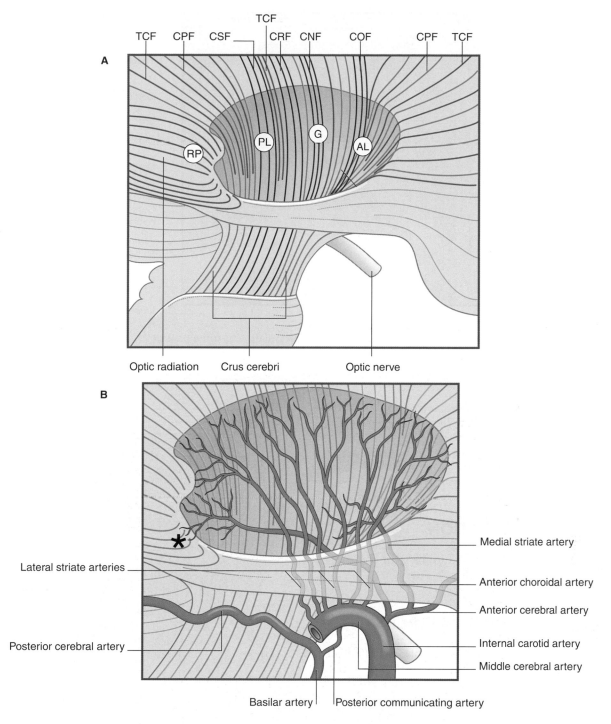

Figure 30.3 Internal capsule.
(A) Pathways. Lateral view of the right cerebral hemisphere showing the oval depression in the white matter following removal of the lentiform nucleus. The internal capsule occupies the floor of the depression. CNF, corticonuclear fibers; COF, cortico-oculomotor fibers; CPF, corticopontine fibers; CRF, corticoreticular fibers; CSF, corticospinal fibers; TCF, thalamocortical fibers. Other abbreviations as in *Figure 30.4*.
(B) Blood supply. The medial striate branch of the anterior cerebral artery is the recurrent artery of Heubner. Only two of the six lateral striate branches of the middle cerebral artery shown are labeled. *Indicates arterial supply from the anterior choroidal artery to the inferolateral part of the lateral geniculate body.

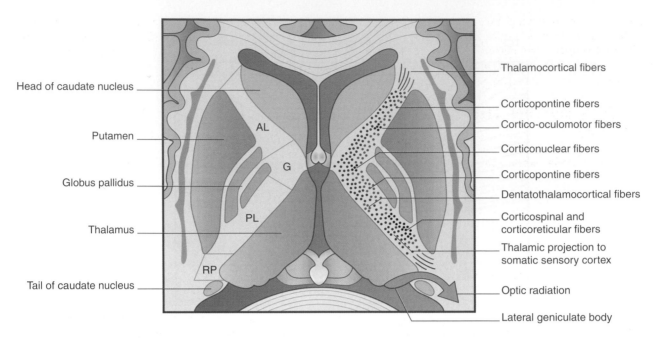

Figure 30.4 Horizontal section of the internal capsule depicting its parts (left) and contents (right). AL, anterior limb; G, genu; PL, posterior limb; RP, retrolentiform part.

The medial striate branch of the anterior cerebral artery (recurrent artery of Heubner) supplies the lower part of the anterior limb and genu of the internal capsule.

The lateral striate arteries penetrate the lentiform nucleus and give multiple branches to the anterior limb, genu, and posterior limb of the internal capsule.

POSTERIOR CIRCULATION

Additional information is confined to the stem branches of the posterior cerebral artery shown in *Figure 30.5*.

TRANSIENT ISCHEMIC ATTACKS

Transient ischemic attacks (TIAs) are episodes of vascular insufficiency that cause temporary loss of brain function, with total recovery within 24 hours. Most TIAs last for less than half an hour, with no residual signs at the time of clinical examination. Diagnosis is therefore usually based upon reported symptoms alone.

Most attacks follow lodgment of fibrin clots or detached atheromatous tissue at an arterial branch point, with subsequent dissolution.

- Transient symptoms originating in the anterior circulation include: motor weakness (a 'heavy feeling') in an arm or leg, hemisensory deficit (a 'numb feeling'), dysphasia, and monocular blindness from occlusion of the central artery of the retina.
- Transient symptoms originating in the posterior circulation include: vertigo, diplopia, ataxia, and amnesia.

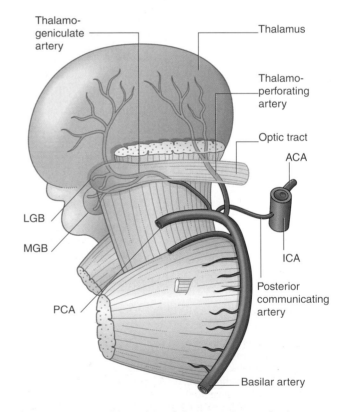

Figure 30.5 Central branches of the posterior cerebral artery (PCA). Although only two arteries are shown, each in fact comprises several branches from the PCA. The thalamoperforating artery shown pierces the posterior perforated substance and supplies the anterior one-third of the thalamus. The thalamogeniculate artery shown supplies the geniculate bodies and the posterior two-thirds of the thalamus. ACA, anterior cerebral artery; ICA, internal carotid artery; LGB, MGB, lateral, medial geniculate bodies.

Recognition of TIAs involving the anterior circulation is important because they serve notice of impending major illness. Without treatment, one person in four will die from a heart attack within 5 years, and one person in six will develop a stroke.

OCCLUSIONS WITHIN THE ANTERIOR CIRCULATION

The symptoms of vascular strokes in the territories of the anterior circulation are summarized in *Clinical Panels 30.1, 30.2* and *30.3*. In the *Clinical Panels*, the term 'occlusion' is used to signify thrombosis or embolism. It should be emphasized that the majority of strokes originate in the territory of the middle cerebral artery.

Aneurysms

Aneurysms are discussed in *Clinical Panel 30.7*.

Clinical Panel 30.1   Anterior choroidal artery occlusion

A complete anterior choroidal artery syndrome is produced by occlusion of the proximal part of the artery, compromising the lower part of the posterior limb and retrolentiform part of the internal capsule. The clinical picture is one of contralateral hemiparesis, hemisensory loss of cortical type (Ch. 26), and hemianopia. Damage to the (crossed)

cerebellothalamocortical pathway may add evidence of intention tremor in the contralateral upper limb, yielding so-called *ataxic hemiparesis*.

Isolated occlusion of the branch to the lateral geniculate body results in a contralateral upper quadrant hemianopia.

Clinical Panel 30.2   Anterior cerebral artery occlusion

Complete interruption of flow in the proximal anterior cerebral artery (ACA) is rare because the opposite artery has direct access to its distal territory through the anterior communicating artery. However, branch occlusions are well recognized, with corresponding variations in the clinical picture:

- *Orbital or frontopolar branch*. The usual result is an apathetic state with some memory loss.

- *Medial striate artery* (recurrent artery of Heubner) occlusion may result in dysarthria owing to compromise of the motor supply to the contralateral nuclei supplying the muscles of the mandible (V), lips (VII) and tongue (XII). Hoarseness and dysphagia are also present if the supranuclear supply to the nucleus ambiguus is interrupted.

- *Callosomarginal*. This branch supplies the dorsomedial prefrontal cortex, the supplementary motor area, and the lower limb and perineal areas of the sensorimotor cortex and the supplementary

sensory area (SSA). The commonest manifestation of occlusion is motor weakness and some cortical-type sensory loss in the contralateral lower limb, as a result of infarction within the paracentral lobule. Urinary incontinence may occur for some days owing to contralateral weakness of the pelvic floor. Damage to the prefrontal cortex results in abulia (lack of initiative). A left-sided infarct of the supplementary motor area (SMA) may produce mutism because SMA normally collaborates with Broca's area in the initiation of speech. Finally, damage to the SSA may result in inability to reach with the contralateral arm toward the side of the lesion.

- *Pericallosal*. Infarction of the anterior part of the corpus callosum may result in ideomotor apraxia. (The lesion would be comparable to lesion 1 in *Figure 27.9*.) Infarction of the midregion may cause tactile anomia owing to blocked transfer of tactile information from right to left parietal lobe.

Clinical Panel 30.3 Middle cerebral artery occlusion

Embolic and lacunar infarcts are frequent in late middle life and in the elderly. Hemorrhage from one of the striate branches is also a frequent event.

Embolism
An embolus may lodge in the stem of the artery, in the upper division, in the lower division, or in a cortical branch of either division.

Stem
Occlusion of the stem affects the central as well as the cortical branches. The complete picture includes contralateral hemiplegia, severe contralateral sensory loss, contralateral homonymous hemianopia, and drifting of the eyes toward the side of the infarct. Left-sided lesions are usually accompanied by global aphasia, right-sided ones with contralateral sensory neglect. Many patients die in coma following midbrain compression by a swollen infarct.

The condition of some patients with stem occlusion improves markedly within days. One explanation is fragmentation of the embolus leading to impaction confined to part(s) of the more distal territory of the artery. Another explanation is the redemption of distal territory via anterior and posterior cerebral branches through the border zone.

Upper division
An embolus occluding the upper division gives rise to contralateral paresis (weakness) and cortical-type sensory loss in the face and arm, together with dysarthria arising from damage to supranuclear pathways involved in speech articulation. Left-sided lesions are usually accompanied by Broca's aphasia, right-sided lesions by contralateral neglect.

Lower division
Embolism of the lower division produces contralateral homonymous hemianopia, and sometimes a confused, agitated state attributed to involvement of limbic pathways in the temporal lobe. Left-sided lesions are also accompanied by Wernicke's aphasia, alexia, and sometimes by ideomotor apraxia (corresponding to lesion 3 in *Figure 27.9*).

Branch embolism
The following isolated deficits are attributable to an embolus lodged in one of the cortical branches:

- Orbitofrontal: elements of a prefrontal syndrome may be present (Ch. 27).
- Precentral (prerolandic): Broca's aphasia (left lesion); monotone speech (right lesion).
- Central (rolandic): contralateral loss of motor and/or sensory function in the face and arm.
- Inferior parietal: contralateral hemineglect (especially with right lesion); tactile anomia.
- Angular: contralateral homonymous hemianopia; alexia with left lesion.

- Posterior/middle temporal: Wernicke's aphasia (left lesion); sensory aprosodia (right lesion).

Lacunar infarcts
In the presence of hypertension, lacunar infarction is suspected where the clinical evidence suggests a small lesion. Well-recognized:

- *pure motor hemiparesis* may be due to a lacuna in the corona radiata or internal capsule (see also pons, later). The weakness is mainly in the lower face and arm and there are no sensory or higher cortical disturbances.
- *pure sensory syndrome* is produced by a lacuna in the ventral posterior nucleus of the thalamus. There is severe impairment of tactile discrimination (Ch. 12) in the contralateral limbs, together with sensory ataxia.
- *dysarthria–clumsy hand syndrome* may be produced by a lacuna among fibers descending to or through the genu of the internal capsule, containing corticonuclear fibers descending to contralateral motor nuclei of pons and medulla oblongata and fibers from the premotor cortex involved in contralateral manual control. The most apparent results are dysarthria owing to paresis of lip, tongue and jaw musculature, and clumsiness of hand movement.

Hemorrhage
The commonest source of a cerebral hemorrhage is one of the lateral striate branches of the middle cerebral artery. The commonest location is the putamen, with spread into the anterior and posterior limbs of the internal capsule. The usual cause is a pre-existing systemic hypertension. The hematoma may be as small as a pea or as big as a golf ball. Large hemorrhages rupture into the lateral ventricle and are usually fatal within 24 hours.

A typical clinical case is one in which a sudden, severe headache is followed by unconsciousness within a few minutes. The eyes tend to drift toward the side of the lesion, as noted in Chapter 26. With recovery of consciousness, there is a complete, flaccid hemiplegia (apart from the upper part of the face). Tendon reflexes are absent on the hemiplegic side and a Babinski sign is present. Conjugate movement of the eyes toward the hemiplegic side may be impossible initially.

Following any kind of stroke involving the left internal capsule, right-handers often notice some initial clumsiness in the left hand. fMRI studies indicate that in healthy right-handers the left motor cortex is more active during movements of the left hand than the right motor cortex is during movements of the right hand. In other words, the left motor cortex has a greater degree of bilateral control.

The end result of capsular stroke is often one of ambulatory spastic hemiparesis with hemihypesthesia (reduced sensation). *Figure CP 30.3.1* shows the typical

Clinical Panel 30.3 *Continued*

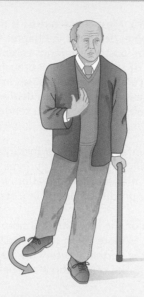

Figure CP 30.3.1 Hemiplegic gait. The patient's right side is affected.

posture during walking: the elbow and fingers are flexed and the leg has to be circumducted during the swing phase (unless an ankle brace is worn) because of the antigravity tone of the musculature. During the early rehabilitation period an arm sling is required in order to protect the shoulder joint from downward subluxation (partial dislocation) This is because the supraspinatus muscle is normally in continuous contraction when the body is upright, preventing slippage of the humeral head.

Figure CP 30.3.2 is from an MR study of a patient who had suffered a right hemiplegia with sensory loss 11 days previously. The picture shows extensive infarction of the white matter on the left side, at the junctional region between the corona radiata and

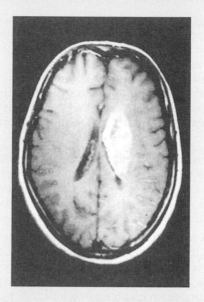

Figure CP 30.3.2 Contrast-enhanced MR image taken from a patient 11 days after an embolic stroke (see text). (Reproduced from Sato, A. et al (1991) Cerebral infarction: early detection by means of contrast-enhanced cerebral arteries at MR imaging. *Radiology* **178**: 433–439 by kind permission of Dr S. Takahashi, Department of Radiology, Tohoku University School of Medicine, Sendai, Japan, and the editors.)

internal capsule, with compression of the lateral ventricle.

Internal carotid artery
In addition to being a source of cerebral emboli, atheromatous plaques may cause partial or complete occlusion of the internal carotid artery itself (see *Clinical Panel 30.4*).

Clinical Panel 30.4 Internal carotid artery occlusion

The lumen of the internal carotid artery may become progressively obstructed by atheromatous deposits. Common sites of obstruction are the point of commencement in the neck, and the cavernous sinus. A slowly progressive obstruction may be compensated for by the opposite internal carotid artery, through the circle of Willis. Additional blood may also be provided through the orbit from the facial artery. At the other extreme, sudden occlusion may cause death from infarction of the entire anterior and middle cerebral territories, and sometimes the posterior cerebral also.

Warning signs of carotid occlusion take the form of

TIAs lasting for up to a few hours. As with TIAs elsewhere, the physician is unlikely to be present during an attack and must interpret the account given by the patient or relative. The territory of the middle cerebral artery is most often affected. Individual symptoms tend to occur in isolation and include any of the following: a feeling of heaviness/weakness/numbness/tingling in one arm or leg, halting or slurring of speech. Disturbance of flow in the ophthalmic artery may cause transient monocular blindness (one eye may be perceived as filled with fog or white steam).

Clinical Panel 30.5 Occlusions within the posterior circulation

The clinical phrase *long tract signs* is most often used in the context of brainstem lesions. It refers to evidence of a lesion in one or more of the three long tracts, namely the pyramidal tract, the posterior column–medial lemniscal pathway, and the spinothalamic pathway. All of the long tract signs occur in the limbs on the side opposite to the lesion.

Small brainstem infarcts may yield the following features:

- *Midbrain.* Ipsilateral third nerve paralysis and/or bilateral cerebellar ataxia caused by damage to the decussation of the superior cerebellar peduncles; 'crossed' third nerve paralysis featuring ipsilateral paralysis combined with contralateral hemiplegia.
- *Pons.* A tegmental infarct may cause ipsilateral facial and/or abducens and/or mandibular nerve paralysis and/or anesthesia of the face. A basilar infarct may produce a contralateral pure motor hemiplegia whose brainstem origin may be indicated by transient ipsilateral functional impairment of the abducens, facial or mandibular nerve passing through the tegmentum.

- *Medulla oblongata.* Most characteristic is the lateral medullary syndrome, described in Chapter 16, caused by occlusion of the posterior inferior cerebellar artery. Occlusion of the labyrinthine branch of the anterior inferior cerebellar artery causes immediate destruction of the inner ear; sudden deafness in that ear is accompanied by vertigo with a tendency to fall to that side.

Large brainstem infarcts in pons or medulla oblongata are usually fatal because of damage to the vital centers of the reticular formation. In the midbrain, they may produce a permanent state of coma.

Cerebellar ataxia of the limbs on one side, without brainstem damage, is more often due to occlusion of the top end of the vertebral artery on that side than to occlusion of one of the three cerebellar arteries.

The posterior cerebral arteries are usually perfused through the basilar bifurcation. Occlusion is more common in branches than in either main stem (*Clinical Panel 30.6*).

Clinical Panel 30.6 Posterior cerebral artery occlusion

A variety of effects may follow occlusion of branches of the posterior cerebral artery. Usually the occlusion is limited to a branch to the midbrain, or to the thalamus, or to the subthalamic nucleus, or to the cerebral cortex.

Midbrain
The classic picture of a unilateral infarct of the midbrain is that of a crossed third nerve palsy, i.e. a complete oculomotor paralysis (Ch. 20) on one side with a hemiplegia on the other side (Weber's syndrome). The hemiplegia is due to infarction of the crus cerebri, which contains corticospinal and corticonuclear fibers in its mid-portion. The hemiplegia usually shows early improvement, but ataxia may appear on that side because of damage to dentatothalamic fibers bypassing the red nucleus.

Thalamus
Occlusion of a thalamogeniculate branch may cause infarction of the posterior lateral nucleus of the thalamus (which receives the spinothalamic tract and medial lemniscus), and sometimes of the lateral geniculate nucleus also. The usual result is a contralateral sense of numbness, perhaps with hemianopia. The rare and unpleasant thalamic syndrome (Ch. 24) may supervene.

Subthalamic nucleus
Occlusion of a thalamoperforating branch may destroy the small subthalamic nucleus and give rise to ballism on the contralateral side, usually affecting the arm (Ch. 28).

Corpus callosum
Infarction of the splenium of the corpus callosum blocks transfer of written information from the right visual association cortex to the left. The result of infarction is alexia for written material presented to the left visual field.

Cortex
Occlusion of the stem of the posterior cerebral artery behind the midbrain gives rise to a homonymous hemianopia in the contralateral field. Macular vision may be spared. One view of 'macular sparing' is that it signifies bilateral representation of the fovea in the primary visual cortex. Another view is that the occipital pole is supplied by a long branch from the middle cerebral artery supplying the angular gyrus.

Occlusion of the left artery also produces alexia, the left visual field being the only area detectable by the patient.

A pure alexia, without agraphia, may follow a lesion of the left lingual gyrus.

Clinical Panel 30.6   *Continued*

Bilateral occlusion

Partial or complete cortical blindness may result from a thrombus arrested where the lumen of the basilar artery normally narrows below the basilar bifurcation, with consequent blockage of both posterior cerebral arteries. It has also been recorded following cardiac arrest with resuscitation.

Temporary cessation of flow in both posterior cerebral arteries sometimes affects only the anterior parts of their territories. If damage is confined to the occipitotemporal junctions, prosopagnosia (inability to identify faces) may occur alone. (Prosopagnosia has been recorded with purely right-sided perfusion failure.) If the entorhinal cortex/hippocampus is compromised on both sides, anterograde and/or retrograde amnesia may follow.

Clinical Panel 30.7   Subarachnoid hemorrhage

Blister-like berry aneurysms 5–10 mm in diameter are a routine autopsy finding in about 5% of people. Most are in the anterior half of the circle of Willis. Spontaneous rupture of an aneurysm into the interpeduncular cistern usually occurs in early or late middle age. The characteristic presentation is a sudden blinding headache, with collapse into semiconsciousness or coma within a few seconds. On physical examination, a diagnostic feature (absent in one-third of cases) is nuchal (neck) rigidity. This is caused by movement of blood into the posterior cranial fossa, where the dura mater is supplied by cervical nerves 2 and 3 (Ch. 4). The term *meningismus* is sometimes used for this sign.

The massive rise in intracranial pressure may be fatal within a few hours or days. Recovery may be impeded by a secondary elevation of intracranial pressure caused by blood clot obstruction of cerebrospinal fluid circulation through the tentorial notch or even within the arachnoid granulations.

About a quarter of all cases develop a neurological deficit 4 to 12 days after the initial attack. The deficit is fatal in a quarter of those who get it. The immediate cause is spasm of the main, conducting segments of the cerebral arteries. The amount of spasm is proportionate to the size of the surrounding blood clot in the interpeduncular cistern.

It is usual practice to define the aneurysm by means of carotid angiography, and to ligate it surgically. Without operation, most aneurysms will leak again at some future date.

Core Information

Etiology of cerebrovascular accidents

The three chief underlying disorders are: atherosclerosis of the internal carotid artery or vertebrobasilar system, thrombi issuing from the left side of the heart, and hypertension. Hypertension may lead either to sudden hemorrhage into the white matter or to the production of small lacunae. Hemorrhage into a tumor may mimic the effects of a vascular stroke. Some 10% of vascular strokes are caused by rupture of a berry aneurysm.

Arterial supply of internal capsule

The anterior choroidal artery supplies the posterior limb and the retrolentiform portion. The medial striate artery supplies the anterior limb and genu. Lateral striate branches supply anterior limb, genu, and posterior limb.

Transient ischemic attacks

TIAs are episodes of vascular insufficiency causing temporary loss of brain function with complete recovery within 24 hours. Anterior circulation TIAs may cause motor and/or sensory deficit and/or dysphasia, sometimes monocular blindness. Posterior circulation TIAs may cause vertigo, diplopia, ataxia, or amnesia.

Arterial occlusion within the anterior circulation

Anterior choroidal artery syndrome results from occlusion of the anterior choroidal artery. The complete syndrome comprises contralateral hemiparesis with upper limb ataxia ('ataxic hemiparesis'), hemihypesthesia and hemianopia.

Clinical effects of anterior, middle and posterior cerebral artery branch occlusion are summarized in *Tables 30.1–30.4*.

The effects of middle cerebral artery occlusion are shown in *Table 30.2*.

Small lacunar infarcts are commonly associated with chronic hypertension. Typical examples are in *Table 30.3*.

Core Information *Continued*

Cerebral hemorrhage most often spreads from the putamen into the internal capsule. Contralateral severe, flaccid hemiplegia results. Sufficient recovery may eventually permit stick-supported spastic ambulation.

Clinical effects of vertebrobasilar arterial occlusion have been summarized in the main text.

Aneurysms
Subarachnoid hemorrhage follows spontaneous rupture of a berry aneurysm at the base of the brain. A typical sequence of clinical effects, in those who survive, is: sudden, blinding headache followed by collapse into unconsciousness and development of neck rigidity. About a quarter of cases develop a neurological deficit within 2 weeks.

Table 30.1 Clinical effects of anterior cerebral artery branch occlusion

Branch	Clinical effects
Orbital/frontopolar	Apathy with some memory loss
Medial striate	Paresis of face and arm
Callosomarginal	Paresis and hypesthesia of face and arm +/− abulia +/− mutism +/− inability to reach across
Pericallosal	Ideomotor apraxia (anterior lesion), tactile anomia (posterior lesion)

Table 30.3 Clinical effects of three common lacunar infarcts

Location	Clinical effects
Genu of internal capsule	Dysarthria–clumsy hand syndrome +/− dysphagia
Posterior limb of internal capsule	Pure motor hemiparesis
Ventral posterior nucleus of thalamus	Pure sensory syndrome +/− sensory ataxia

Table 30.2 Clinical effects of middle cerebral artery occlusion

Segment	Clinical effects
Either stem	Hemiplegia, hemihypesthesia, hemianopia
Left stem	Same + global aphasia
Right stem	Same + sensory neglect
Either upper division	Paresis and hypesthesia of face and arm, dysarthria
Left upper division	Same + Broca's aphasia
Right upper division	Same + hemineglect or expressive aprosodia
Either lower division	Hemianopia +/− agitated state
Left lower division	Same + Wernicke's aphasia, alexia, ideomotor apraxia
Branches	
Orbitofrontal	Prefrontal syndrome
Left precentral	Broca's aphasia
Right precentral	Motor aprosodia
Central	Loss of motor +/− sensory function in face and arm
Inferior parietal	Hemineglect
Either angular	Hemianopia
Left angular	Alexia
Left temporal	Wernicke's aphasia
Right temporal	Receptive aprosodia

Table 30.4 Clinical effects of posterior cerebral artery occlusion

Stem	Clinical effects
Either	Homonymous hemianopia
Left	Alexiain visible field
Both	Cortical blindness +/− amnesia
Branch	
Midbrain	Ipsilateral 3rd nerve palsy + contralateral hemiplegia
Thalamus	Contralateral numbness +/− hemianopia +/− thalamic syndrome
Subthalamic nucleus	Contralateral ballism
Corpus callosum	Alexia in contralateral visual field

REFERENCES

Adams, R.D. and Victor, M. (1989) *Principles of Neurology*, 4th edn. New York: McGraw-Hill.

Amarenco, P., Caplan, L.R. and Pessin, M.S. (1998) Vertebrobasilar occlusive disease. In *Stroke: Pathophysiology, Diagnosis and Management*, 3rd edn (Barnett, H.J.M., Mohr, J.P., Stein, B.M. and Yatsu, F.M., eds), pp. 513–598. New York: Churchill Livingstone.

Betz, A.L., Goldstein, G.W. and Katzman, R. (1989) Blood-brain-cerebrospinal fluid barriers. In *Basic Neurochemistry: Molecular, Cellular, and Medical Aspects*, 4th edn (Siegel, G.J. et al, eds), pp. 591–605. New York: Raven Press.

Brazis, P.W., Masdeu, J.C. and Biller, J. (1996) Vascular syndromes of the cerebrum. In *Localization in Clinical Neurology* (edited by the authors). New York: Little Brown.

Brust, J.C.M. (1998) Anterior cerebral artery disease. In *Stroke: Pathophysiology, Diagnosis and Management*, 3rd edn (Barnett, H.J.M., Mohr, J.P., Stein, B.M. and Yatsu, F.M., eds), pp. 401–426. New York: Churchill Livingstone.

Duus, P. (1983) *Topical Diagnosis in Neurology*. New York: Thieme-Stratton.

Georgiadis, A.L., Yamamoto, Y., Kwan, E.S., Pessin, M.S. and Caplan, L.R. (1999) Anatomy of sensory findings in patients with posterior cerebral artery territory infarction. *Arch. Neurol.* **56**: 835–838.

Mohr, J.P., Lazar, R.M., Marshall, R.S. Gautier, J.C. and Hier, D.B. (1998) Middle cerebral artery disease. In *Stroke: Pathophysiology, Diagnosis and Management*, 3rd edn (Barnett, H.J.M., Mohr, J.P., Stein, B.M. and Yatsu, F.M., eds), pp. 427–480. New York: Churchill Livingstone.

Mohr, J.P. and Pessin, M.S. (1998) Middle cerebral artery disease. In *Stroke: Pathophysiology, Diagnosis and Management*, 3rd edn (Barnett, H.J.M., Mohr, J.P., Stein, B.M. and Yatsu, F.M., eds), pp. 481–502. New York: Churchill Livingstone.

Glossary

Abbreviations: Ch. Chapter containing main reference. *Fr.* Signifies French origin. *Gr.* Signifies Greek origin; *L.* Signifies Latin origin.

Abducens *L.* 'leading away'. Abducens nerve stimulates lateral rectus muscle to abduct the direction of gaze (Ch. 20).

Abulia *Gr.* 'lack of will'. Loss of willpower associated with prefrontal cortical disorders (Ch. 27).

Accommodation Focusing light by allowing the lens to become more convex (Ch. 20).

Active zone Site of release of neurotransmitter through the presynaptic membrane (Ch. 6).

Adaptation Attenuation of response to a sustained sensory stimulus (Ch. 9).

Adrenaline Synonym for epinephrine (Ch. 10).

Affective disorder A disorder of mood, e.g. major depression (Ch. 23).

Afferent *L.* 'carrying toward'. Strictly, applies to nerve impulses traveling toward CNS along sensory fibers; is loosely applied within CNS, e.g. afferent connections of the cerebellum (Ch. 22). See also Centripetal.

Agnosia *Gr.* 'without knowledge'. Inability to interpret sensory information (Ch. 26).

Agraphia *Gr.* 'without writing'. Inability to express oneself in writing owing to a central lesion (Ch. 27).

Akinesia *Gr.* 'without movement'. Refers to immobility often seen in Parkinson's disease (Ch. 25).

Alexia *Gr.* 'without reading'. Inability to read (Ch. 30).

Allocortex *Gr.* 'other cortex'. Phylogenically old, three-layered cortex in the temporal lobe (Ch. 26).

Alpha (α) motor neuron The motor neuron that innervates extrafusal fibers of skeletal muscle (Ch. 8).

Alveus *Gr.* 'trough'. Refers to the thin layer of white matter on the surface of the hippocampus (Ch. 26).

Alzheimer's disease A form of dementia (Ch. 23).

Amnesia Loss of memory (Ch. 29).

Amygdala *Gr.* 'almond'. Nucleus at the tip of the inferior horn of the lateral ventricle (Ch. 26).

Analgesia *Gr.* 'without pain'. Absence of perception of a noxious stimulus (Ch. 12).

Aneurysm *Gr.* 'widening'. Localized dilation of an artery (Ch. 30).

Angiogram Image of blood vessels obtained by intra-arterial injection of radio-opaque fluid (Ch. 5).

Anomia *Gr.* 'without names'. Inability to name common objects (Ch. 27).

Anopsia *Gr.* 'without vision' (Ch. 25).

Anterograde amnesia Inability to lay down new memories (Ch. 29).

Anterograde transport Axonal transport from soma to nerve terminals (Ch. 6).

Antidromic *Gr.* 'running against'. Usually refers to nerve impulses which, traveling proximally along one branch of a Y-shaped sensory nerve fiber, arrive at the junction and travel distally along the other branch (Ch. 9).

Aphasia *Gr.* 'without speech,' e.g. motor aphasia, sensory aphasia (Ch. 27).

Apraxia *Gr.* 'without movement'. Inability to carry out voluntary movements in the absence of paralysis (Ch. 27).

Arachnoid *Gr.* 'spider like'. Refers to the web-like delicacy of the arachnoid mater (Ch. 4).

Archi- (arche-) *Gr.* 'beginning'. Refers to oldest areas, e.g. archicerebellum (Ch. 14).

Area postrema *L.* 'back end area'. Refers to the posterior tip of the fourth ventricle (Ch. 19).

Arnold–Chiari malformation Maldevelopment of the posterior cranial fossa (Ch. 11).

Ascending reticular activating system (ARAS) A polysynaptic chain of reticular formation neurons involved in maintaining the conscious state (Ch. 21).

Assistance reflex During voluntary movement, positive feedback from actively stretched neuromuscular spindles assists the movement (Ch. 13). Compare with Resistance reflex.

Association cortex Area of cortex receiving afferents from one or more primary sensory areas (Ch. 26).

Astereognosis *Gr.* 'without knowledge of solid'. Refers to inability to identify common objects by touch alone (Ch. 26).

Astrocyte The 'star-like' neuroglial cell (Ch. 5).

Ataxia *Gr.* 'without order'. Describes the uncoordinated movements associated with posterior column (Ch. 12) or cerebellar (Ch. 22) disease.

Atherosclerosis Arterial degenerative disorder associated with fatty subintimal plaques capable of detachment with consequent embolism within the arterial territory (Ch. 30).

Athetosis *Gr.* 'without stability'. Describes the continuous writhing movements sometimes associated with damage to the basal ganglia (Ch. 28).

Autogenetic inhibition Negative feedback from Golgi tendon organs causing a muscle to relax (Ch. 8).

Autonomic Self-regulating (Ch. 10).

Autoreceptor A presynaptic receptor acted upon by the transmitter released at the same nerve ending (Ch. 10).

Axolemma *Gr.* 'husk' covering the central part or 'axis' of a nerve fiber (Ch. 6).

Axoplasm *Gr.* 'substance' (i.e. cytoplasm) of the axon (Ch. 6).

Axoplasmic transport Orthograde or retrograde transport of materials within an axon (Ch. 6).

Babinski sign Reflex fanning of the toes with extension of the great toe, following a scraping stimulus to the lateral part of the sole; sign of corticospinal tract disorder (Ch. 13).

Ballism *Gr.* 'throwing,' with reference to the flailing movements that follow damage to the subthalamic nucleus (Ch. 28).

Baroreceptor *Gr.* 'weight' receptor. Refers to the blood pressure receptors of the carotid sinus and aortic arch (Ch. 21).

Baroreceptor reflex Reflex increase of sympathetic vascular tone in response to a fall in intracranial blood pressure, e.g. on assuming the upright position (Ch. 14).

Barosympathetic reflex Reflex reduction of sympathetic tone in response to a rise of arterial blood pressure (Ch. 14).

Barovagal reflex Reflex reduction of heart rate in response to a rise of arterial blood pressure (Ch. 14).

Bell's palsy Peripheral facial nerve paralysis caused by swelling of the nerve followed by its compression against the wall of the bony facial nerve canal (Ch. 19).

Benign essential tremor A tremulous disorder commonly, attributed to Parkinson's disease (Ch. 28).

Berry aneurysm Blister-like aneurysm on or near the Circle of Willis (Ch. 30).

Binocular visual field The visual field common to both eyes (Ch. 25).

Bitemporal hemianopia Lateral visual field defects resulting from pressure on cross-over optic nerve fibers in the midregion of the optic chiasm, usually by a pituitary adenoma (Ch. 25).

Blindsight Patients with cortical blindness may perceive movement in the peripheral field without being able to see anything there (Ch. 26).

Blinking-to-light reflex Reflex blinking in response to a flash of bright light (Ch. 19).

Blinking-to-noise reflex Acousticofacial reflex causing the orbicularis oculi to twitch in response to a loud sound (Ch. 19).

Body schema Consciousness of the relative position of body parts; a function of (mainly right) area 40 (inferior parietal lobe) (Ch. 27).

Bradykinesia *Gr.* 'slow movement' characteristic of Parkinson's disease (Ch. 28).

Brain Intracranial CNS.

Brain attack Stroke (Ch. 30).

Brain-derived neurotrophic factor (BDNF) A 'nourishing' factor that promotes survival and normal functioning of cortical neurons (Ch. 6).

Brainstem Comprises midbrain, pons and medulla oblongata (Ch. 3). In the embryo, also includes the diencephalon (Ch. 1).

Broca's aphasia Aphasia caused by damage to the motor speech area (Ch. 27).

Broca's area Pars triangularis (area 44) and pars anterior (area 45) of the frontal operculum, involved in generating speech (Ch. 27).

Brown–Sequard syndrome The constellation of signs that follows hemisection of the spinal cord (Ch. 13).

Bulbar *L.* 'bulb' of the brain. A discredited term usually meaning medulla oblongata.

Calcar avis *L.* 'spur of a bird'. Refers to the elevation produced by the calcarine sulcus in the medial wall of the atrium of the lateral ventricle (Ch. 2).

Catecholamines The neurotransmitters, dopamine, norepinephrine, and epinephrine (Ch. 6), comprising amines attached to catechol rings.

Cauda equina *L.* 'horse's tail'. Refers to the leash of spinal nerve roots below the level of the spinal cord (Ch. 11).

Caudal anesthesia Pelvic/perineal anesthesia produced by injection of local anesthetic through the sacral hiatus into the epidural space (Ch. 11).

Caudate *L.* having a tail (caudate nucleus, Ch. 2).

Center-surround receptive field A visual receptive field having a center surrounded by a ring of opposite sign (Ch. 25).

Central pattern generator A neural circuit giving rise to rhythmic motor activity.

Centrifugal *L.* 'fleeing the center'. See Efferent.

Centripetal *L.* 'seeking the center'. See Afferent.

Cerebellar ataxia Ataxia of cerebellar origin (Ch. 22).

Cerebellar cognitive affective syndrome Constellation of symptoms associated with cerebellar pathology (Ch. 22).

Cerebellar signs Ataxia/intention tremor (in particular) associated with cerebellar pathology (Ch. 22).

Cerebellum *L.* 'little brain'.

Cerebrovascular accident Thrombosis, embolism or hemorrhage in or around the brain (Ch. 30).

Cerebrum *L.* 'brain,' comprising cerebral hemispheres and diencephalon (Ch. 2).

Cervical spondylosis A form of vertebral arthritis accompanied by bony outgrowths around the margins of cervical facet joints resulting in compression of cervical nerve roots (Ch. 11).

Cervicogenic headache Headache caused by pressure on cervical nerves (Ch. 11).

Chemical synapse Distinguished from electrical synapses by release of neurotransmitter (Ch. 6).

Chemoreceptor A sensory receptor (e.g. carotid body) selective for a chemical substance (Ch. 21).

Chiasma *Gr.* 'crossing'. Refers mainly to the optic chiasma (chiasm) (Ch. 2).

Chorea *Gr.* 'dance'. Involuntary movements representing fragments of motor programs (Ch. 28).

Choroid plexus *Gr.* 'membranous network' of capillaries invested with choroidal epithelium, within the ventricles of the brain (Ch. 2).

Chromatolysis *Gr.* 'dissolution of color' in the perikaryon, following axotomy (Ch. 5).

Cingulotomy Section/excision of anterior cingulate cortex, usually for relief of pain (Ch. 29).

Cingulum *L.* the 'girdle' of white matter within the cingulate gyrus.

Claspknife rigidity Initial resistance to passive movement followed by collapse of resistance; a sign of upper motor neuron disease (Ch. 13).

Claustrum *L.* the 'barrier' of gray matter between insula and lentiform nucleus (Ch. 2).

Clonus *L.* 'turmoil'. Rapid beating movement at ankle or wrist produced by sudden passive extension; associated with upper motor neuron disease (Ch. 13).

Coactivation (a) Simultaneous activation of α and γ motor neurons; (b) simultaneous activation of motor neurons supplying prime movers and antagonists (Ch. 8).

Co-contraction Simultaneous contraction of prime movers and antagonists.

Cognition Information-processing associated with thinking (Ch. 27).

Cognitive style Subtle differences in left vs right cerebral function (Ch. 27).

Cogwheel rigidity Ratchety response of muscles to passive movement of joints; associated with Parkinson's disease (Ch. 28).

Colliculus *L.* 'little hill'. Four colliculi comprise the tectum of the midbrain (Ch. 3).

Column A term used interchangeably for the posterior funiculus of the spinal cord (Ch. 12).

Commissure *L.* 'link' between the two sides of the nervous system, e.g. white commissure of the spinal cord (Ch. 3), anterior commissure of the brain, corpus callosum (Ch. 2).

Compensation reflex Vestibulo-ocular reflex compensating for movement of the head; associated with fixation/foveation (Ch. 16).

Complex spikes Complex response of Purkinje cells to stimulation of olivocerebellar fibers (Ch. 22).

Concussion Brief cortical dysfunction resulting from a blow to the head (Ch. 4).

Conduction aphasia Aphasia caused by damage to the arcuate fasciculus (Ch. 27).

Conductive deafness Deafness caused by disease in the outer ear canal or middle ear (Ch. 17).

Conjugate movement Movement in parallel, e.g. ocular saccades (Ch. 20).

Conscious proprioception Perceived sensations arising within the body, notably from muscle spindles (Ch. 12).

Consolidation The process of storing information in long-term memory (Ch. 29).

Continuous conduction Mode of impulse conduction along unmyelinated nerve fibers (Ch. 6).

Contralateral *L.* Refers to opposite side of the body (compare with ipsilateral, same side).

Convolution *L.* a gyrus (Ch. 2).

Cordotomy Incision of the spinal cord for pain relief (Ch. 12).

Corneal reflex Blinking in response to corneal contact (Ch. 19).

Corona radiata *L.* 'radiating crown' of white matter extending from cerebral cortex to internal capsule and vice versa (Ch. 2).

Corpus callosum *L.* 'hard body'. Refers to the great transverse commissure of white matter interconnecting like areas of the cerebral hemispheres (Ch. 2).

Corpus striatum *L.* 'striated body' comprising caudate and lentiform nuclei (Ch. 2).

Cortex *L.* the 'bark' of gray matter at the surface of the cerebrum and cerebellum (Ch. 2).

Cortical blindness Blindness owing to damage to the primary visual cortex (Ch. 26).

Cortical mosaic Mosaic arrangement created by interdigitation of cortical modules of different kinds (Ch. 26).

Cortical type sensory loss Diminution of tactile perception associated with damage to the primary sensory cortex (Ch. 26).

Crossed hemiplegia Follows unilateral brainstem lesion affecting one or more motor cranial nerve nuclei (resulting in ipsilateral paralysis) together with corticospinal fibers (resulting in contralateral hemiplegia/hemiparesis) (Ch. 30).

Crus *L.* 'leg', e.g. c. of fornix (Ch. 2), c. of midbrain (Ch. 2).

Cuneate *L.* 'wedge-like', e.g. cuneate fasciculus (Ch. 11).

Cuneus *L.* 'wedge', e.g. the gyrus of that shape in the occipital lobe (Ch. 2).

Declarative memory Memory for facts and events (Ch. 26).

Decussation *L.* from Roman numeral X. Refers to X-shaped crossing of nerve bundles at junctional regions, e.g. pyramidal decussation (brain–spinal cord, Ch. 3), decussation of superior cerebellar peduncles (pons–midbrain, Ch. 3).

Déjà vu *Fr.* Epileptic aura where a novel visual field seems familiar (Ch. 28).

Dementia Loss of cognitive abilities in the presence of intact motor and sensory systems (Ch. 29).

Dendrite(s) *Gr.* 'tree(s)'. Refers to the neuronal processes receiving the axons of other neurons (Ch. 5).

Dentate *L.* 'toothed', e.g. dentate nucleus of cerebellum (Ch. 2), dentate gyrus in the temporal lobe (Ch. 29).

Denticulate *L.* 'little-toothed', e.g. denticulate ligament of pia mater anchoring the spinal cord (Ch. 4).

Depolarization block Conduction block produced by high frequency stimulation (Ch. 28).

Depolarize Make the membrane potential of the neuron less negative (Ch. 6).

Detrusor instability 'Unstable bladder' characterized by spontaneous expulsion of urine despite conscious attempts at restraint (Ch. 10).

Developmental dyslexia Pronounced reading difficulty in children who are the match of their peers in other respects (Ch. 27).

Diabetes insipidus Hypothalamic disorder characterized by polyuria and polydypsia (Ch. 23).

Diencephalic amnesia Amnesia associated with shrinkage of the mammillary bodies (Ch. 29).

Diencephalon *Gr.* 'between-brain', comprising epithalamus (Ch. 22), thalamus (Ch. 22), and hypothalamus (Ch. 21).

Diffuse noxious inhibitory controls Appropriate neural connections whereby painful stimulation of one part of the body may produce pain relief in all other parts (Ch. 21).

Diplopia *Gr.* 'double vision' (Ch. 20).

Discriminative touch Fine touch sensibility (Chs 12, 26).

Disinhibition Release of excitatory neurons by inhibition of inhibitory neurons (Chs 6, 28).

Dissociated sensory loss Loss of one sensory modality with preservation of others (Ch. 12).

Dopa Dihydroxyphenylalanine, a precursor of dopamine, norepinephrine, and epinephrine (Ch. 6).

Dopamine Catecholamine neurotransmitter synthesized from dopa.

Dura mater *L.* 'hard cover'. Outermost meninx (Ch. 4).

Dynamic (kinetic) labyrinth The semicircular canals (Ch. 16).

Dynamic posturography Testing postural reflex responses to sudden tilting (Ch. 22).

Dys- *Gr.* 'difficult'.

Dysarthria *Gr.* 'difficult articulation' (Ch. 30).

Dysarthria–clumsy hand syndrome Syndrome associated with a vascular lesion of the genu of the internal capsule (Ch. 30).

Dysdiadochokinesia *Gr.* 'difficult successive movements'. Refers to difficulty in performing rapid pronation–supination sequences (Ch. 22).

Dyskinetic cerebral palsy Movement problems associated with damage to the basal ganglia associated with cerebral palsy (Ch. 28).

Dyslexia *Gr.* 'difficult reading'. Reading difficulty (Ch. 27).

Dysmetria *Gr.* 'difficult measurement'. Refers to reduced motor control in cerebellar disease (Ch. 22).

Dysphagia *Gr.* 'difficult eating/swallowing,' e.g. following paralysis of pharyngeal constrictors (Ch. 15).

Dysphasia Mild/moderate expressive aphasia (Ch. 27).

Dysphonia Hoarseness of speech (Ch. 15).

ECT (Electroconvulsive therapy) A treatment for epilepsy (Ch. 29).

Ectoderm *Gr.* 'outer skin'. Refers to the outer germ layer giving rise to the nervous system and to the epidermis of the skin (Ch. 1).

EEG (Electroencephalography) Taking a record of brain waves (Ch. 26).

Efferent *L.* 'carrying away'. Strictly, applies to nerve impulses traveling away from the CNS; also used regionally, e.g. cerebellar efferents. See also Centrifugal.

Ejaculation *L.* 'throwing'. Expelling semen into the vagina (Ch. 10).

Electrical potential Voltage.

Electrical synapse Synapse consisting of gap junctions (Ch. 6).

Electrotonus A decremental voltage change passing over the neuronal soma following receptor activation (Ch. 6).

Emboliform *Gr.* 'plug like,' e.g. emboliform nucleus of cerebellum (Ch. 20).

Embolus *Gr.* 'plug', e.g. cerebral embolus formed by a blood clot breaking away from the internal carotid artery (Ch. 27).

EMG Electromyography (Ch. 8).

Emission Expulsion of semen into the urethra (Ch. 10).

Endocytosis Vesicular uptake of material from the extracellular space (Ch. 6).

Endogenous opioids Brain-derived neuropeptides (Ch. 21).

Endoneurium *Gr.* 'within nerve'. Refers to the connective tissue sheath surrounding individual nerve fibers (Ch. 7).

Engram The chemical intraneuronal representation of a memory.

Enteroception *L.* 'reception from inside'. Refers to stimuli transduced within the alimentary tract (Ch. 10).

Entorhinal *Gr.* 'in nose'. Refers to entorhinal cortex of the temporal lobe (Ch. 29).

Ependyma *Gr.* 'upper garment'. Refers to the epithelium lining the ventricular system of brain (Ch. 2) and the central canal of the spinal cord (Ch. 3).

Epidural anesthesia Anesthesia procured by injecting analgesic solution into the epidural space, usually in the lumbar region (Ch. 11).

Epinephrine Catecholamine hormone synthesized in adrenal medulla (Ch. 10); also a neurotransmitter synthesized in the brainstem (Chs 14, 21). Also known as adrenaline.

Epineurium *Gr.* 'on nerve'. Refers to loose connective tissue investment of peripheral nerves (Ch. 7).

Episodic memory Ability to recollect episodes of one's own earlier life (Ch. 29).

Epithalamus *Gr.* 'above thalamus,' includes pineal gland (Ch. 22).

Excitotoxicity Toxic effects on target neurons, of excessive glutamatergic activity (Ch. 29).

Expressive aphasia Loss of motor speech (Ch. 27).

Extensor plantar response See Babinski sign.

Exteroception *L.* 'reception from outside'. Refers to stimuli transduced at the body surface, rather than within the body wall/limbs (proprioception) or alimentary tract (enteroception).

Extrapyramidal *L.* 'nonpyramidal'. Refers to pathways involving the basal ganglia (Ch. 28).

Facilitation Increasing the likelihood of depolarization (Ch. 6).

Falx *L.* 'sickle'. Refers to shape, e.g. falx cerebri, falx cerebelli (Ch. 4).

Familial tremor Benign essential tremor (Ch. 28).

Far response Sympathetic activity causing flattening of the lens for far vision (Ch. 20).

Fascicle *L.* 'small bundle' of nerve or muscle fibers (Ch. 7).

Fasciculation Involuntary twitching of muscle fascicles; often associated with lower motor neuron disease (Ch. 13).

Fasciculus *L.* 'small bundle' of nerve fibers within CNS, e.g. fasciculus gracilis, fasciculus cuneatus (Ch. 12).

Fastigial *L.* 'apex of a roof,' e.g. fastigial nucleus in roof of fourth ventricle (Ch. 20).

Feature extraction Separate simultaneous analysis of individual features of the scene by the visual association cortex (Ch. 26).

Fibrillation Minute skeletal muscle contractions resulting from denervation supersensitivity (Ch. 13).

Fimbria *L.* 'fringe'. Refers to the fringe of white fibers along the edge of the hippocampus (Ch. 26).

Finger-to-nose-test A test of cerebellar function (Ch. 22).

Fixation Visual targeting of an object; compare with foveation (Ch. 20).

Flatness of affect Dearth of emotional expression (Ch. 27).

fMRI Functional magnetic resonance imaging (Ch. 26).

Foramen *L.* 'opening'.

Forceps *L.* 'pair of tongs,' e.g. the forceps minor and forceps major of the corpus callosum (Ch. 2).

Fornix *L.* 'arch'. Refers to the efferent projection of the hippocampal formation (Chs 2, 28).

Fovea *L.* 'pit', e.g. fovea centralis of the retina (Ch. 23).

Foveation Visual targeting so that the center of the scene is aligned with the fovea (Ch. 22).

Functional electrical stimulation Muscle rehabilitation by electrical stimulation at the motor point (Ch. 8).

Functional sympathectomy Preganglionic sympathetic nerve section (Ch. 10).

Funiculus *L.* 'small cord' (Ch. 3).

Fusimotor Motor to intrafusal muscle fibers (Ch. 8). See Gamma motor neuron.

GABA Gamma aminobutyric acid; the main inhibitory neurotransmitter (Ch. 8).

Gag reflex Reflex contraction of the pharyngeal constrictors in response to stroking the oropharynx (Ch. 15).

Gait ataxia Staggering gait associated with posterior column disease (Ch. 12) and cerebellar disease (Ch. 22).

Gamma (γ) motor neuron Fusimotor neuron supplying the intrafusal muscle fibers of a muscle spindle (Ch. 8).

Ganglion *Gr.* 'knot'. Refers (a) to spinal and peripheral autonomic ganglia (Chs 7, 10); (b) to the basal ganglia (Ch. 28).

Gating Controlling ease of passage of impulses from one set of neurons to another, e.g. from primary to secondary sensory neurons (Ch. 21).

Geniculate *L.* 'knee-form,' meaning bent.

Genu *L.* 'knee,' meaning a bend.

Giant motor unit potential Abnormally large motor unit potential seen in EMG records of aging muscle (Ch. 8).

Glia *Gr.* 'glue'. Refers to the supporting neuroglial cells of the CNS (Ch. 6).

Gliosis Scarring produced by astrocytes (Ch. 6).

Globose *L.* 'ball-like'. Refers to the globose nucleus of the cerebellum (Ch. 22).

Globus *L.* 'ball'. Usually refers to the globus pallidus in the cerebral white matter (Ch. 2).

Glomerulus *L.* 'little ball of yarn,' e.g. synaptic glomeruli in the cerebellum (Ch. 22) and olfactory bulb (Ch. 28).

Glossopharyngeal *G.* 'lingual–pharyngeal,' with reference to the sensory distribution of the glossopharyngeal nerve (and to its motor supply to stylopharyngeus) (Ch. 15).

Glutamate The most common excitatory neurotransmitter in the CNS (Ch. 6).

Gracilis *L.* 'slender,' e.g. gracile fasciculus in the spinal cord (Ch. 12).

Grapheme A written syllable (Ch. 27).

Growth cone The conical tip of a growing axon (Ch. 7).

Gustation/gustatory Having to do with taste sensation (Ch. 19).

Gyrus *L.* convolution of the cerebral cortex (Ch. 2).

Head-righting reflex A reflex, engaging the static labyrinth and medial vestibulospinal tract, designed to keep the head upright (Ch. 16).

Heel-to-knee-test A test of cerebellar function (Ch. 22).

Hemi- *Gr.* 'half'.

Hemianopia *Gr.* 'half-blindness,' caused by a lesion of the geniculocalcarine pathway or primary visual cortex (Ch. 25).

Hemiballism *Gr.* 'half-throwing,' refers to involuntary, 'throwing' movements of arm and/or leg on one side, associated with damage to the subthalamic nucleus (Ch. 28).

Hemiparesis *Gr.* 'half-weakness'. Weakness of one side of the body associated with upper motor neuron disease (Chs 13, 30).

Hemiplegia *Gr.* 'half-struck'. Refers to paralysis of one half of the body following a major stroke (Ch. 28).

Hering–Breuer reflex Reflex inhibition of the dorsal respiratory center by pulmonary stretch receptors (Ch. 15).

Hertz (Hz) Cycles per second (Ch. 28).

Hippocampus *Gr.* 'sea horse'. Part of the limbic system (Chs 2, 28).

Histaminergic system Widespread histaminergic innervation of cerebral cortex by the tuberoinfundibular nucleus of hypothalamus (Chs 23, 26).

Homonymous *Gr.* 'matching'. (a) Matching motor neurons (Ch. 8); (b) matching parts of the binocular visual field (Ch. 25).

Horner's syndrome Signs of cervical sympathetic paralysis, the complete syndrome comprising miosis, ptosis, and anhidrosis (Chs 10, 20).

Huntington's disease A hereditary hyperkinetic disorder (Ch. 28).

Hydrocephalus *Gr.* 'water-head,' meaning increased volume of cerebrospinal fluid (Ch. 4).

Hyper- *Gr.* 'excessive'.

Hyperacusis Excessive perception of sound (Ch. 17).

Hyperhidrosis *Gr.* 'too much watering'. Excessive sweating (Ch. 10).

Hyperkinetic states Disorders associated with involuntary movements (Ch. 28).

Hyperreflexia Exaggerated tendon reflexes; associated with upper motor neuron disease (Ch. 13).

Hypo- *Gr.* 'below,' e.g. hypoglossal (Ch. 15), hypothalamus (Ch. 23).

Idiopathic Pathology of unknown origin.

Impotence Inability to maintain an erection (Ch. 10).

Incontinence Involuntary voiding of urine/feces (Chs 10, 21).

Infarction *L.* 'stuffed into'. Refers to blood-stuffed necrotic tissue resulting from vascular occlusion (Ch. 30).

Infranuclear lesion Lesion of the trunk of a cranial nerve (Ch. 15).

Infundibulum *L.* 'funnel,' leading down to the hypophysis (Ch. 23).

Insula *L.* 'island' of cerebral cortex covered by the opercula (Ch. 2).

Intention tremor Tremor appearing during performance of purposive movements; associated with cerebellar disease (Ch. 22).

Internuncial *L.* 'messenger between'. Refers to small connecting neurons (Ch. 6).

Intra- *L.* 'within,' e.g. intralaminar nucleus of thalamus (Ch. 24).

Ipsilateral *L.* 'on same side'.

Iso- *Gr.* 'equal,' e.g. isocortex, uniformly containing six layers of neurons (Ch. 26).

Isofrequency stripes Bands of primary auditory cortex responding to particular tonal frequencies (Ch. 26).

Jamais vu *Fr.* 'never seen'. Epileptic aura where a familiar scene appears novel (Ch. 28).

Jargon aphasia Jumbled speech associated with a lesion of Wernicke's area (Ch. 27).

Joint sense The sense of direction of passive movement of a joint; affected in posterior column disease (Ch. 12).

Joint stiffness 'Active' joint stiffness is the element of resistance to movement introduced by autogenetic inhibition and designed to prevent oscillation (Ch. 8). 'Passive' joint stiffness is a progressive resistance to passive movement caused by intramuscular collagen accumulation following an upper motor neuron lesion (Ch. 13).

Jugular foramen syndrome Constellation of symptoms and signs associated with injury to the glossopharyngeal, vagus, and accessory nerves related to the jugular foramen (Ch. 15).

Kindling ('lighting a fire') Progressively increasing group response of hippocampal neurons to a repetitive stimulus of uniform strength (Ch. 29).

Kinesthesia *Gr.* 'perception of movement' (Ch. 12).

Kinetic/dynamic labyrinth The semicircular canals (Ch. 15).

Kluver–Bucy syndrome Constellation of personality changes following anterior temporal lobectomy (Ch. 29).

Korsakoff's psychosis State of anterograde amnesia associated with shrinkage of the mammillary bodies (Ch. 29).

Lacuna *L.* 'little lake'. See below.

Lacunar infarct Brain infarct in the form of a lacuna, associated with hypertension (Ch. 30).

Lateral medullary syndrome Characteristic symptoms and signs following thrombosis of the vertebral or posterior inferior cerebellar artery (Ch. 16).

Lead pipe rigidity Uniform resistance to passive joint movement; characteristic of Parkinson's disease (Ch. 28).

Lemniscus *Gr.* 'ribbon'. Used with reference to several afferent pathways (tracts) in the brainstem (Ch. 14).

Lentiform *L.* Lens-shaped nucleus, part of the corpus striatum (caudate and lentiform nuclei) (Ch. 2).

Leptomeninges *Gr.* 'thin membranes' comprising the arachnoid and pia mater (Ch. 4).

Lesion *L.* 'wound'. Refers to tissue damage of any kind.

Limbic *L.* 'marginal'. Refers to limbic structures at the inner margin of the cerebral hemisphere (Ch. 26).

Locus ceruleus *L.* 'dark blue place' in the (fresh) floor of fourth ventricle (Ch. 19). See Cerulean nucleus.

Long tract signs Signs indicative of damage to major sensory and motor pathways, especially in relation to brainstem vascular lesions (Chs 16, 20).

Lower motor neuron signs Signs of lower motor neuron disease (Ch. 13).

LTD Long-term (prolonged) depression of neuronal responsivity following conditioning stimuli (Ch. 22).

LTP Long-term potentiation of neuronal responsivity following conditioning stimuli (Ch. 29).

Lumbar puncture Needle puncture of the lumbar cistern to obtain a sample of cerebrospinal fluid (Ch. 11).

Macula *L.* 'spot', e.g. macula of utricle (Ch. 16), macula lutea (yellow) of retina (Ch. 23).

Major depression Prevalent psychiatric disorder associated with depressed mood (Ch. 23).

Mammillary *L.* 'nipple-like'. Refers to the mammillary bodies (Ch. 23).

Marche à petit pas *Fr.* 'walk with small steps'. Hesitant gait associated with frontal lobe disease (Ch. 27).

Mechanoreceptor Sensory receptor sensitive to mechanical stimuli, e.g. muscle spindles and tendon organs (Ch. 8), some cutaneous receptors (Ch. 9), carotid sinus receptors (Ch. 14) and inner ear hair cells (Chs 15, 16).

Medulla *L.* 'marrow'. Refers to the marrow-like appearance of the fresh brain and spinal cord within their bony shells.

Medulla oblongata *L.* 'oblong' (elongate) part of the hindbrain (Ch. 3).

Membrane potential The voltage across a cell membrane (Ch. 6).

Meningism Neck retraction characteristic of meningitis (Ch. 4) and subarachnoid hemorrhage (Ch. 30).

Meningomyelocele A form of spina bifida accompanied by a cyst protruding from the vertebral canal (Ch. 11).

Mesencephalon *Gr.* 'midbrain' (Ch. 1).

Mesocortical fibers Dopaminergic fibers projecting to the prefrontal cortex from the ventral tegmental nuclei of the midbrain (Ch. 29).

Mesoderm *Gr.* 'middle skin'. Refers to the middle germ layer (Ch. 1).

Mesolimbic fibers Dopaminergic fibers projecting to the limbic system from the ventral tegmental nuclei (Ch. 29).

Metencephalon *Gr.* 'after the brain'. Comprises embryonic pons and cerebellum (Ch. 1).

Microglia *Gr.* small glial cells (Ch. 6).

Microzone A 'beam' of excitation of Purkinje cells by granule cells (Ch. 22).

Miosis *Gr.* 'constriction' of the pupil (Ch. 20).

Mnemonic *Gr.* 'memory related'. Having to do with memory (Ch. 29).

Modality See Sensory modality.

Modulation Effect of neurotransmitters, notably the catecholamines and serotonin, in altering the response of neurons to classic transmitters (Ch. 6).

Module A cell column in the cerebral cortex (Ch. 26).

Monocular blindness Blindness in one eye (Ch. 25).

Monocular crescent The C-shaped monocular visual field (Ch. 25).

Monoplegia Paralysis of one limb resulting from upper motor neuron disease (Chs 13, 30).

Monosynaptic reflex Term applied to the tendon reflex (Ch. 8).

Motor learning Learning of a motor skill (Ch. 22).

Motor neuron disease Disease of spinal cord/brainstem motor neurons (Chs 13, 15).

Motor point The point of entry of a motor nerve into muscle (Ch. 8).

Motor set Posture adopted prior to movement (Ch. 26).

Motor unit An α motor neuron together with the squad of muscle fibers it supplies (Ch. 8).

Movement synergy Manner of operation of the primary motor cortex (Ch. 26).

MRI Magnetic resonance imaging (Ch. 26).

Multimodal association cortex See polymodal association cortex.

Multiple sclerosis Demyelinating disease associated with multiple areas of sclerosis (hardening) caused by glial scarring (Ch. 6).

Multisystem atrophy A neurological disorder frequently misdiagnosed as Parkinson's disease (Ch. 28).

Muscarinic receptor A subtype of acetylcholinergic (ACh) receptor; historically, activated by muscarine (Ch. 10).

Myasthenia *Gr.* 'muscle weakness' (Ch. 8).

Myelencephalon *Gr.* 'marrowbrain'. Refers to the embryonic medulla oblongata (Ch. 1).

Myelin *Gr.* 'marrow'. Refers to the myelin sheath of axons (Chs 6, 7).

Myelocele A form of spina bifida associated with an open neural tube (Ch. 11).

Myelogram Image of the spinal subarachnoid space produced by injection of a radio-opaque substance into the lumbar cistern (Ch. 4).

Myotatic reflex *Gr.* 'muscle touching'. Tendon reflex (Ch. 8).

Near response Passive thickening of the lens, miosis, and convergence, combined for close-up viewing (Ch. 20).

Neglect Neglect of contralateral personal/extrapersonal space associated with inferior parietal lobe disease (Ch. 27).

Neo- *Gr.* 'new', e.g. neocerebellum (Ch. 20), neocortex (Ch. 24).

Neurite *Gr.* process of a neuron, whether axon or dendrite (Ch. 6).

Neuroblast *Gr.* 'nerve germ'. Refers to embryonic neuron (Ch. 1).

Neurofibril *L.* Refers to matted neurofilaments seen by light microscopy (Ch. 6).

Neurofibrillary tangles Tangles of neurofibrils, most numerous in Alzheimer's disease (Ch. 29).

Neurofilament *L.* The fine filaments seen in neurons by electron microscopy (Ch. 6).

Neurogenic inflammation See Triple response.

Neurohumoral reflex Reflex with neural afferent limb and hormonal efferent limb, e.g. the milk ejection reflex (Ch. 23).

Neurolemma *Gr.* 'nerve sheath', comprising chains of Schwann cells (Ch. 7).

Neuron *Gr.* 'nerve'. Refers to the complete nerve cell (Ch. 6).

Neurotoxicity Refers to damage inflicted on target neurons by excess glutamate (Ch. 26).

Neurotransmitter A chemical liberated at a nerve terminal which activates postsynaptic and/or presynaptic receptors (Ch. 6).

Nicotinic receptor An acetylcholine receptor, historically activated by nicotine (Ch. 10).

Nociceptive *L.* 'taking injury'. Responsive to noxious stimulation (Ch. 9).

Nonconscious proprioception Sensory signals arising within the body that are not perceived, e.g. spinocerebellar tracts (Ch. 12).

Noradrenergic Neurons using norepinephrine (noradrenaline) as transmitter, e.g. postganglionic sympathetic (Ch. 10), cerulean nucleus (Ch. 14).

Norepinephrine (Also called noradrenaline.) Hormone released by the adrenal medulla (Ch. 10); also a brainstem neurotransmitter (Ch. 14).

Nuclear lesion Lesion of a motor nucleus in the brainstem.

Nucleus *L.* 'nut'. Refers either to the trophic center of a cell, or to a group of neurons within the CNS (Ch. 6).

Nystagmus *Gr.* 'nodding'. Refers to involuntary oscillation of the eyes (Ch. 16).

Occupational deafness Deafness brought on by noise in the workplace (Ch. 17).

Ocular dominance columns Cell columns in the primary visual cortex activated by geniculostriate neurons (Ch. 26).

Oculomotor *L.* 'eyemoving'. Refers to the oculomotor nerve (Ch. 20).

Oculomotor hypokinesia Inadequate saccades associated with Parkinson's disease (Ch. 28).

Olfactory aura Epileptic aura accompanied by illusion of an odor (Ch. 28).

Oligodendrocyte *Gr.* 'few tree cell'. A myelin-forming neuroglial cell with few processes (Ch. 6).

Operculum *L.* 'cover'. Refers to any of the three opercula covering the insula (Ch. 2).

Ophthalmoplegia *Gr.* 'eye stroke'. Signifies paralysis of extrinsic ocular muscles (Ch. 20).

Orthodromic Impulse conduction in a centrifugal direction, as distinct from antidromic conduction (Ch. 9).

Orthograde transneuronal degeneration Neuronal degeneration in a proximodistal direction (Ch. 7).

Orthograde transport Proximodistal axoplasmic transport (Ch. 6).

Orthography Processing of letter shapes by the visual cortex (Ch. 27).

Osteophytes Bony excrescences associated with spondylosis (Ch. 11).

Otitis media Middle ear disease (Ch. 17).

Otosclerosis Ear disease associated with ankylosis of the footplate of stapes (Ch. 17).

Ototoxic Term referring to drugs causing sensorineural deafness (Ch. 17).

Pachymeninx *Gr.* 'thick membrane'. The dura mater (Ch. 4).

Paleo- *Gr.* 'old,' e.g. paleocerebellum (mainly the anterior lobe, Ch. 21), paleocortex (olfactory, Ch. 26), paleostriatum (globus pallidus, Ch. 28).

Pallidotomy Surgical lesion of globus pallidus, a treatment for Parkinson's disease (Ch. 28).

Pallidum *L.* 'pale'. Refers to globus pallidus (Ch. 25).

Pallium *Gr.* 'cloak'. The cerebral cortex.

Papez circuit An 'emotional' circuit of the limbic system first described by Papez (Ch. 29).

Papilledema Swelling of the optic papilla, usually in association with raised intracranial pressure (Ch. 4).

Para- *Gr.* 'beside'.

Paralysis *Gr.* 'disablement'. Loss of voluntary movement.

Paralysis agitans See Parkinson's disease.

Paraplegia *Gr.* 'paralysis'. Refers to paralysis of both lower limbs.

Paresis *Gr.* 'weakness'. Incomplete paralysis.

Paresthesia *Gr.* 'side feeling'. A sense of numbness or tingling.

Parkinson's disease Disorder of the basal ganglia associated with one or more characteristic features (Ch. 28).

Peduncle *L.* 'little foot'. Refers to stem, e.g. cerebral peduncle (Ch. 2).

Peri- *Gr.* 'around'.

PET Positron emission tomography (Ch. 26).

Phasic motor neurons α Motor neurons innervating squads of fast, glycolytic muscle fibers (Ch. 14).

Phoneme A syllable of sound corresponding to a grapheme (Ch. 27).

Phonemic paraphrasia In Wernicke's aphasia, the use of incorrect but similar-sounding words (Ch. 27).

Phonology The sounds of words (Ch. 27).

Pia mater *Gr.* 'soft cover'. The innermost layer of the meninges (Ch. 4).

Pineal *L.* 'pine cone'. Pineal gland is part of the epithalamus (Ch. 21).

Plasticity Capacity of neurons to adapt to a changed environment (Chs 22, 26).

Plexus *L.* 'interwoven'. Interwoven nerves or blood vessels.

Polymodal afferent Afferent neuron receptive to more than one sensory modality, e.g. touch and pain (Ch. 9).

Polymodal association cortex Association cortex processing signals in more than one sensory modality (Ch. 26).

Pons *L.* 'bridge'. Part of brainstem in the interval between midbrain and medulla oblongata (Ch. 2).

Position sense Perception of the position of body parts (Ch. 12).

Positron emission tomography (PET) Imaging technique identifying radioactive atoms that emit positrons (Ch. 26).

Posterior circulation The vertebrobasal arterial system (Ch. 5).

Postsynaptic inhibition Inhibition of a target neuron (Ch. 6).

Postural fixation Fixation of axial musculature prior to voluntary movement of a limb (Ch. 13).

Postural hypotension Fall of arterial blood pressure on assuming the upright posture (Ch. 13).

Posture The position adopted between movements (Ch. 13).

Pressure coning Displacement of the cerebellar tonsils into the foramen magnum with compression of the medulla oblongata (Ch. 6).

Presynaptic inhibition Inhibition of conduction along the axon terminal of a target neuron (Ch. 6).

Priapism Persistent involuntary erection of the penis (Ch. 10).

Procedural memory 'How to do' memory (Ch. 29).

Progressive bulbar palsy Rapidly lethal medullary variant of progressive muscular atrophy (Ch. 15).

Projection *L.* 'forward throw'. Target of a neuronal pathway, e.g. spinothalamic tract projecting to the thalamus (Ch. 12).

Prolapsed intervertebral disc Herniation of the nucleus pulposus into the vertebral canal with consequent pressure on spinal nerve roots (Ch. 11).

Proprioception *Gr.* 'self perception'. Conscious or nonconscious reception by the brain, of information from muscles, tendons, and joints (Ch. 12).

Pros- *Gr.* 'before,' e.g. prosencephalon, the embryonic forebrain (Ch. 1).

Prosody Tonal variations during speech having emotional attributes (Ch. 27).

Prosopagnosia *Gr.* 'face-no-knowledge'. Inability to recognize faces (Ch. 26).

Pseudobulbar palsy Term given to the clinical picture arising from compromise of the corticonuclear supply to motor cranial nuclei in pons and medulla oblongata (Ch. 15).

Psychogenic impotence Impotence probably caused by excessive sympathetic activity (Ch. 10).

Psychosis Mental disorder involving a distorted sense of reality, e.g. schizophrenia (Ch. 27).

Ptosis *Gr.* 'falling'. Drooping of the upper eyelid (Ch. 20).

Pulvinar *L.* 'cushion'. Refers to posterior bulge of thalamus above the midbrain (Ch. 3).

Pure motor syndrome Syndrome associated with a lacuna in the posterior limb of the internal capsule (Ch. 30).

Pure sensory syndrome Syndrome associated with a lesion of the ventral posterior nucleus of the thalamus (Ch. 30).

Putamen *L.* 'shell'. Refers to outer part of lentiform nucleus (Ch. 2).

Quadrantic hemianopia Blindness in one quadrant of the visual field (Ch. 25).

Quadriplegia *L./Gr.* 'four-stroke'. Paralysis of all four limbs (Ch. 13).

Raphe *Gr.* 'seam'. Refers to the midline. Greek genitive case is used in nucleus raphes magnus (Ch. 19).

Raynaud phenomenon Painful blanching of the fingers in cold weather (Ch. 10).

Receptor A term with two distinct meanings: (a) sensory receptors, e.g. photoreceptors, neuromuscular spindles, transduce sensory stimuli; (b) molecular receptors on or within cells are protein molecules acted upon by messenger molecules, e.g. hormones, neurotransmitters.

Receptor blocker A drug that can occupy a membrane receptor without activating it (Ch. 10).

Referred pain Perception of pain at a site distant from the locus of nociceptive activity (Ch. 10).

Reflex reversal Term used to signify the 'change of sign' accompanying a switch from reflex resistance to reflex assistance (Ch. 13).

Reflexive impotence Impotence caused by damage to reflex arcs (Ch. 10).

REM sleep Rapid eye movement sleep (Ch. 21).

Resistance reflex Resistance to passive movement, notably at the knee joint, produced by passive stretching of neuromuscular spindles (Ch. 13). Compare with Assistance reflex.

Resting tremor Tremor at rest; characteristic of Parkinson's disease (Ch. 28).

Reticular *L.* 'netlike', e.g. reticular formation (Ch. 21).

Retrieval Calling up items from memory stores (Chs 27, 29)

Retrograde amnesia Amnesia for past events (Ch. 29).

Rhinencephalon *Gr.* 'nosebrain'. Refers to olfactory areas (Ch. 26).

Rhombencephalon *Gr.* 'rhomboid-brain' containing the rhomboid fourth ventricle. Embryologically, the hindbrain vesicle (Ch. 1).

Rostral limbic system The anterior cingulate cortex and related areas (Ch. 29).

Rostrum *L.* 'beak'. Rostrum of corpus callosum extends from genu to lamina terminalis (Ch. 2).

Rubro- *L.* 'red'. Refers to projections from red nucleus (Ch. 14).

Saccade Scanning movement of the eyes (Ch. 20).

Saltatory conduction *Gr.* 'jumping'. Mode of impulse conduction along myelinated fibers (Ch. 6).

Satellite *L.* 'attendant', e.g. the satellite cells in spinal ganglia.

Schizophrenia *Gr.* 'split mind'. Psychiatric state with variable manifestations (Ch. 27).

Scotoma Blind spot (Ch. 25).

Segmental antinociception Relief of pain at segmental level, e.g. by 'rubbing the sore spot' (Ch. 21).

Semantic Having to do with meaning (Ch. 27).

Semantic retrieval Retrieving the meaning of a word from memory stores (Ch. 27).

Senile tremor Benign essential tremor, often mistaken for a sign of Parkinson's disease (Ch. 28).

Sensorineural deafness Deafness caused by disease of the cochlea or of the cochlear nerve (Ch. 17).

Sensory competition An explanation for cortical sensory plasticity (Ch. 26).

Sensory modality A distinct mode of sensation, e.g. touch vs pain (Ch. 9).

Sensory unit A cutaneous nerve fiber together with all of its sensory terminals (Ch. 9).

Septal rage A rage attack thought to originate in the septal nuclei (Ch. 29).

Septum pellucidum *L.* 'transparent partition' separating the frontal horns of the lateral ventricles (Ch. 2).

Sign An objective indicator of a disorder, e.g. Babinski sign (Ch. 13).

Soma *Gr.* The cell body of a neuron (Ch. 6).

Somatic *Gr.* 'body-related'. Implies body wall as distinct from viscera.

Somatotopic Containing a body map.

Somesthetic Somatic sensory, e.g. s. cortex (Ch. 26).

Sound attenuation Dampening of sound by contraction of stapedius or tensor tympani (Ch. 17).

Sound field The peripheral field of sound perception by one ear (Ch. 17).

Spastic State of increased muscle tone induced by an upper motor neuron lesion (Ch. 13).

Spastic diplegia A form of cerebral palsy involving corticospinal fibers destined for lower limb motor neurons (Ch. 28).

Sphincter-detrusor dyssynergia Failure of the urethral sphincter to relax at the onset of micturition; a feature of spinal cord injury (Ch. 14).

Spina bifida Varying degrees of failure of the embryonic neural arches to unite in the posterior midline (Ch. 11).

Spinal tap See Lumbar puncture.

Splanchnic *Gr.* 'visceral'.

Splenium *L.* 'pad'. Refers to posterior end of corpus callosum (Ch. 2).

Startle response Generalized muscle twitch in response to sudden loud noise (Ch. 17).

Static labyrinth The utricle and saccule (Ch. 17).

Static posturography Study of postural responses on an unstable platform. Compare with Dynamic posturography.

Stellate *L.* 'starlike,' e.g. stellate ganglion (Ch. 10).

Stereopsis Three-dimensional vision (Ch. 26).

Stimulus-induced analgesia Analgesia induced by electrical stimulation of the peri-aqueductal gray matter (Ch. 21).

Strabismus *Gr.* 'squinting' (Ch. 20).

Stria *L.* 'narrow band,' e.g. stria terminalis originating in the amygdala (Ch. 26).

Striatum *L.* 'furrowed'. Refers to caudate nucleus and putamen taken together (Ch. 2).

Stroke A disorder of brain function following a cerebrovascular accident that does not disappear within 24 hours (Ch. 30).

Subfalcal herniation Displacement of brain tissue beneath the falx cerebri (Ch. 6).

Subiculum *L.* 'little layer'. Refers to transitional zone between six-layered parahippocampal gyrus and three-layered hippocampus (Ch. 26).

Substantia *L.* 'substance,' e.g. substantia gelatinosa of the spinal gray matter (Ch. 12), and substantia nigra of the midbrain (Ch. 14).

Sulcus *L.* 'groove'.

Supraspinal antinociception Pain suppression by pathways descending to the posterior horn gray matter from the brainstem (Ch. 21).

Sympathetic *Gr.* 'with-feeling', i.e. responsive to emotional state.

Symptom Clues about a disorder derived from the patient's account.

Synapse *Gr.* 'contact'. Refers to sites of contact between neurons (Ch. 6).

Syndrome *Gr.* 'running together'. A characteristic group of symptoms/signs.

Syringomyelia *Gr.* 'marrow-tube'. Refers to central cavitation of the spinal cord (Ch. 12).

Tactile agnosia Inability to identify common objects by touch alone (Ch. 27).

Tandem Romberg sign A toe-the-line test for presence of ataxia (Ch. 12).

Tapetum *L.* 'carpet'. Refers to sheet of callosal fibers above the lateral ventricles (Ch. 2).

Tectum *L.* 'roof' of midbrain (Ch. 14).

Tegmentum *L.* 'covering'. Refers to intermediate region of midbrain and pons (Ch. 14).

Tela choroidea *L.* 'membranous web', consisting of vascular pia-ependyma (Ch. 2).

Telencephalon *Gr.* 'endbrain', comprising the embryonic cerebral hemispheres (Ch. 1).

TENS Transcutaneous electrical nerve stimulation (Ch. 21).

Tentorium *L.* 'tent', e.g. tentorium cerebelli (Ch. 4).

Tetanus *Gr.* 'taut'. Spasmodic state of musculature, especially those of the face and lower jaw, following infection with *Clostridium tetani* (Ch. 6).

Tetraplegia *Gr.* 'four-paralysis'. Synonymous with quadriplegia.

Thalamic syndrome Syndrome including contralateral intractable pain, following occlusion of the thalamogeniculate artery (Ch. 30).

Thalamus *Gr./L.* 'bridal meeting place'.

Thermosensitive neurons Peripheral sensory neurons having sensory receptors activated by heat (Ch. 9).

Theta rhythm Slow-wave temporal lobe rhythm associated with the septohippocampal cholinergic pathway (Ch. 29).

Thrombus *Gr./L.* 'clot' (of blood, Ch. 27).

TIA Transient ischemic attack (Ch. 30).

Tinnitus A ringing/booming/buzzing sound heard in one or both ears (Ch. 17).

Tonic motor neuron α Motor neuron innervating a squad of slow, oxidative-glycolytic muscle fibers (Ch. 8).

Tonic–clonic convulsions Convulsions characteristic of temporal lobe epilepsy (Ch. 28).

Tourette's syndrome Involuntary exclamations associated with anterior cingulate cortex dysfunction (Ch. 29).

Tracking Smooth visual pursuit of a moving object (Ch. 20).

Tract *L.* tractus, 'district'. A group of CNS axons having the same origin and destination.

Transduction *L.* 'leading across'. Refers to conversion of sensory stimuli into trains of nerve impulses.

Transient ischemic attack (TIA) Episode of vascular insufficiency causing focal loss of brain function, with total recovery within 24 hours (Ch. 30).

Transneuronal atrophy Atrophic neuronal degeneration passing from one neuron to another, in either an orthograde or a retrograde manner (Ch. 7).

Trapezoid *L.* 'diamond-shaped'. Collection of second-order auditory fibers in the pons (Ch. 15).

Tremor Involuntary trembling of one or more body parts; may accompany cerebellar (Ch. 22) or basal ganglionic disease (Ch. 28).

Trigeminal *L.* 'triplet'. Refers to the ophthalmic, maxillary, and mandibular divisions of the trigeminal nerve (Ch. 17).

Triple response The line-flare-wheal response to a sharp stroke to the skin, involving an axon reflex (Ch. 9).

Trochlear *L.* 'pulley'. Transferred epithet: tendon of superior oblique muscle passes through a fascial pulley, and the name is applied to the nerve of supply (trochlear) (Ch. 18).

Trophic *Gr.* 'nourishing'.

Tropic *Gr.* 'turning'. Chemotropic substances attract ('turn') axonal growth cones (ch. 7).

Truncal ataxia Inability to maintain the upright position; a feature of midline cerebellar disease (Ch. 22).

Two-point discrimination A test used to assess discriminative touch (Ch. 12).

Uncal herniation Displacement of the uncus through the tentorial notch (Ch. 6).

Unconscious proprioception See Nonconscious proprioception.

Uncus *L.* 'hook'. In the anterior temporal lobe (Chs 2, 28).

Unimodal sensory cortex Primary somatic sensory, visual or auditory cortex (Ch. 26).

Unstable bladder See Detrusor instability.

Upper motor neuron Corticonuclear/corticospinal neuron.

Upper motor neuron signs Physical signs indicating presence of upper motor neuron disorder (Ch. 13).

Upregulation Increase in the number of membrane receptors (Chs 28, 29).

Urinary retention Inability to void urine (Ch. 10).

Uvula *L.* 'little grape'. A lobule of the cerebellum (Ch. 22).

Vagus *L.* 'wandering' with reference to the tenth cranial nerve (Ch. 15).

Vallecula *L.* 'little valley' between the cerebellar hemispheres (Ch. 22).

Ventricle *L.* 'little belly'.

Verbal paraphrasia In Wernicke's aphasia, the use of words of allied meaning (Ch. 27).

Vergence Convergence of gaze for close-up viewing (Ch. 20).

Vermis *L.* 'worm'. Refers to the segmented appearance of the vermis of the cerebellum (Ch. 22).

Vestibular nystagmus Nystagmus resulting from vestibular disorder (Ch. 16).

Vibration sense A test of posterior column function, using a tuning fork placed on a bone, e.g. shaft of tibia (Ch. 12).

Volume transmission Nonsynaptic release of neuropeptides into the extracellular space (Ch. 6).

Wallerian degeneration Orthograde degeneration of a peripheral nerve (Ch. 7).

Warm caloric test A test of kinetic labyrinthine function (Ch. 16).

Withdrawal reflex Reflex retraction of a limb in response to a noxious stimulus; includes the flexor reflex (Ch. 11).

Working memory Holding relevant memories briefly in mind while performing a task (Ch. 29).

Index